Current Methods in Physical Education and Sport Science

Current Methods in Physical Education and Sport Science

Edited by Edward Osborne

SYRAWOOD
PUBLISHING HOUSE
New York

Published by Syrawood Publishing House,
750 Third Avenue, 9th Floor,
New York, NY 10017, USA
www.syrawoodpublishinghouse.com

Current Methods in Physical Education and Sport Science
Edited by Edward Osborne

International Standard Book Number: 978-1-64740-002-6 (Hardback)

Cataloging-in-Publication Data

Current methods in physical education and sport science / edited by Edward Osborne.
p. cm.
Includes bibliographical references and index.
ISBN 978-1-64740-002-6
1. Sports sciences. 2. Physical education and training. 3. Physical education and training--Methodology.
4. Sports. I. Osborne, Edward.
GV558 .C87 2020
613.711--dc23

Printed in China.

TABLE OF CONTENTS

PREFACE

This book has been a concerted effort by a group of academicians, researchers and scientists, who have contributed their research works for the realization of the book. This book has materialized in the wake of emerging advancements and innovations in this field. Therefore, the need of the hour was to compile all the required researches and disseminate the knowledge to a broad spectrum of people comprising of students, researchers and specialists of the field.

Physical education aims to develop physical competence in students. It also aims to provide knowledge of movement and safety as well as the ability to use these skills for performing a wide range of activities connected to the development of an active and healthy lifestyle. Sports science refers to the discipline which studies the working of the human body during exercise as well as the effect of physical activity and sports upon health. It involves the use of tools from a range of disciplines such as physiology, sports psychology, anatomy and biomechanics. It also plays a vital role in improving the athletic performance of sportsmen. This book unfolds the innovative aspects of physical education and sport science which will be crucial for the progress of this field in the future. It presents researches and studies performed by experts across the globe. Those with an interest in these fields would find this book helpful.

At the end of the preface, I would like to thank the authors for their brilliant chapters and the publisher for guiding us all-through the making of the book till its final stage. Also, I would like to thank my family for providing the support and encouragement throughout my academic career and research projects.

Editor

1

ANALYSIS OF OLYMPIC EDUCATION THEORETICAL READINESS OF FUTURE PHYSICAL CULTURE TEACHERS

Bondar A.A.
Kamenetz-Podolsk National University

Abstract. *Purpose:* analysis of Olympic knowledge system in future physical culture teachers. *Material:* in the research 180 4 year students of physical culture faculties participated. *Results:* it was found that students' theoretical knowledge level in the sphere of Olympic movement corresponds to low. It was confirmed that system of Olympic knowledge is an integral part of future physical culture teachers' readiness for Olympic education of schoolchildren. It was found that in the process of knowledge formation in students it is necessary to consider theoretical material on Olympic education, acting academic programs for pupils of comprehensive educational establishments. *Conclusions:* students have low level of knowledge in sphere of Olympic movement (general indicator was 57.4%). It weakens effectiveness of skills, knowledge and motivation's formation in realization of schoolchildren's Olympic education.
Key words: Olympic education, knowledge, students, test.

Introduction

At the beginning of 21st century one of the most important directions of modern Olympic movement Olympic education of children and students became. In our country, for recent decade the system of Olympic education has powerfully developed and formed; it is directed at formation of harmoniously developed personality. All it is achieved by acquiring of knowledge, skills and abilities, development of interests, value orientations. The received knowledge is based on humanistic ideals and values of Olympic movement and is a part of general education.

Implementation of Olympic education elements in educational process is studied in works of domestic authors [7, 8]. Besides, Olympic education is reflected in State standard of primary comprehensive education, in which there are requirements to the level of comprehensive education of pupils. The requirements envisage pupils' mastering of Olympic topics' problems [State standard of primary comprehensive education. (Approved by Cabinet of ministers of Ukraine, № 462, dt. April 20th, 2011).]. Analysis of existing academic programs for 1- and 5-11 forms shows that questions of Olympic education are a part of chapter "theoretical-methodic knowledge' on discipline "Physical culture". They are compulsory for pupils of every form [18].

Alongside with it results of foreign and domestic scientists (G. Polikarpov, G. Ragozin, V. Sergeyev, V. Yermolovaq) witness about low level of pupils' knowledge of Olympic topics. This fact is explained by insufficient quantity of qualified specialists in the field of children and students' Olympic education. [8, 11, 12, 14,]. This problem is mentioned not only in domestic but also in foreign scientific literature [19, 20, 21, 22, 23, 24]. Most of foreign authors are sure that effective realization of Olympic education is possible only with presence of highly qualified specialists. Such specialists shall have proper knowledge and skills in attracting of a personality to ideals and values of Olympic movement. Leading specialists [7, 8, 10, 11] note that main pedagogic specialists on implementation of Olympic movement's ideology in comprehensive educational establishments are graduates of specialized higher educational establishments and physical culture faculties of HEEs.

In such situation the problem of future physical culture knowledge of Olympic movement acquires first importance as well as their readiness for realization of Olympic education in the frames of future professional functioning. As on to day one of main criteria of future physical culture readiness for effective realization of Olympic education is formation level of their knowledge system in the field of Olympic movement. For confident assessment of physical culture faculties graduates' Olympic knowledge system alongside with analysis of special literature we carried out this research.

Purpose, tasks of the work, material and methods

The purpose of the research is to analyze Olympic knowledge system in future physical culture teachers.

The methods of the research: theoretical analysis and generalization of scientific-methodic literature data, testing, methods of mathematical analysis.

Knowledge level of students was determined with the help of test tasks, which were composed on the base of theoretical material on Olympic education. This material is a part of acting academic programs for 1-4 and 5-11 forms' pupils of comprehensive educational establishments [18].

Topics of test tasks consisted of three parts. The first part contained questions on history and development of Olympic Games in ancient Greece, the second – history and development of modern Olympic Games, the third – questions on history of Olympic movement in Ukraine [15].

The researches were conducted on the base of physical culture faculties of the following higher educational establishments of Ukraine: Kamenets-Podolskiy national university, named after Ivan Ogniyenko, Ternopol national pedagogic university, named after Vladimir Gnatiuk, Chernovitskiy national university, named after Yuriy Fedkovych, Kharkov national pedagogic university, named after Grygoriy Skovoroda. In the research 180 4 year students participated.

Results of the research

The received testing results showed low level of Students' knowledge about origin of Olympic Games. For example 57.7% of students knew when the first Olympic Games took place and only 42.8% knew in what town they were conducted.

Only 43.3% of the questioned knew the program of Olympic Games of ancient Greece and 61. 6% of students knew what were the awards of winners.

54.2% of respondent gave correct answer to question "who had right to participate in Olympic Games of ancient Greece?".

The reasons of prohibitions of ancient Olympic Games were known only to 20.7% of students.

Analyzing the answers to the second part of questionnaire we noted that 67.9% of students knew who founded modern Olympic Games.

It was interesting that the place of first modern Olympic Games was known to 88.8% of students. Among them only 62.6% pointed the years of their conduct correctly.

Only 23.7% of students could call correctly the name of first president of International Olympic committee. Alongside with it the name of acting president was known only to 58.8% of the questioned.

The questioning showed that students know Olympic symbolism quite good. For example 88.3% knows the meaning of five bound rings on Olympic flag. Formulation of Olympic motto was known to 87.3% of students.

Conception "Olympism" is familiar only to 19.9% of the questioned. Such low indicator witnesses about students' unawareness of ideals and values, which are the basis of Olympic movement.

Students' questioning also showed that only 51.9% knew about existence of the Olympic Charter.

The question "where the next summer and winter Olympic Games will be conducted?" was answered correctly by accordingly 52.9% and 51.2% of students. Only 24.8% of students knew how long modern Olympic Games last.

Analyzing students' answers to the third part of the questionnaire we noted high level of students' knowledge about history of Olympic movement in Ukraine.

The questioning results witness that most of students knew when National Olympic committee of Ukraine was formed; who was its first president (accordingly 74.8% and 70.3%). Acting president of NOC of Ukraine was known to 79.2% of students.

When Ukrainian team participated as teams of independent country in summer and winter Olympic Games for the first time was known to accordingly 51.6% and 68.1% of students.

The name of the first Ukrainian, who won gold Olympic medal, was pointed correctly by 74.5% of the questioned. Alongside with it the first Olympic champion of winter Games was known only to 57.9% of students.

General indicator of correct answers in the sphere of history and modern state of Olympic movement was less than 60% (table 1).

Table 1 Formation of Olympic knowledge system in students

№	Questions to be answered	Respondents' answers by HEEs, %				General indicator %
		Kamenets-Podolskiy	Ternopol	Chernovtsy	Kharkov	
1.	Which year is considered to be the birth year of ancient Greece Olympic Games?	62,3	58,2	53,1	57,2	**57,7**
2.	In what city ancient Olympic Games were conducted?	49,8	32,6	40,7	46,1	**42,8**
3.	Name please main competitions of Olympic Games in ancient Greece	45,8	36,4	44	47,1	**43,3**
4.	What awards the Olympic Games winners received?	62,1	63,9	59,3	61,2	**61,6**
5.	Who had right to participate in ancient Olympic Games?	62,8	43,7	51,9	58,4	**54,2**
6.	Why Olympic Games were prohibited?	20,3	21,8	16,8	24	**20,7**

№	Questions to be answered	Respondents' answers by HEEs, % Kamenets-Podolskiy	Ternopol	Chernovtsy	Kharkov	General indicator %
7.	Who is considered to be the founder of modern Olympic Games?	74,2	69,3	54,1	73,9	**67,9**
8.	Where the first modern Olympic Games were conducted?	89,3	91,3	86,2	88,4	**88,8**
9.	Ion what year the first Olympic Games were conducted?	68,3	55,8	64,2	62,2	**62,6**
10.	Who was the first president of IOC?	24,5	21,3	19,8	29,1	**23,7**
11.	Point the name of acting president of IOC	57,7	67,1	58,3	52,0	**58,8**
12.	What is the meaning of Olympic rings?	89,1	92,3	84,5	87,4	**88,3**
13.	Write please Olympic motto	88,3	92,4	81,2	87,1	**87,3**
14.	What is the meaning of concept "Olympism"?	19,4	21,3	18,8	20,1	**19,9**
15.	What is Olympic Chart?	55	43,4	57,2	52,1	**51,9**
16.	Where will the next summer Olympic Games be conducted?	47,9	61,1	52,7	50	**52,9**
17.	Where will the next winter Olympic Games be conducted?	57,2	44,7	48,9	54,2	**51,2**
18.	What is the maximal duration of summer Olympic Games?	28	36,1	16,3	19,1	**24,8**
19.	In what year was NOC of Ukraine formed?	80,3	65,4	74,7	78,9	**74,8**
20.	Who was the first president of NOC of Ukraine?	73,2	70,7	63,1	74	**70,3**
21.	Write please the name of acting president of NOC of Ukraine	84,2	72,1	82,1	78,3	**79,2**
22.	When team of independent Ukraine took part in summer Olympic Games for the first time?	58,3	49,4	52,8	45,3	**51,6**
23.	When team of independent Ukraine took part in summer Olympic Games for the first time?	68	65,2	71,3	67,8	**68,1**
24.	Who became the first Olympic champion of independent Ukraine at summer Olympic Games?	79,1	72,3	64,2	82,2	**74,5**
25.	Who became the first Olympic champion of independent Ukraine at winter Olympic Games?	58,3	52,1	62,4	57,3	**57,9**
	General indicator %	**60,1**	**56,0**	**55,1**	**58,1**	**57,4**

Analyzing general indicators of correct answers by HEEs we noted the following results: Kamenets-Podolskiy national university, named after Ivan Ogniyenko – 60.1%, Ternopol national pedagogic university, named after Vladimir Gnatiuk - 56%, Chernovitskiy national university, named after Yuriy Fedkovych - 55,1%, Kharkov national pedagogic university, named after Grygoriy Skovoroda - 58,1%. It should be noted that difference between indicators is rather insignificant. It confirms low knowledge level of all higher educational establishments' students.

Discussion

The results of our research supplemented the data of other authors [7, 8, 11, 12] that main pedagogic specialists in schools' Olympic education system are graduates of specialized higher educational establishments and physical culture faculties of higher educational establishments.

We confirmed the data that system of knowledge in the field of "Olympism" and Olympic movement is an integral part of future physical culture teachers' readiness for schoolchildren's Olympic education.

It brings better results in formation of skills, knowledge and motivation in realization of Olympic education in comprehensive educational establishments.

We confirmed the data about students' low theoretical readiness in the field of Olympic movement [7, 8, 11, 12].

In the process of formation of future physical culture teachers' knowledge system in the field of Olympic education it is necessary to consider theoretical material on Olympic education, which is a part of acting academic programs for 1-4 and 4-11 forms of comprehensive educational establishments.

Conclusions

Results of our research showed low level of Olympic knowledge system in future physical culture teachers. General indicator of correct answers in the field of history and modern state of Olympic movement was only 57.4%.

Comparison of general indicators of correct answers by every HEE showed that difference between them is insignificant. It confirms insufficient level of students' knowledge in all HEEs, in which the research was conducted. That is why it is rather early to state that training of future physical culture teachers for realization of Olympic education in comprehensive educational establishments is effective.

The further researches will be oriented on perfection of physical culture faculties students' theoretical readiness in the field of Olympism and Olympic movement by introduction of new informational technologies and modern means of education in educational process.

Conflict of interests

The author declares that there is no conflict of interests.

References:

1. Bulatova MM. Olimpizm iak universal'na koncepciia vikhovannia ta osviti molodi [Olympism as versatile conception of youth's education and teaching]. *Fizichne vikhovannia v shkoli* 2008;1(51):40–43. (in Ukrainian)
2. Bulatova MM. Sistema olimpijs'koi osviti v Ukraini ta novi formi ii vprovadzhennia [System of Olympic education in Ukraine and new forms of its implementation]. *IX Mizhnarodnij naukovij kongres «Suchasnij olimpijs'kij sport i sport dlia vsikh»* [9th International scientific congress "Modern Olympic sports and sports for all"]. Kiev: Olympic Literature; 2005. (in Ukrainian)
3. Bulatova MM. Olimpijs'ka osvita [Olympic education], Kiev; 2002. (in Ukrainian)
4. Bulatova MM. Sistema Olimpijskogo obrazovaniia v Ukraine (1991–2006) [System of Olympic education in Ukraine (1991–2006)]. *X Mezhdunarodnoj nauchnyj kongress "Sovremennyj olimpijskij sport i sport dlia vsekh"* [10th International scientific congress "Modern Olympic sports and sports for all"], Gdansk; 2006. 38–41. (in Russian)
5. Vaceba OM, Iukhimchuk VP. Aktual'nye voprosy olimpijskogo obrazovaniia v uchebno-vospitatel'nom processe uchenikov obshcheobrazovatel'nykh shkol [Current issues of Olympic education in educational process of comprehensive schools' pupils]. *Nauka v olimpijskom sporte* 2007;2:87–92. (in Russian)
6. Georgiadis K. Teoreticheskie osnovy olimpijskogo obrazovaniia [Theoretical principles of Olympic education]. *Nauka v olimpijskom sporte* 2007;2:2–5. (in Russian)
7. Dudkin VIu. Olimpijs'ka osvita v procesi pidgotovki fakhivciv sferi «Fizichne vikhovannia i sport» u specializovanikh vishchikh navchal'nikh zakladakh Ukraini [Olympic education in training of specialists in "Physical education and sports" in specialized higher educational establishments of Ukraine]. *Moloda sportivna nauka Ukraini* 2009;4:57–61. (in Ukrainian)
8. Iermolova VM. *Olimpijs'ka osvita* [Olympic education]. Kiev; 2011. (in Ukrainian)
9. Kudriavceva N. Novye formy raboty po olimpijskomu obrazovaniiu detej i molodezhi [New forms of work on Olympic education of children and youth]. *Mezhdunarodnyj forum «Molodezh' – Nauka – Olimpizm», Moskva, 14–18 iiulia 1998 g.* [International forum "Youth – Science – Olympism", Moscow, July 14-18, 1998], Moscow; 1998. P. 131. (in Russian)
10. Platonov VN, Bulatova MM, Bubka SN. *Olimpijskij sport* [Olympic sports], Kiev: Olympic Literature; 2009;2. (in Russian)
11. Polikarpova GM. *Olimpijskoe obrazovanie i vospitanie kak predmet pedagogicheskogo issledovaniia. Doct. Diss.* [Olympic education as the subject of pedagogic study. Doct. Diss.], Velikiy Novgorod; 2003. (in Russian)
12. Ragozina GA. *Tekhnologiia podgotovki kadrov dlia realizacii olimpijskogo obrazovaniia detej i uchashchejsia molodezhi. Cand. Diss.* [Technology of specialists' training for realization of children and students' Olympic education. Cand. Diss.], Sankt Petersburg; 2002. (in Russian)

13. Sergeev VN. Olimpijskoe obrazovanie [Olympic education]. *Mezhdunarodnyj forum «Molodezh' – Nauka – Olimpizm», Moskva, 14–18 iiulia 1998 g*. [International forum "Youth – Science – Olympism", Moscow, July 14-18, 1998], Moscow; 1988. P. 217–218.
14. Sergeev VN. *Gumanisticheskaia napravlennost' realizacii olimpijskogo obrazovaniia. Cand. Diss.* [Humanistic orientation of Olympic education realization. Cand. Diss.], [Volgograd; 2000. (in Russian)
15. Solopchuk MS, Bodnar AO. *Olimpijs'ka osvita* [Olympic education]. Kamenets Podolsky; 2013. (in Ukrainian)
16. Stoliarov VI. Aktual'nye problemy teorii i praktiki olimpijskogo obrazovaniia detej i molodezhi [Current issues of theory and practice of children and youth's Olympic education], *Fizicheskaia kul'tura* 1998;4:13–19. (in Russian)
17. Diatlenko SM. *Fizichna kul'tura v shkoli: 5–11 klasi* [Physical culture at school: 5-11 forms], Kiev: Litera; 2011. (in Ukrainian)
18. Diatlenko SM. *Fizichna kul'tura v shkoli: navchal'na programa dlia 1–4, 5–9 klasiv* [Physical culture at school: 1-4, 5-11 forms], Kiev: Litera; 2013. (in Ukrainian)
19. Binder DL. *Teaching Olympism in schools: Olympic Education as a focus on values education: university lectures on the Olympics*. Bellaterra: Centre d'EstudisOlimpics (UAB). International Chair in Olympism (IOC UAB); 2005. Binder DL. *Teaching Olympism in schools: Olympic Education as a focus on values education:university lectures on the Olympics*. Bellaterra: Centre d'EstudisOlimpics (UAB). International Chair in Olympism (IOC UAB); 2010.
20. Francisco N. Olympic Education in Africa. *5 International Special Session for Presidents and Directors of NOA and Officials of NOC*. Ancient Olympia: Greece; 2000. P. 15.
21. Georgiadis K, Syrigos A. *Olympic truce sport as a platform for peace*. Athens; 2009.
22. Grammatikopoulos V, Hassandra M, Koustelios A,Theodorakis Y. Evaluating the olympic education program: A qualitative approach. *Studies in Educational Evaluation*, 2005;31(4):347–357.
23. Naul R. Olympism' and education: a critical review. *Quest*. 2012;64:3:261–264.

2

APPLICATION OF MOBILIZING EXTRA-TRAINING MEANS IN PROCESS OF PRE-START MARTIAL ARTS SPORTSMEN'S TRAINING (ON EXAMPLE OF FENCING)

Lopatenko G.O., Tumanova V.N., Gatsko E.V.
Borys Grinchenko Kyiv University

Abstract. *Purpose:* to test experimentally influence of worked out extra-training means' complex on functional potentials of elite fencers. *Material:* in the research 12 qualified sportsmen participated. Changes in cardio-respiratory system's responses were detected by training impulse. *Results:* application of experimental complex resulted in increase of training impulse by 1.94 conv.un., than traditional sportsmen's warming up. With usage of experimental complex sportsmen fulfilled, in average, 64.4% of work in zones of sub-maximal and maximal intensity. Restoration of heart beats rate of all sportsmen was within standard requirements (restoration of 120 b.p.m. during 3 minutes). In conditions of traditional warming up sportsmen fulfilled, in average, 71.2% of work with low or moderate intensity. *Conclusions:* the offered complex of extra-training influences increase effectiveness of pre-start warming up, raise organism's potentials for realization of available functional potential.
Key words: martial arts, fencing, training, extra-training means, competitions.

Introduction

Sportsmen's workability and effectiveness of their organisms' functional systems in competitions to large extent are determined by rationally built pre-start training [8, 12]. In sport practice pre-start training is regarded as one of the most important factors of formation of functions' high mobilization, which influence on realization of available motor potential and determine achievement of high sport result [10, 13, 15].

In modern fencing intensification of sportsmen's training suggests still wider purposeful application of extra-training means and development of new technologies of special (mobilizing) influences for perfection of special workability and rising of competition functioning's effectiveness [5, 9]. One of sides of such mobilization is preliminary stimulation of workability before competitions.

Alongside with it, analysis of special literature, devoted to training of qualified fencers, points at certain contradiction of existing pre-start training system and modern system of fencing competitions. Contest has grown greatly at present in fencing; duels have become more tensed and dynamic, Requirements to realization of special workability in initial duels, at the end of tournament and in conditions of tiredness have also increased [17, 18, 19, 20]. All these reduce opportunities for realization of organism's reserves and ensuring of optimal competition functioning's structure.

In this connection research and working out of special means, ensuring rising of pre-start training's effectiveness in fencing, are rather important and urgent.

Purpose, tasks of the work, material and methods

The purpose of the research is to experimentally test influence of the worked out extra-training means on functional potentials of qualified fencers.

We used the following *methods of the research:* theoretical analysis and generalization of scientific-methodic literature data, pedagogic observation, pedagogic experiment, radio-telemetric pulse metering, methods of mathematical statistics.

Results of the research

Among specific features of modern stage of fencing competitions there exists deficit of attention to seeking of special means, which could be used in pre-start-training for increasing of special workability and effectiveness of sportsmen's competition functioning. In this connection we worked out special complex for increasing of qualified fencers' special workability. This complex consists of extra-0training means to be fulfilled with partner's resistance and special fencers' exercises [5, 6]. In the process of our researches we found that application of experimental means positively influences on indicators of spoirtsmen's neuro-dynamic functions. It also permits to optimize the structure of fencers' pre-start training [6].

For determination of the worked out experimental means' influence on organism's functional potentials we carried out assessment of cardio-respiratory system's (CRS) responses to fulfillment of the worked out complex of pre-start influences. The received results were compared with CRS indicators, registered in the process of fencers' traditional warming up.

Changes in CRS responses in process of control and experimental tasks' fulfillment were assessed by indicators of training impulse – integral indicator of training work's tension [7]. This indicator is an integral characteristic of power, kinetics, stability of cardio-respiratory system and determines correlation "doze-effect" of load.

As a result of fulfilled series of experiments we received data, which permitted to compare influence of traditional warming up and warming up with the help of experimental complex of pre-start influences on indicators of sportsmen's CRS. Indicators of CRS responses in fulfillment of control and experimental tasks are presented in table 1.

Table 1

Indicators of cardio-respiratory system's responses in fulfillment of control and experimental tasks

Statistical indicators	Indicators of cardio-respiratory system's responses					
	Experimental complex (n=12)			Traditional warming up (n=12)		
	HBR av. b.p.m. $^{-1}$	HBR max.b.p.m. $^{-1}$	TI** conv.un.	HBR av.b.p.m. $^{-1}$	HBR max.b.p.m. $^{-1}$	TI** conv.un.
$\overline{x}$	151.2	177.4	9.92*	115.4	150	7.98
S	14.61	13	0.65	9.2	14.4	0.52

Notes: * – differences are statistically significant, comparing with recived after traditional warming up (in compliance with Wilkinson's criterion at level of $p<0.05$); ** TI– training impulse; HBR – heart beats rate

Results of analysis witness about presence of differences in responses of sportsmen's organisms under influence of traditional warming up and experimental complex of pre-start influence. After experimental complex of pre-start influences indicator of training impulse was confidently higher ($p<0.05$), than after traditional warming up (see table 1). Difference, comparing with indicators, received in traditional warming up, was 1.94 conventional units. It witnesses that application of experimental complex influences more expressively on sportsman's organism. It can be noticed by confident increase of training impulse, "doze-effect" indicator's effect in response to fulfilled work. Increase of "doze-effect' influence is connected with increasing of HBR indicators in the process of fulfillment of pre-start tasks.

Analyzing indicators of fulfillment of pre-start experimental complex we can see that mean HBR indicator in group was 1512 b.p.m.$^{-1}$, maximal HBR indicator in group was, in average, 1774 b.p.m.$^{-1}$ (see table 1).

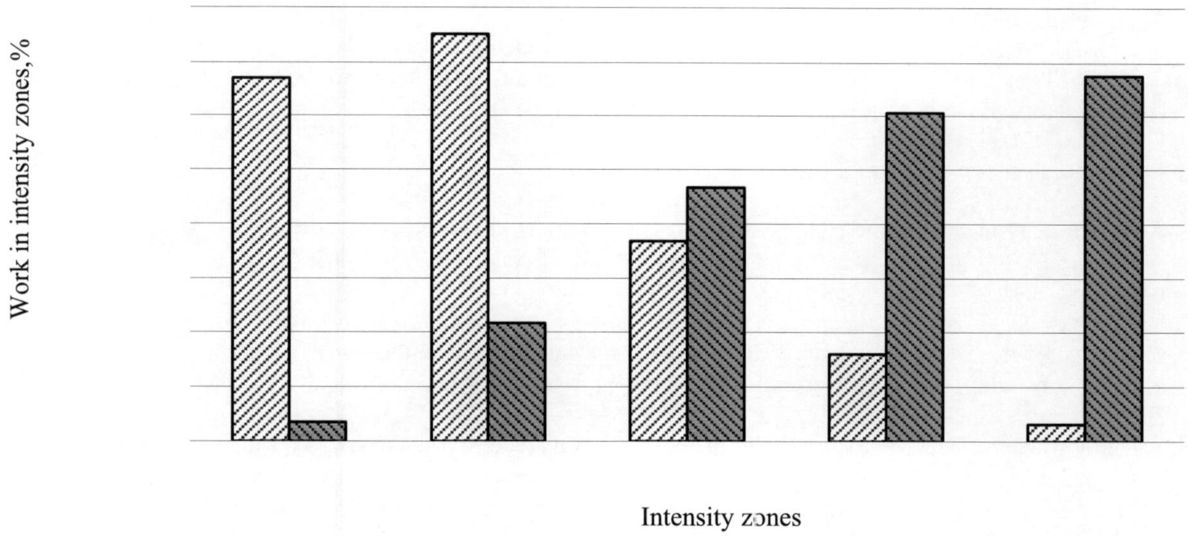

Fig.1. Percentage of work in different intensity zones:

1 – zone of middle intensity; 2 – zone of moderate intensity;

3 – zone of high intensity; 4 – zone of sub-maximal intensity; 5 – zone of maximal intensity;

▨ – traditional warming up;

▩ – application of experimental complex of pre-start means

In fig.1 we can see that with application of experimental complex of extra-training means sportsmen, mainly, fulfilled work in sub-maximal intensity zone (30.5% of total scope of work) and maximal (33.9% of total scope of work) In the process of traditional warming up sportsmen were in the mentioned zones only 8% and 1.6% of total scope of work.

It is evident that work in zones of low and moderate intensity is not effective in conditions of pre-start training. Such work does not cause required functional changes in sportsmen's organisms. As a result sportsman can not achieve optimal readiness by the moment of competition's beginning.

The worked out complex of pre-start influences implies highly intensive work, lasting up to 20 minutes, mainly in zones of sub-maximal and maximal intensity. Such approach facilitates effective mobilization of all organism's functions and permits to effectively fulfilled tasks of pre-start training.

The results, presented above permit to speak about purposeful application of the worked out complex of pre-start influences in the process of qualified fencers' competition functioning.

Discussion

The conducted research proved results of some authors' works, devoted to complex and rational application of training and extra training means in system of sport perfection that result in increasing of competition functioning's effectiveness in general [2, 3, 4, 11]. Besides, we supplemented theoretical principals of realization of existing functional potential of qualified sportsmen in the process of direct preparation for competitions [1, 2, 14, 16]. Besides, we supplemented information about modern approaches to optimization or pre-start training of qualified fencers with the help of extra training means [9, 17, 18].

Alongside with it, the conducted research permitted to substantiate purposefulness of application of experimental means' complex in sportsmen's pre-start training. The received results permit to say that the offered complex of extra training means increase effectiveness of pre-start training, sportsmen's potentials for realization of their skills. For the first time the data about influence of extra training complex means on cardio-respiratory systems' indicators were obtained. The received results witness about positive impact of experimental complex on functional potentials of qualified fencers.

Conclusions:

1. Analysis of research's results showed that application of experimental complex influences more expressively on sportsman's organism. It was shown that worked out complex of extra-training means positively influences on CRS indicators in the process of pre-start training of qualified fencers.
2. Increasing of CRS responses was registered by integral indicator - training impulse: after application of experimental complex training impulse was in average by 1.94 conv. un. ($p<0.05$) higher than after usage of traditional warming up of fencers.
3. Using experimental complex, sportsmen fulfilled in average by 64.4% more work in zones of sub maximal and maximal intensity. With it restoration of HBR of all sportsmen was within standard (restoration of HBR up to 120 b.p.m^{-1} within 3 minutes). Fulfilling traditional warming up, sportsmen realized in average 71.2% of work with low and moderate intensity.

Acknowledgement

The research has been fulfilled in compliance with "Combined plan of SRW in sphere of physical culture and sports for 2011-2015" by topic 2.10 "Control of training loads in conditions of intensive competition functioning in yearly cycle of qualified sportsmen's training" (state registration number 0106U0107769).

Conflict of interests

The authors declare absence of any conflict of interests.

References:

1. Ankina L. I. Osobennosti predstartovoj razminki i massazha plovcov vysokoj kvalifikacii [Peculiarities of pre-start warming up and massage of highly qualified swimmers]. *Teoriia i praktika fizicheskoj kul'tury*, 1997, vol.2, pp. 12-19.
2. Vinogradov V. E. *Stimuliaciia rabotosposobnosti i vosstanovitel'nykh processov v trenirovochnoj i sorevnovatel'noj deiatel'nosti kvalificirovannykh sportsmenov* [Stimulation of workability and recreational processes in training and competition functioning of qualified sportsmen], Kiev, "APF" Slavutich-Dolphin ", 2009, 367 p.
3. Vinogradov V.E., D'iachenko A.Iu., Efremenko A.N. Sovershenstvovanie sredstv trenirovki, napravlennykh na vosstanovlenie i stimulirovannie rabotosposobnosti v sovremennom piatibor'e [Perfection of training means, oriented on recreation and stimulation of workability in modern pentathlon]. *Nauka v olimpijskom sporte,* 2009, vol.2, pp. 62-69.
4. Golec V. I. *Kompleksnoe ispol'zovanie fizicheskikh sredstv vosstanovleniia s cel'iu upravleniia parametrami trenirovochnykh i sorevnovatel'nykh nagruzok vysokokvalificirovannykh sportsmenov (na primere plavaniia i velosporta), Cand. Diss.* [Complex application of physical recreation means for control of parameters of qualified sportsmen's training and competition loads (on example of swimming and bicycle sport)] Cand. Diss.], Kiev, 1987, 22 p.
5. Lopatenko G. O. Vikoristannia pozatrenuval'nikh zasobiv pidvishchennia special'noi pracezdatnosti kvalifikovanikh sportsmeniv, shcho specializuiut'sia v fekhtuvanni [Application of extra training means of increasing of fencers' special workability]. *Aktual'ni problemi fizichnoi kul'turi i sportu,* 2012, vol.24(2), pp. 43–47.
6. Lopatenko G.O., Kosik N.S., Kosik N.L., New approaches to the organization of prestart preparation of qualified athletes in single combats (on an example of fencing). *Pedagogics, psychology, medical-biological problems of physical training and sports,* 2015, vol.4, pp. 33-37. http://dx.doi.org/10.15561/18189172.2015.0406
7. Mak-Dugall Dzh. *Fiziologicheskoe testirovanie sportsmenov vysokogo klassa* [Physiological testing of elite sportsmen], Kiev, Olympic Literature, 1998, 430 p.
8. Matveev L. P. *Osnovy obshchej teorii sporta i sistemy podgotovki sportsmenov* [Principles of general theory of sports and system of sportsmen's training] Kiev, Olympic Literature, 1999, 320 p.
9. Mirzoev O. M. *Vosstanovitel'nye sredstva v sisteme podgotovki sportsmenov* [Recreational means in system of sportsmen's training], Moscow, Physical Culture and Sport,, 2005, 220 p.

10. Pavlenko Iu.A. *Neposredstvennaia podgotovka k sorevnovaniiam kvalificirovannykh sportsmenov v sovremennom piatibor'e, Cand. Diss*. [Direct preparation of qualified sportsmen for competitions in modern pentathlon], Cand. Diss.], Kiev, 1991, 170 p.
11. Planida E.V. Primenenie uprazhnenij na rastiazhenie (stretching) dlia srochnogo vosstanovleniia [Application of stretching exercises for urgent recreation], *Mir sporta,* 2005, vol.3(20), pp. 30-35.
12. Platonov V. N. *Sistema podgotovki sportsmenov v olimpijskom sporte* [System of sportsmen's training in Olympic sport]. Kiev, Olympic Literature, 2004, pp. 327–352.
13. Platonov V.N. *Teoriia periodizacii sportivnoj trenirovki* [Periodization theory in sports training], Kiev, Olympic Literature, 2013, 624 p.
14. Rybachok R. A. *Povyshenie special'noj rabotosposobnosti kvalificirovannykh bokserov vnetrenirovochnymi sredstvami v processe sorevnovatel'noj deiatel'nosti. Cand. Diss.* [Increasing of qualified boxers' special workability by extra training means in process of competition functioning. Cand. Diss.], Kiev, 2011, 23 p.
15. Sur'enkov I. A. *Rabotosposobnost' tkhekvondistov na predsorevnovatel'nom etape pri ispol'zovanii stimuliacionno-vosstanovitel'nogo kompleksa. Cand. Diss*. [Workability of thaequandoists at pre-competition stage with usage of stimulating-recreational complex. Cand. Diss], Moskva, 2000, 112 p.
16. Turmanidze V.G. *Differencirovannoe ispol'zovanie fizicheskikh sredstv vosstanovleniia na etape predsorevnovatel'noj podgotovki i v period sorevnovanij kvalificirovannykh badmintonistov. Cand. Diss.* [Differential usage of physical recreational means at stage of pre-competition training and in period of qualified badminton players' competitions. Cand. Diss.], Omsk, 2005, 24 p.
17. Tyshler D. A., Movshovich A. D. Dvigatel'naia podgotovka fekhtoval'shchikov [Motor training of fencers], Moscow, Academic Project, 2007, 153 p.
18. Tyshler G. D. *Tekhnika peredvizhenij fekhtoval'shchikov v mnogoletnej trenirovke i sorevnovaniiakh* [Techniques of fencers' movements in many years' training and in competitions], Moscow, Academic Project, 2009, 186 p.
19. Sowerby A. *Fencing: Skills, Tactics, Training (Crowood Sports Guides).* Crowood Press; 2012, June 1, p. 96.
20. Wayne H. *Fencing Techniques*. Amazon Digital Services, 2013, 99 p.

3

OPTIMIZATION OF PHYSICAL TRAINING OF STUDENTS OF HIGH SCHOOL WITH REGARD TO QUANTITATIVE FEATURES MUSCULAR COMPONENTS OF THEIR BODIES

Kolokoltsev M.M.[1], Cieslicka Miroslawa[2], Muszkieta Radoslaw[2]
National Research Irkutsk State Technical University, Russia[1]
Kazimierz Wielki University in Bydgoszcz, Poland[2]

Annotation. *Purpose*: to provide a quantitative description of the muscle component of students" body with regard to their motor characteristics to improve training in the discipline "Physical Education". *Material*: a study of muscular component of the body in 1937 students aged 17-20 years old of age living in the Baikal region. Motor quality students were evaluated by tests. Problem analysis was conducted based on the data of Polish authors. *Results*: the dependence of the amount of content in muscle mass in the body of the frequency of physical training in high school. Also found significantly higher levels of performance in motor tests in the group of students with a high level of expression of muscle mass. *Conclusions*: the studies have shown a direct relationship content of lean body mass of locomotor activity. Set better indicator values in tests of physical fitness with a high content of muscle tissue. Lack of exercise training on older years is recommended to compensate for self-manage motor activities.
Keywords: students, muscle mass, physical, preparedness, physical culture.

Introduction

Among environmental factors, which influence on formation of body"s componential composition, practicing of physical culture and sports are rather important. In this connection significance of studying of body"s componential composition, considering motion characteristics in complex studying of organism, is scientifically grounded and demanded [8].

It has been proved that componential composition of body reflects level of physical condition. At the same time it is a criterion of health and motion functioning [2, 5].

Thus, modern ideas, theories and methodic of physical education and medicine are single in opinion that it is necessary to consider individual specificities of person"s development and condition [1, 11, 13, 15, 20]. Seeking of methods of physical load"s individualization has been carrying out for long time, but mainly on the base of personification of methodic, pointed at achievement of mean-statistical standards of motion functioning. However, such approach weakens individual abilities of a person, because it requires their uniformity [10]. In opinion of V.V. Zaytseva [4], it is possible to significantly increase effectiveness of trainings and strengthen motivation for practicing of physical culture and sports with the help of methods and means, pointed at achievement of individual standards by every person on the base of his (her) constitutional-typological belonging. With it, level of indicators of body composition and their dynamic completely depends on structure of trainings, scope and intensity of physical loads [5, 14, 16-19].

Recent years, in Irkutskaya region there have been conducting researches on evaluation and analysis of only type-morphological status of 17-20 years old girls [6]. That is why it is important to fulfill additional researches for determination of composition and characteristic of interconnection between indicators of physical fitness and quantity of muscular component in girl students" bodies (girl student of technical HEE in Baykal district).

Purpose, tasks of the work, material and methods

The purpose of the research is to provide quantitative characteristics of girl students" muscular component, (Baykal district) considering their motion abilities, for perfection of "Physical culture" lessons.

The methods and organization of the research. We have examined*Методы и организация исследования.* 1937 girl students of National research Irkutsk state technical university. Mean age of the girls was 18.5 years and varied from 17 to 20 years. In our work we used standard anthropometrical methodic of V.V. Bunak (1941), considering requirements of anthropological scientific research institute of MSU (1982), and with the help of standard devices. Our measurements were carried out in medical office of HEE, considering volunteer character of participation, considering rights and freedom of a personality, guaranteed by Cl. 21 and 22 of Constitution of RF. The research was fulfilled in compliance with principles of Helsinki Declaration (2008). All tested were informed about character and purposes of the research and gave written permission for participation in it.

From all, mentioned in literature methodic of determination of body"s component composition we chose and used methodic of R.N. Dorokhov and V.G. Petrukhin (1989) [3], which was tested in clinical and pedagogic practice. This scheme is highly informative and has significant advantages in comparison with subjective schemes of diagnostic; besides, it is the most convenient for application in evaluation of morphological characteristics. Componential level of variation of properties (CLP) was determined by content of fat (FM), muscular (MM) and bone (BM) masses. Evaluation of MM was fulfilled by summing of four circumferences (shoulder and hip (upper and lower) and by deduction of FM, multiplied by 3.13 from this sum:

$$MM=(CUS + CLS + CUH + CLH) - FM \times 3.14.$$

Content of body"s muscular component (in %) was divided by 5 sigma classes: M±0.67s–«mean»value of indicators for sample. If they are in interval from ±0.67s to ±1.34s; content of muscular mass was evaluated as "above middle" or "below middle". If it was in interval from ±0.67s to ±1.34s, content was characterized as "above middle" or "below middle"[7]. If the data are out of limits ±1.34s, muscular component was evaluated as "high" or "low".

First and second year girl students attended physical culture lessons twice a week; third and forth year girl students – once a week. Every lesson lasted for 90 minutes; the training were conducted in compliance with governmental educational standards of second generation (approximate academic program for higher educational establishments in "physical culture" discipline, 2000), mainly with using of fitness-aerobics system, oriented on education of all main motion abilities.

Motion abilities were evaluated by tests, worked out in scientific-research institute of physical culture of RF. For evaluation of quickness we used *20 meters run from walking (sec);* speed endurance and dexterity – *shuttle run 10 times by 5 meters (sec.);* strength and power endurance of upper girdle muscles – *hanging (sec.);* speed-power endurance of muscular, bending torso – *torso raising (times);* flexibility – *torso bending (cm);* dynamic power of lower limbs" muscles – *long jump from the spot (cm);* endurance – *5 minutes run (meters).*

We calculated mean arithmetic value of indicators, *M,* mean square deviation, *s,* and standard error *m.* According to recommendations of O.Yu. Rebrova [9], we used in our work parametric methods of material"s processing, considering normal Gauss distribution of the studied quantitative characteristics. Evaluation of differences" confidence of independent samples" mean values was fulfilled with the help of *t*-criterion of Student. Differences between indicators with level $P<0.05$ was considered as statistically significant. Calculation of indicators was conducted with the help of applied programs Statistica 6.0. For optimization of primary digital material"s analysis we developed authors" program complex "Analysis of data of population"s physical health" (state registration of program for computers, №2010612275, dt. 26.03.2010).

Results of the research

It was determined that muscular mass (MM) of girls from Baykal district (17-20 years old age) in average was 23.7±0.08 kg that was 42.4±0.1 % of body mass (in the range from 25.7 to 59.4%) , and expressiveness of MM – 0.49±0.002 (in the range from 0.18 to 0. 68). Dispersion of girls" MM indicator was from minimal value 14.5 kg to maximal – 44.9 kg.

Studying of quantitative MM content in componential composition of girls" bodies during four years of their study at physical culture department witnesses, that the highest content of muscular tissue was in groups of first and second year girl students, when trainings practiced twice a week. Absolute content of MM in girls „bodies in this period was in average 24.8±0.1kg (44.6 %). When trainings started to be practiced once a week (3rd – 4th years) there was reduction of MM content characteristics up to 23.3±0.2 kg (40.2%) and. against this background, increase of fat mass ($P < 0.05$).

It is interesting to analyze dependence of motion tests" results on quantitative MM content (see table). For example in speed endurance and dexterity test (shuttle run 10x5) the best time 20.5±0.1 sec. was shown by girls with high level of MM content ($P < 0.05$). In other levels no dependence were found. In test for quickness (20 meter run from walking) we registered the same dependence of indicator"s dynamic. The best result (3.78±0.1 sec.) was shown by girls with high MM content and the lowest result (4.03±0.1 sec.) was shown by girls with MM expressiveness of "below middle" ($P < 0.05$).

Table

Dynamic of dependence of motion tests' results on level of muscular mass's expressiveness and anthropometrical parameters of girls (17-20 years old age)

Anthropometrical parameters and motion tests	Content of muscular mass (% from body mass)				
	Low (less than -1.34s)	Below middle (from -0.67s to -1.34s)	Middle M±0,67s	Above middle (from +0.67s to +1.34s)	High (more than +1.34s)
	Values of indicators and tests				
Body length, cm	165.8±0.4	165.4±0.3	164.9±0.1	165.0±0.3	166.1±0.4
Body mass, kg	56.9±0.6	54.9±0.3	55.8±0.1	56.09±0.4	56.6±0.6
Chest circumference, cm	78.7±0.1	82.4±0.04	86.1±0.05	90.7±0.05	90.6±0.4
Shuttle run 10 x 5m, sec.	21.3±0.1	21.3±0.1	21.2±0.06	21.1±0.1	20.5±0.1
Run from walking 20 m, sec.	3.97±0.04	4.03±0.1	3.97±0.04	3.98±0.1	3.78±0.1

Anthropometrical parameters and motion tests	Content of muscular mass (% from body mass)				
	Low (less than -1.34s)	Below middle (from -0.67s to -1.34s)	Middle M±0,67s	Above middle (from +0.67s to +1.34s)	High (more than +1.34s)
	Values of indicators and tests				
5 minutes run, meters	837.8±20.5	880.2±5.9	914.2±11.9	918.0±11.1	918.7±14.0
Hanging, sec.	8.8±0.3	9.6±0.3	9.7±0.1	10.3±0.3	11.3±0.6
Torso raising during 30 sec., times	22.7±0.5	23.2±0.4	23.2±0.2	23.8±0.6	24.7±0.2
Torso bending, cm	8.9±0.1	15.0±0,5	14.9±0.2	21.3±0.1	28.2±0.2
Long jump from the spot, cm	119.9±0.5	133.5±0.2	151.2±0.2	168.9±0.2	183.3±0.5

Characteristic of general endurance (test 5 minutes run) witnesses that the best result was shown by girls with high and "above high" level of muscular mass content. With it, girls with such MM content run distance by 80.9 meter longer during 5 minutes than girls with "low" level ($P < 0.05$).

In power tests (hanging and torso raising) we also registered that girls with high MM expressiveness showed better results.

Similar dynamic was registered during testing of sportsmen and not sportsmen in Lithuania [5], as well as persons, who trained weight lifting as a part of physical culture program at HEE [12].

Analysis of such characteristic as flexibility witnesses that in group of girls with high MM content indicators of "torso bending" was 3.2 times higher than in groups with low muscular mass (28.2±0.2 and 8.9±0.1 cm) accordingly, $P < 0.05$).

In test for dynamic strength of lower limbs (long jump from the spot) girls with high MM content showed result by 52.8% higher than girl students with low MM level.

Conclusions

1. Quantity of muscular mass in componential composition of girls is higher in first two years of physical culture (with lessons being conducted twice a week) (24.8±0.1kg). With passing to "once a week lessons" there happens reduction of MM content in girls" bodies by from 4.4% to 23.3±0.2 kg % and increase of fat mass against this background ($P < 0.05$).
2. In group of girls with high MM content results of all motion tests were better than in groups with "low" and "below middle" MM content.
3. Deficit of girl students" motion functioning shall be compensated with controlled independent trainings.

References:

1. Bal'sevich V.K., Lubysheva L.I. [New technologies of formation of physical culture of the schoolchild]. *Problemy sovershenstvovaniia fizicheskogo vospitaniia uchashchikhsia obshcheobrazovatel'nykh shkol. Mezhdunarodnyj seminar* [Problems of improving physical education pupils of comprehensive schools. International workshop]. Moscow, 1993, pp. 42–50. (in Russian)
2. Bujkova O.M., Tristan V.G. Vliianie zaniatij razlichnymi vidami aerobiki na komponentnyj sostav tela studentok [Effect of different types of aerobic training on body composition component of students]. *Vestnik Iuzhno-Ural'skogo gosudarstvennogo universiteta*. 2010, vol.19, no.195, pp. 131-134. (in Russian)
3. Dorokhov R. N., Petrukhin V. G. *Mediko-pedagogicheskie aspekty podgotovki iunykh sportsmenov* [Medical and pedagogical aspects of training young athletes]. Smolensk, 1989, pp. 4-14. (in Russian)
4. Zajceva V.V. *Metodologiia individual'nogo podkhoda v ozdorovitel'noj fizicheskoj kul'ture na osnove sovremennykh informacionnykh tekhnologij. Dokt.dis.* [Methodology individual approach in improving physical training on the basis of modern information technologies. Dokt. Diss.]. Moscow, 1995, 48 p. (in Russian)
5. Zuoziene I.J., Peculiarities of physical fitness and body composition of students engaged and not engaged in sports. *Physical Education of Students*, 2013, no.6, pp. 15-19. doi:10.6084/m9.figshare.840494
6. Kolokol'cev M.M., Lumpova O.M. Konstitucional'naia tipologiia organizma studentov Pribajkal'ia [Constitutional typology of students" organism of Pribaikal region]. *Vestnik Irkutskogo gosudarstvennogo tekhnicheskogo universiteta.* 2013, no.7, pp. 267–273. (in Russian)
7. Nikolaev V.G. *Metody ocenki individual'no-tipologicheskikh osobennostej fizicheskogo razvitiia cheloveka* [Methods for assessing individual typological features of physical development of a man] Krasnoyarsk, KrasGMA Publ., 2005, 111 p. (in Russian)

8. Nikolaev V.G., Sindeeva L.V. Opyt izucheniia formirovaniia morfofunkcional'nogo statusa naseleniia Vostochnoj Sibiri [The experience of studying the formation of morphofunctional status of Eastern Siberia population]. *Saratovskij nauchno-medicinskij zhurnal*. 2010, vol.6, no.2, pp. 238–241. (in Russian)
9. Rebrova O.Iu. *Statisticheskij analiz medicinskikh dannykh. Primenenie paketa prikladnykh programm STATISTICA* [Statistical analysis of medical data. Application software package STATISTICA]. Moscow, Mediasphere, 2002, 305 p. (in Russian)
10. Khodakovski-Mal'cevich L. *Zavisimost' sportivnogo rezul'tata ot razvitiia fizicheskikh kachestv i morfologicheskikh pokazatelej iunoshej na etapakh predvaritel'noj podgotovki k begu. Kand. dis.* [The dependence of the sports results from the development of physical qualities and morphological parameters of boys during the preliminary preparation for the run. Cand. Diss.]. 1992, 18 p. (in Russian)
11. Khristovaia T.E. Vliianie fizicheskikh nagruzok na obmen veshchestv i gormonal'nyj status liudej s raznym somatotipom [The influence of physical activity on the metabolism and hormonal status of people with different somatotipom]. *Fizicheskoe vospitanie studentov*. 2011, no.6, pp. 131-135. (in Russian)
12. Chernozub A.A. Kharakter izmenenij pokazatelej sostava tela u studentov v processe zaniatij fizicheskoj kul'turoj s ispol'zovaniem kompleksov atletizma [The nature of changes in body composition of students in the physical training complexes with athleticism]. *Fizicheskoe vospitanie studentov*. 2011, no.3, pp. 99-102. (in Russian)
13. Gautier G., Thouvarecq R., Larue J. Influence of Experience on Postural Control: Effect of Expertise in Gymnastics. *Journal of Motor Behavior*. 2008, vol.40, no.5, pp. 400–408.
14. Kruk J. Intensity of lifetime physical activity and breast cancer risk among Polish women. *Journal of Sports Sciences*. 2009, vol.27, no.5, pp. 437–445.
15. McPherson J., Anderson B., Blown E., Kirkland J., McLachlan-Smith C. Non-individual approaches to understanding human development. *Early Child Development and Care*. 1990, vol.55, no.1, pp. 51–57.
16. Mota J., Silva P., Santos M.P., Ribeiro J.C., Oliveira J., Duarte J.A. Physical activity and school recess time: Differences between the sexes and the relationship between children"s playground physical activity and habitual physical activity. *Journal of Sports Sciences*. 2005, vol.23, no.3, pp. 269–275.
17. Rhodes R.E., de Bruijn G-J. Automatic and Motivational Correlates of Physical Activity: Does Intensity Moderate the Relationship? *Behavioral Medicine*. 2010, vol.36, no.2, pp. 44–52.
18. Scott F., Rhodes R.E., Downs D.S. Does Physical Activity Intensity Moderate Social Cognition and Behavior Relationships? *Journal of American College Health*. 2009, vol.58, no.3,pp. 213–222.
19. Sobko I.N., Kozina Zh.L., Iermakov S.S., Muszkieta Radosław, Prusik Krzysztof, Cieślicka Mirosława, Stankiewicz Błażej. Comparative characteristics of the physical and technical preparedness of the women's national team of Ukraine and Lithuania basketball (hearing impaired) before and after training to Deaflympic Games. *Pedagogics, psychology, medical-biological problems of physical training and sports*, 2014, no.10, pp. 45-51. http://dx.doi.org/10.5281/zenodo.10490
20. Szalma J.L., Individual differences in human–technology interaction: incorporating variation in human characteristics into human factors and ergonomics research and design. *Theoretical Issues in Ergonomics Science*. 2009, no.10, pp. 381–397. http://dx.doi.org/10.1080/14639220902893613

RATIONALE SET OF INDICATORS AND PRIORITIZE RELEVANT TO ASSESS COMPETITIVE ACTIVITY OF HOCKEY PLAYERS OF HIGH QUALIFICATION OF DIFFERENT ROLES

Mikhnov A.P.
National University of Physical Education and Sport of Ukraine

Annotation. *Purpose:* organize technical and tactical actions and determine their priority importance for high-end players of different roles. Establish their priority importance for the success of competitive activity hockey with the game roles. *Material*: the study involved 54 experts on hockey coaches and players of high class. The significance of technical and tactical actions evaluated for players of different roles. *Results*: systematic account of technical and tactical actions of athletes and prioritize them to assess the significance of competitive activity. Three groups of technical and tactical actions: 1) active attacks; 2) - active safety; 3) - organizational and maneuvering. Set priorities for technical and tactical actions for players of different roles. *Conclusions*: the proposed technical and tactical actions can be recommended for the evaluation of the effectiveness of competitive activity players. In the process of estimating the action game players need to consider their role playing. Identification of priority in the implementation of technical and tactical actions in the game can be used in integrated assessment of actions players different roles.
Keywords: competitive, activities, technique, tactics, reliability index, indicator of success.

Introduction

Perfection of management of competition functioning on the base of objectification of knowledge about its structure and provisioning components is one of the most important tasks of sportsmen training system's formation in game kinds of sports [5,6,7,11,17,20].

Prestige character and popularity of sport games, their high level of competitiveness at international sport arena and importance of sport result are so evident that urgency of questions, connected with increasing of competition functioning's effectiveness is out of the question [1-3,12-15,19].

One of the most important problems in sport games in general and in hockey in particular is evaluation of competition functioning. Total sport result of a collective does not always permits to reflect competition functioning of separate players [4,8,9,18].

Active counter action of adversary requires instant change of previously worked out plan of individual hockey player's and team's actions. Sportsmen have to act in conditions of expressed deficit of time with changes of game situation and demand in adequate response [10].

For evaluation of actions in match specialists consider qualitative and quantitative characteristics of technical tactic actions. Such actions are means of realization of sport duel's tasks and they also serve as the most informative criteria, permitting to reflect sportsman's behavior in match and effectiveness of his actions [8,16]. However, with it, it is necessary to consider the fact that hockey players of different roles have different priorities in realization of different tasks in match.

Thus, in present research we have tried to systemize technical tactic actions, fulfilled by hockey players in competition functioning and to determine their priority importance for hockey players of different roles. The work has been fulfilled in the frames of scientific research topic 2.4. "Theoretical methodic principles and individualization of training process in game kinds of sports" in compliance with combined plan of SRW in sphere of physical culture and sports for 2011-2015.

Purpose, tasks of the work, material and methods

The purpose of the work is to systemize technical tactic actions and determine of their priority significance for highly qualified hockey players of different roles.

The tasks of the research were to determine and systemize technical tactic actions, offered by specialists for evaluation of competition functioning, determination of their priority significance for successful competition functioning of highly qualified hockey players, considering their roles in match.

The methods of the research: pedagogic observation and generalization of special scientific-methodic literature data, expert questioning, analysis of Internet data. In researches 54 experts participated, who, in order of priority, determined significance of technical tactic actions for hockey players of different roles.

Results of the research

Analysis of special scientific-methodic literature and questioning of hockey experts showed that in competition functioning hockey players fulfill great number of different technical-tactic actions and every of them influence on sport duel's process and can, to some or other extent, influence on its result.

In total more than thirty separate match actions were marked out, which can be conventionally divided (for systemizing) into three main groups (see fig.1) Detail grouping and differentiation were determined by sense similarity of actions and their relation to different phases of match.

So, in separate group we can mark out those technical-tactic actions, which are oriented on active attack of adversary's net and sharpening of attacking phase – group of active attacking actions.

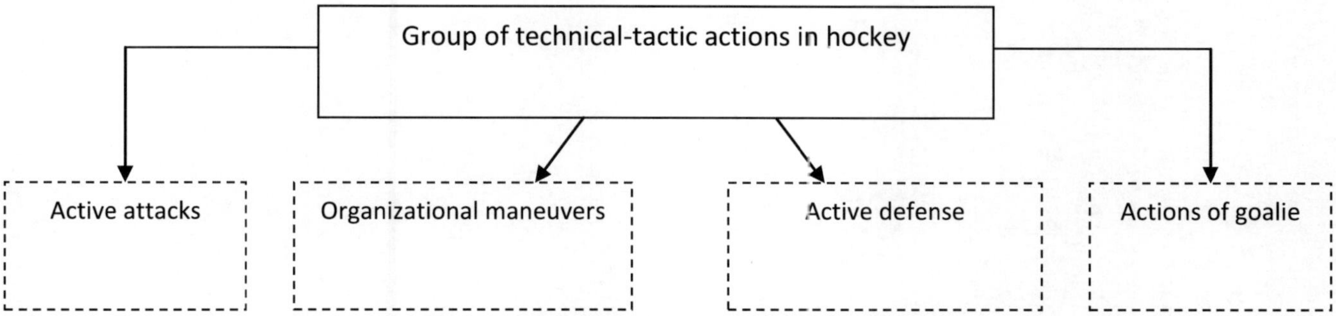

Fig.1. Groups of technical tactic actions in hockey

The second group contains technical-tactic actions, oriented on organization of hockey players' actions and their skating on field, maneuvering and current interaction, i.e. organizational-maneuvering actions.

The third group (active defensive actions) consists of hockey players' actions, oriented on defense of net and active picking up of puck.

Technical-tactic actions, fulfilled by goalie can be marked out in separate group – game of hockey goalie.

So, among active attacking actions experts offer to mark out throws in hockey net, thrown in pucks, efficient passes, duels with adversary's goalie. Besides, to day indicator of gained scores (sum of thrown in pucks) is used as important indicator for highly qualified hockey players.

Group of organizational-maneuvering actions contains the most of actions, which can be fulfilled both in phase of defense and in phase of attack.

In this group, among main technical–tactic actions the following can be marked out: dribbling of puck, maneuvering on skates, cheating of adversary (by long trajectory, short, with strength), passes of puck (excluding efficient), catching of puck by body, coming out of adversary's guiding, choosing of position and etc.

This group can also include fight of hockey players at throw of puck on field because successful or unsuccessful start can influence on further organizational actions of team.

The third group – active defensive actions - includes the following: picking up of puck, power fight, repelling of puck and etc.

Besides, specialists offer to mark out a number of indicators, which characterize effectiveness of competition functioning of goalie. These indicators in general characterize successfulness of repelling of pucks from net. As informative indicators they mark out the following: quantity of throws in net, quantity of missed pucks, percentage of missed pucks, index of reliability (integral index of match's effectiveness).

As a result of questioning experts marked out and offered to use in our further researches the following informative technical-tactic actions and indicators of hockey players: fulfilled throws in net; thrown in pucks; percentage of throws' realization; quantity of power techniques; penalty minutes for violation of rules; efficient passes, successful throws of puck on field; pucks, repelled from net; picking ups of pucks; realized obstacles for goalkeeper; support of partner; loss of puck; gained scores; indicator of successfulness +/-.

Separately for evaluation of competition functioning of goalie experts marked out the following technical-tactic actions and indicators: missed pucks; repelled pucks; percentage of repelled pucks; index of reliability (integral indicator, conv. un.).

In order to determine the most significant technical-tactic actions for highly qualified hockey players of different roles we conducted questioning of experts, hockey specialists (see fig.2). Concordance coefficient was W=0.76, that witnesses about high concordance of experts, hockey specialists.

For example for winger experts related to the most significant technical tactic actions the following: thrown in pucks– 15%, gained scores in match– 15 %, percentage of throws' realization– 14 % total quantity of throws in net– 10 %. For center forward, in opinion of experts, technical-tactic actions of priority are: thrown in pucks – 16%, gained scores – 14%, percentage of throws' realization – 13 %.

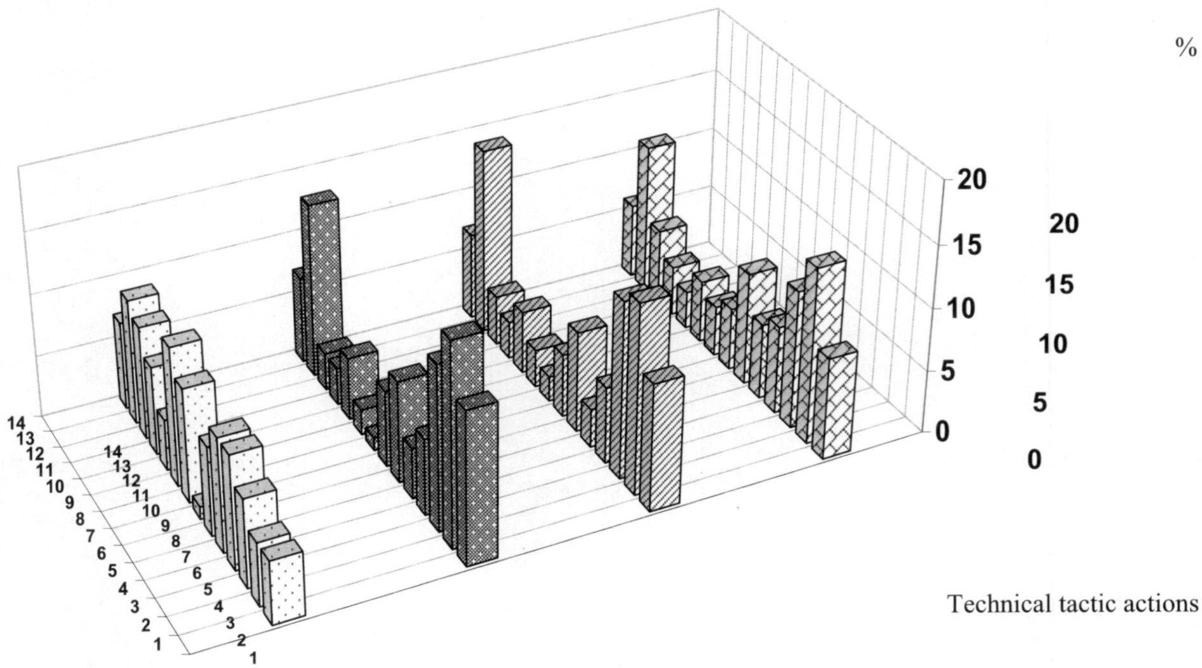

Fig.2. Significance of technical-tactic actions for highly qualified hockey players of different roles (in experts' opinion, n=54):

Without consideration of role; winger; center forward; back

1 – Throws in netl; 2 – thrown in pucks; 3 – percentage of throws' realization; 4 – power techniques; 5 – penalty minutes; 6 – efficient passes; 7 – successful throws on field; 8 – repelled pucks; 9 – picking ups of puck; 10 – obstacle to goalkeeper; 11 – support of partner; 12 –loss of puck; 13 – the gained scores; 14 – indicator of successfulness +/-.

Among the most significant technical-tactic actions of a back, experts marked out the following: picking up of puck - 10%, gained scores– 10 %, power techniques– 9 %, losses of puck repelled from net pucks – 9 %, indicator of successfulness (+/-) - 7 %. One of main tasks of backs is defense of own net, repelling of adversary's pucks, directed to net. During match backs shall conduct personal duels, use power techniques.

Also we separately conducted expert questioning about significance of actions in match for goalie. This way or another all technical-tactic actions and match indicators, which are used at present for evaluation of hockey goalie competition functioning, are connected with his skills in repelling throws to goal. From the offered by experts indicators the most significant are: missed pucks – 32 %, index of reliability – 25 points, percentage of repelled pucks – 22 %, repelled throws in net– 21 % (see fig.3).

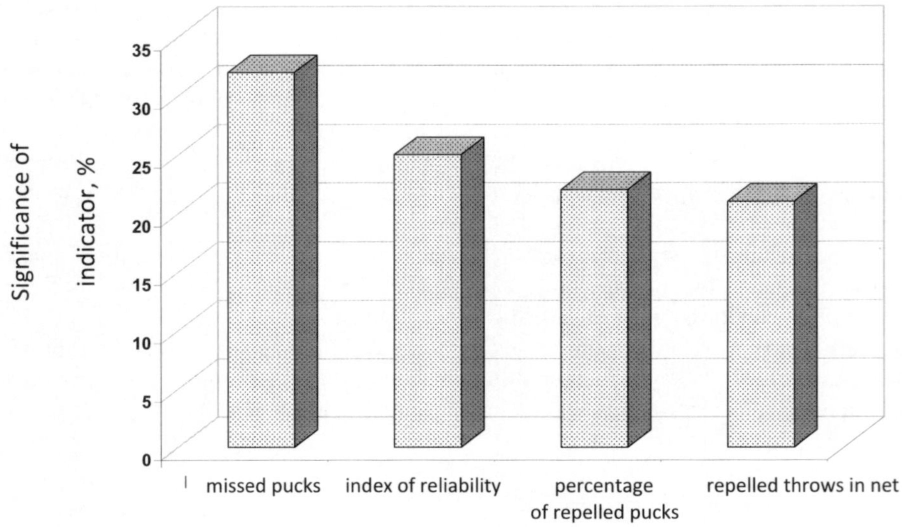

Fig.3. Significance of match indicators for highly qualified hockey goalkeeper (in experts' opinion, n=54):

In specialists' opinion, good goalie shall have perfect reaction, ability to take correct position in front of hockey net and organize coordinated actions of partners in defense. Important qualities in hockey goalkeeper's actions are abilities for instant responding and anticipation.

Conclusions:

1. The conducted analysis of literature sources, pedagogic observations and questioning of experts permitted to systemize technical tactic actions, fulfilled by highly qualified hockey players in match and conventionally divide them into three relatively independent groups: 1) active attacking actions; 2) organizational-maneuvering actions; 3) active defensive actions; 4) actions of hockey goalie.
2. As a result of conducted exerts' questioning we determined the most informative indicators, which are recommended to be used for control and evaluation of hockey players' competition functioning: fulfilled throws in hockey net; thrown in pucks;, percentage of realization of throws in net; fulfilled power techniques; penalty minutes for violation of rules; efficient passes of puck; successful throws on field;, repelled from hockey net pucks; picked up pucks; obstacles for hockey goalie; support of partner; loss of puck; gained scores; indicator of successfulness (+/-). For hockey players of different roles expert marked out as technical tactic actions of first priority the following: for winger they are thrown in net pucks – 15%, gained in match scores– 15 %, percentage of throws' realization– 14 %. For center forward: thrown in net pucks - Для 16%, gained scores– 14%, percentage of realization of throws in hockey net– 13 %. For backs: picking up of pucks– 10%, gained scores– 10 %, power techniques– 9 %, потери шайбы – 9 %, repelled from net pucks– 9 %

The prospects of further researches imply working out of model characteristics of technical tactic actions of different roles' highly qualified hockey players as well as analysis of influence of personality's psychological features on hockey players' competition functioning.

References:

1. Ajrapet'ianc L.G. *Pedagogicheskie osnovy planirovaniia i kontrolia uchebno-trenirovochnoj i sorevnovatel'noj deiatel'nosti v sportivnykh igrakh. Dokt.diss.* [Pedagogical bases of planning and control for training and competitive activity in sports. Dokt. Diss.]. Moscow, 1992, 41 p. (in Russian)
2. Babushkin V.Z. *Specializaciia v sportivnykh igrakh* [Specialization in sports games]. Kiev, 1991, 161 p. (in Russian)
3. Bezmylov N.N. Obosnovanie kompleksa informativnykh pokazatelej i opredelenie ikh prioritetnoj znachimosti dlia otbora kvalificirovannykh basketbolistov v komandu [Justification complex informative indicators and determining their priority importance to the selection of qualified basketball team]. *Fizicheskoe vospitanie studentov*, 2010, no.2, pp. 18-23. (in Russian)
4. Godik M.A., Skorodumova A.P. *Kompleksnyj kontrol' v sportivnykh igrakh* [Complex control in sports games]. Moscow, 2010, 336 p. (in Russian)
5. Keller V.S. *Sorevnovatel'naia deiatel'nost' v sisteme sportivnoj podgotovki. Sovremennaia sistema sportivnoj podgotovki* [Competitive activity in the athletic training]. Moscow, 1995, pp. 41–50. (in Russian)
6. Kozina Zh.L. *Individualizaciia podgotovki sportsmenov v igrovykh vidakh sporta* [Individualization of training of athletes in team sports]. Kharkov, 2009, 396 p. (in Russian)
7. Kostiukevich V. Integral'naia ocenka tekhniko-takticheskoj deiatel'nosti vysokokvalificirovannykh igrokov v khokkee na trave [Integral assessment of technical and tactical activity of highly skilled players in field of hockey]. *Nauka v olimpijskom sporte*, 2008, no.1, pp. 32-40. (in Russian)
8. Krasnikov A.A. *Osnovy teorii sportivnykh sorevnovanij* [Fundamentals of the theory of sports competitions]. Moscow, 2005, 160 p. (in Russian)
9. Latyshkevich L.A., Vorob'ev M.I., Bukhtij L.G. Problema povysheniia effektivnosti sorevnovatel'noj deiatel'nosti v sportivnykh igrakh [The problem of increasing the efficiency of competitive activity in sports games], *Nauka v olimpijskom sporte,* 1997, no.2, pp. 13-16. (in Russian)
10. Platonov V.N. *Sistema podgotovki sportsmenov v olimpijskom sporte* [The system of preparation of sportsmen in Olympic sport], Kiev, Olympic Literature, 2004, 808 p. (in Russian)
11. Portnov Iu.M. *Teoreticheskie i nauchno-metodicheskie osnovy podgotovki kvalificirovannykh sportsmenov v igrovykh vidakh sporta. Dokt.diss.* [Theoretical and methodological bases of preparation of qualified athletes in team sports. Dokt. Diss.]. Moscow, 1989, 51 p. (in Russian)
12. Savenkov G.I. *Psikhologicheskaia podgotovka sportsmena v sovremennoj sisteme sportivnoj trenirovki* [Psychological training of athlete in the modern system of sports training]. Moscow, Physical Culture and Sport, 2006, 96 p. (in Russian)
13. Temchenko V.A. Registraciia, obrabotka i analiz pokazatelej sorevnovatel'noj deiatel'nosti v sportivnykh igrakh [Registration, processing and analysis of competitive activity in sports games]. *Fizicheskoe vospitanie studentov tvorcheskikh special'nostej,* 2006, no.2, pp. 37–48. (in Russian)
14. Shinkaruk O.A., Bezmilov M.M. Teoretiko-metodichni zasadi rozrobki ta vikoristannia model'nikh kharakteristik tekhniko-taktichnikh dij basketbolistiv visokoi kvalifikacii [Theoretical and methodological basis for the development and use of model performance technical and tactical basketball skill]. *Teoriia i metodika fizichnogo vikhovannia i sportu,* 2013, no.2, pp. 35-44. (in Ukrainian)

15. Shustin B.N. *Model'nye kharakteristiki sorevnovatel'noj deiatel'nosti. Sovremennaia sistema sportivnoj podgotovki* [Model characteristics of competitive activity]. Moscow, 1995, pp. 226 – 237.
16. Bompa T.O., Carrera M. *Periodization training for sports*. Chapmaign, Human Kinetics, 2005, 259 p.
17. Enciu S.L. Hockey. *For children and juniors. Quidde book for young coaches*. Romanicu Field Hockey Federation. 2001, 272 p.
18. Trninić S., Dizdar D. Performance Evaluation Criteria. *Coll. Antropol.* 2000, vol.24, no.1, pp. 217–234.
19. Platonov V.N. *Qualified Sportsmen Training*. Moscow, Physical Culture and Sports, 1986, 255 p.

INFLUENCE EMPLOYMENT BY IMPROVING AEROBICS ON MOTOR READINESS OF GIRLS

Shypulo I. P.
Chernihiv National Pedagogical University

Annotation. *Purpose*: substantiate the effect of employment by improving aerobics on motor readiness of girls in extracurricular educational institutions. *Material*: the study involved 90 women aged 16-18 years old. Classes are held 3 times a week for 1 hour each. *Results*: defined state and the most informative indicators motor fitness girls. Built analytical model of graph model for forecasting and conducting quantitative and qualitative control of motor fitness girls. The degree of severity of each of the parameters studied motor fitness girls. *Conclusions*: the possibilities of predicting outcomes. Recommended method of aerobics classes, which has five stages. Its main feature - the constant objective control efficiency of employment.
Keywords: classes, aerobics, motion, training, girls.

Introduction

Worsening of health and insufficient motion fitness of school age children is undoubtedly a serious problem [15]. That is why, at present, one of main tasks is control of strengthening of youth's health, formation of their demand in motion perfection and healthy life style.

Unfortunately, as on to day traditional physical culture lesson ensures, in average, up to 11% of required weekly motion functioning; about 50% of children have no steady interest to physical culture [5]. Most of specialists think that accent on increasing of physical culture-physical education work shall be realized in out of school forms of trainings.

Hat is why at present there is active implementation of innovative methodic in out of school educational establishments in order to achieve and maintain children's optimal physical condition, their motivation and individual features [1, 2, 14].

These problems were reflected in Conception of out of school education and learning, in Laws of Ukraine "On education", "On physical culture and sports", in National doctrine of development of education, in National doctrine of physical culture and sports development, in decree of Council of Ministries of Ukraine "On approval of nomenclature of national educational establishments' types; principles of out of school educational establishments and National strategy of development of education in Ukraine for 2011-2016. The state ensures creation of all conditions for children's involvement in sports and motion functioning.

It is known that just motion fitness influences substantially on physical condition of a person. For example, it can improve health and mental state of a person (reduce risk of many diseases, strengthen "life tonus", activity and workability, regulate organism's functioning, improve mood, everyday self-feeling and so on). It improves physical condition (increases strength and endurance, flexibility and coordination); it improves posture (reduces quantity of fat, increase or reduce volume of muscles and etc.). Alongside with it motion fitness is interpreted as result of comprehensive development of motion abilities, functional potentials of organism's organs and systems, their coordination in process of muscular functioning [6, 9, 15, 20].

Analysis of health related practices witnesses that among girls one of the most popular kinds of health related physical culture is aerobic. Analysis of scientific methodic literature showed that high health related effect is reached exactly with aerobics' exercises [3, 5, 11, 12].

As on to day there have been researched and worked out great number of methodic and programs of aerobics' traininga [4, 7, 8, 10, 13, 16-19]; but the problem of demand in aerobics' trainings of 16-18 years old girls in out of school educational establishments has been still remaining urgent and insufficiently studied.

The work has been fulfilled in compliance with priority direction of scientific researches of Chernigov national pedagogic university, named after T.G. Shevchenko: Didactic principles of motion functions' formation of persons, practicing physical culture and sports", (state registration number 0108U000854, dt. February 19th, 2008), "Pedagogic ways of formation of healthy life style of different age groups' schoolchildren" (state registration number 0112U001072 dt. 18.01.2012).

Purpose, tasks of the work, material and methods

The purpose of the work is to analyze influence of health related aerobics' trainings on girls' motion fitness in out of school educational establishments.

The research was conducted on the base of methodic center of vocational training in Chernigov region and in Regional public organization "Federation of aerobics of Chernigovschina", Federation of aerobics in Odessa, studio of dance and aerobics "VerDikt", dancing center "5th element" and on the base of Chernigov national pedagogic university, named after T.G. Schevchenko.

For solution of our tasks, in academic health related process on aerobics at out of school educational establishment we introduce and carried out forming pedagogic experiment (we created experimental and control groups). Experimental (EG) group of girls was trained by offered by us methodic, control group (CG) – by traditional.

Trainings were conducted trice a week; 1 hour every training. Total scope and intensity of loads in both groups were equal. Trainings in CG were conducted in compliance with recommendations [4, 8, 10].

The worked out by us structure of process of girls' motion development at aerobics' trainings at out of school educational establishments included: purpose; certain tasks, model indicators of development of motion abilities, health and motion progress; principles; control; scope of load; forms of trainings' organization; methods; system of pedagogic influences; practical application; health related result.

Exactly methodic of aerobic training of girls at out of school educational establishments includes five stages, which differ by particular tasks and purposes.

We conducted the following tests: 1 – long jump, cm; 2- "Shuttle run", sec.; 3- chin ups, q-ty of times; 4- pressing ups in lying position, q-ty of times; 5 – taking sitting position from lying one (during 1 minute); 6- hanging on bent arms, sec.; 7- forward torso bending, cm; 8- dynamometry of backbone, kg.

Testing was fulfilled at the beginning and at the end of experiment. Experiment lasted for three years.

Results of the research

Research of girls' (who train aerobics) motion fitness is very important for practice of training and education of rising generation. Exactly such researches permit to reveal all problems at aerobics' trainings and in changing of girls' individual abilities under influence of trainings, as well as to reveal motivation and interest to trainings.

By results of tests we determined girls' motion fitness in special health group (SHG) and in sport group (SG).

We found that in SHG, in comparison with SG (see fig.1) indicators of motion fitness were much worse. For example:

- In long running jump SHG girls' indicators: 121.30±5.17 cm and 198.52±7.28 cm;
- In "Shuttle run": 16.84±1.43 sec. and 10.55±1.04 min.;
-In chin ups, SHG groups' girls had 2.58±0.27 times and 5.04±0.51 timers;
- In pressing ups in lying position SHG indicators were 16.77±1.71 times and in SG 30.53±3.15 times;
- Taking sitting position from lying one (during 1 minute) in SHG – 23.52±2.42 times and in SG – 45.00±3.94 times;
- Indicators of hanging on bent arms in SHG were 22.28±2.51 sec. and in SG – 41.68±4.31 sec;
- Indicators of forward torso bending in SHG were 13.93±1.41 cm and 26.68±2.70 cm;
- Indicators of backbone dynamometry were in SHG 32.79±3.34 kg and in SG - 59.74±6.10 kg.

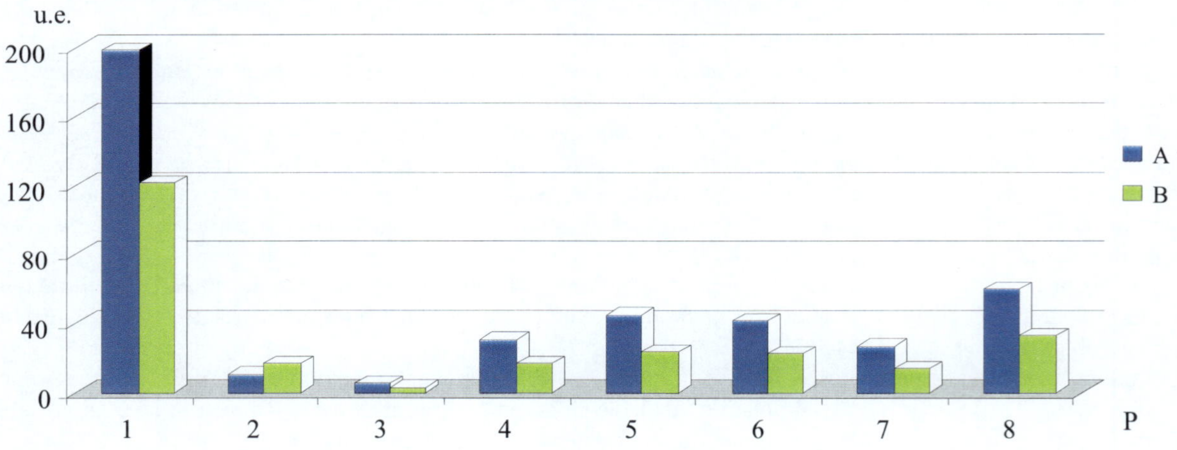

P – indicators; u.e. – conventional units.

Fig.1. Mean statistical results of motion fitness of SHG (A) SG(B)girls:

1 – long jump, cm; 2 – "Shuttle run", sec.; 3 – Chin ups, q-ty of times; 4 – Pressing ups in lying position, q-ty of times; 5 – Taking sitting position from lying one (during 1 minute); 6 – Hanging on bent arms, sec.; 7 – Forward torsi bending, cm; 8 – Back dynamometry, kg.

It was determined that girls of sport group had better motion fitness. The received data permit to rather objectively prognosticate results with purposeful, comprehensive girls' trainings of aerobics.

Correlation analysis permitted to determine the most informative girls' indicators. The received indicators are interconnected and influence on girls' physical fitness.

On the base of the obtained data we built graphic analytic model for quantitative and qualitative control, which also permits to prognosticate development of girls' motion fitness (see fig.2).

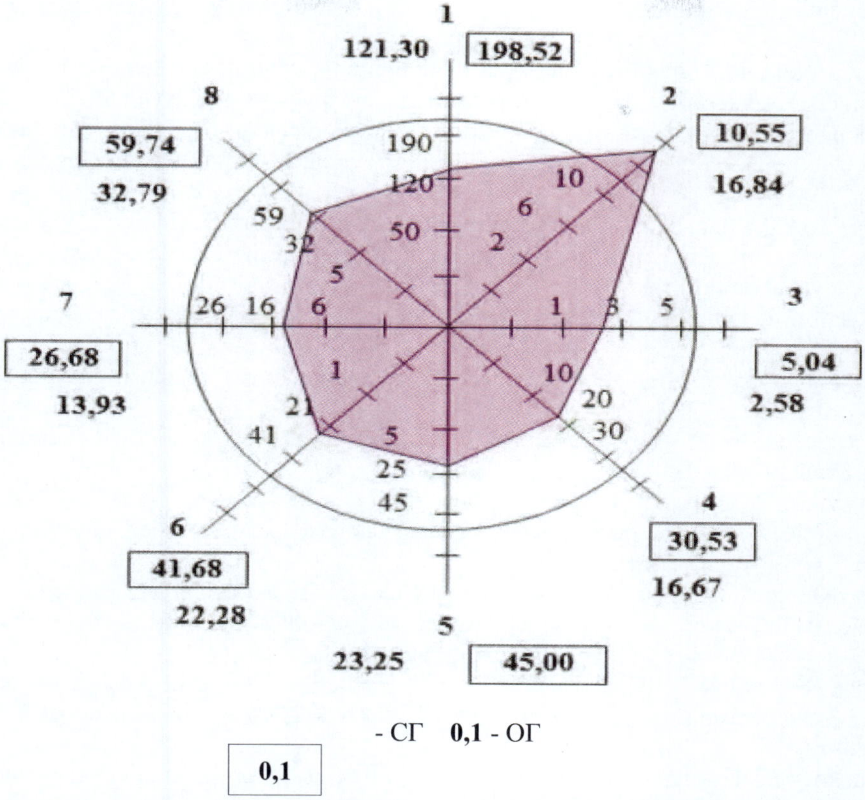

Fig.2. Graphic analytical model of motion fitness of health related (SHG) group's girls and sport group's (SG) girls: 1 – shuttle run; 2 – forward torso bending; 3 – taking sitting position from lying one during 1 minute; 4 – backbone dynamometry (torso); 5 – long jump; 6 – chin ups; 7 – hanging on bent arms; 8 – pressing ups in lying position.

Analysis of aerobic trainings' influence on girls' motion fitness showed that in EG it improved by 37%, and in CG – by 23% (see fig.3).

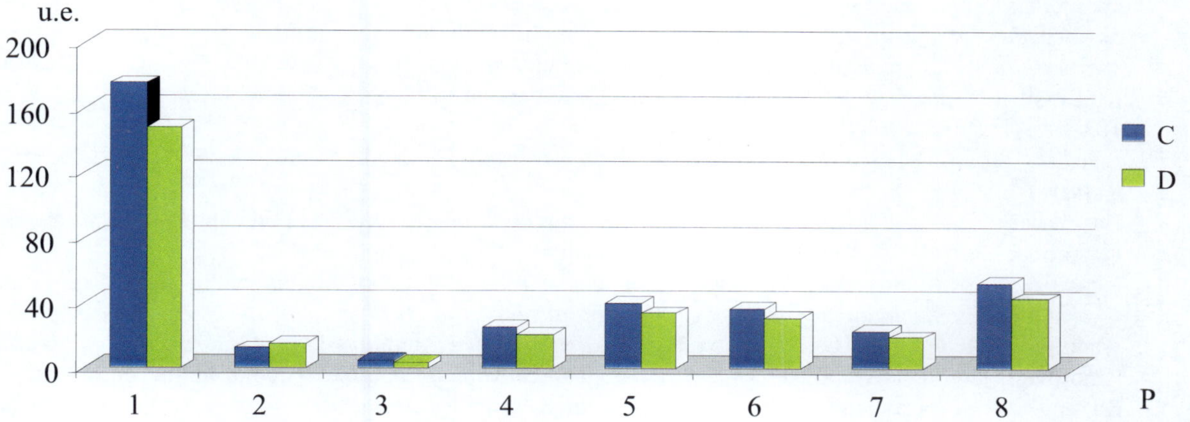

P -indicators; u.e. – conventional units.

Fig.3. Comparison of motion fitness of experimental group's girls (C) and control group's girl (D): 1 – shuttle run; 2 – forward torso bending; 3 – taking sitting position from lying one during 1 minute; 4 – backbone dynamometry (torso); 5 – long jump; 6 – chin ups; 7 – hanging on bent arms; 8 – pressing ups in lying position.

The received EG indicators are much better than indicators of CG and witness that introduction of experimental methodic was rather useful.

Discussion

In the whole, in context of improvement of girls' motion fitness our data are accorded quite satisfactory with ideas of other authors [4, 7, 8, 10, 13, 16- 19]. Alongside with it approaches, recommended by us, differ a little from commonly accepted by the following:

- complex approach to application of aerobics for comprehensive girls' development;
- at aerobics' trainings we used new and variable means and methods;

- development of girls' motion skills was realized with accurate dozing of loads' parameter and their control at every training;

- realization of health, functional state and motion fitness control контроль took place at every training, every week, every month for determination of loads' parameters and diagnostic of dynamic of indicators' change;

- in power part of every training we paid attention to development of legs', arms' and torso muscles;

- we also paid attention to perfection of coordination, videlicet: dexterity, jumping ability, balance, rhythm and etc.;

- in warming up and final parts of every training we paid attention to flexibility;

- trainings were conducted with application of aerobics' health related exercises, which were based on prognostic graphic analytical models;

- for evaluation of initial data of girls' motion fitness we used bio-mechanical indicators except generally accepted characteristics;

- correction of girls' motion fitness at aerobics' trainings was realized on the base bio-mechanical monitoring.

In general results of pedagogic experiment completely prove our opinion about solution of increasing of girls' motion fitness at out of school educational establishments.

Conclusions:

1. Testing of effectiveness of pedagogic experiment showed that purposeful education-learning process of health related aerobics improves girls' motion fitness.
2. The received indicators of girls' motion fitness are maximally close to model indicators.
3. Application of the newest means and methods will vary aerobics' trainings of 16-18 years' old girls.

References:

1. Bulatova M.M. Fitnes i dvigatel'naia aktivnost': problemy i puti resheniia [Fitness and physical activity: problems and decision ways]. *Teoriia i metodika fizicheskogo vospitaniia i sporta*, 2007, no.1, pp. 3-7. (in Russian)
2. Zinchenko V.B., Usachev Iu.A. *Fitnes-tekhnologii v fizicheskom vospitanii* [Fitness technology in physical education], Kiev, NAU, 2011, 152 p. (in Russian)
3. Ivlev M.P. *Soderzhanie i metodika zaniatij ritmicheskoj gimnastikoj s zhenshchinami zrelogo vozrasta. Kand.dis.* [Content and methodology of employment by rhythmic gymnastics with women of mature age. Kand.dis.], Moscow, 1987, 23 p. (in Russian)
4. Krivoruchko S.N., Panasejko Iu.G., Belous N.S. *Aerobika na zaniatiiakh po fizicheskom vospitaniiu* [Aerobics on physical education classes], Kharkov, KHAI, 2012, 56 p. (in Russian)
5. Krucevich T.Iu., Bezverkhniaia G.V. [Formation of motivation in physical education and sport at school age]. *Olimpijskij sport i sport dlia vsekh. Problemy zdorov'ia, rekreacii, sportivnoj mediciny i reabilitacii, IV Mezhdunarodnyj nauchnyj kongress* [Olympic sport and sport for all. Health problems, recreation, sports medicine and rehabilitation. IV International Scientific Congress], Kiev, 2000, pp. 385. (in Russian)
6. Kuzemko L.M. *Razvitie fizicheskikh kachestv* [Development of physical qualities], Chernigov, 2008, pp. 108-146. (in Russian)
7. Lisickaia T.S., Sidneva L.V. *Aerobika* [Aerobics]. Moscow, Federation aerobics, 2002, no.2, 232 p. (in Russian)
8. Bachinskaia N.V., Lapuga G.V. *Uchebnye zaniatiia po aerobike* [Teaching aerobics classes], Dnepropetrovsk, RVVDNU, 2011, 52 p. (in Russian)
9. Nosko N.A., Arkhipov A.A. [Quality motor as the main criteria of human motor function]. *Vestnik Chernigovskogo nacional'nogo pedagogicheskogo universiteta*. 2013, no.2, pp. 25-29. (in Russian)
10. Abdullin M.G., Gimranova L.V., Lopatina Z.F., Rylova E.V., Khalitova O.Iu. *Ozdorovitel'naia aerobika* [Improving aerobics], Ufa, Bashkir State Pedagogical University Publ., 2010, 64 p. (in Russian)
11. Rajcina L.P. [Sports and dance aerobics in high school]. *Materialy IY mezhvuzovskoj nauchno-prakticheskoj konferencii «Fizicheskoe vospitanie i sport uchashchejsia molodezhi»*. [IY Interuniversity Scientific and Practical Conference "Physical education and sport students."]. Moscow, MGIU, 1998, pp. 12 – 13. (in Russian)
12. Rostovceva M.Iu. *Povyshenie fizicheskoj rabotosposobnosti zhenshchin molodogo vozrasta sredstvami ritmicheskoj gimnastiki. Kand.dis.* [Increase physical performance young women by means of rhythmic gymnastics. Kand.dis.], Malahovka, 1990, 24 p. (in Russian)
13. Sinica S.V., Shesterova L.E. *Ozdorovitel'naia aerobika* [Improving aerobics], Poltava, PNPU, 2011, 236 p. (in Russian)
14. Usachev V.I. *Sposob kachestvennoj ocenki funkcii ravnovesiia* [A method of qualitative evaluation of balance function]. Patent UA, no. 2175851, 2001. (in Ukrainian)
15. Khoroshukha M.F. *Osnovy zdorov'ia iunykh sportsmenov* [Health basics of young athletes], Kiev, NUBiP Ukraine, 2014, 722 p. (in Russian)

16. Shevchenko O.Iu. [Influence of improving aerobics on the functional state]. *Olimpijs'kij sport i sport dlia vsikh. 14 Mizhnarodnij naukovij kongres* [14 International Scientific Congress. Olympic sport and sport for all], Kiev, 2010, pp. 639. (in Ukrainian)
17. Céline Aguer, Olivier Gavarry, Yoann Gole, Alain Boussuges, Pierre Doyard, Guy Falgairette. A 5-month weight-reduction programme has a positive effect on body composition, aerobic fitness, and habitual physical activity of severely obese girls: A pilot evaluation study. *Journal of Sports Sciences*. 2010, vol.28, no.3, pp. 281-289.
18. Marcus Wayne Kilpatrick, Amy Lynn Bortzfield, Lisa Marie Giblin. Impact of aerobic exercise trials with varied intensity patterns on perceptions of effort: An evaluation of predicted, in-task, and session exertion. *Journal of Sports Sciences*. 2012, vol.30, no.8, pp. 825-832.
19. Melitta McNarry & Andy Jones. The influence of training status on the aerobic and anaerobic responses to exercise in children: A review. Journal: *European Journal of Sport Science*. 2014, vol.14, no.1, pp. S57-S68.
20. Stuart J.H. Biddle, Rock Braithwaite, Natalie Pearson. The effectiveness of interventions to increase physical activity among young girls: A meta-analysis. *Preventive Medicine*, 2014, no.62, pp. 119-131.

6

POSITION OF MEDICAL COLLEGES' STUDENTS IN RESPECT TO SIGNIFICANCE OF PHYSICAL EXERCISES' PRACTICING AND RESONS, CONDITIONING IT

Kubaj G.V.
Vasyl Stefanyk Precarpathian National University

Abstract. *Purpose:* to create pre-conditions for rising effectiveness of physical exercises' practicing by increasing of appropriate medical colleges students' motivation and attitude to role of such trainings in health strengthening and protection. *Material:* in the research 221 students (105 boys and 116 girls) participated; all they were 3rd year students. *Results:* Extra curriculum physical exercises' training is much more interesting for boys. With it 50% of boys and girls like in-college physical culture lessons. The content of such trainings does not facilitate formation of students' position in respect to role of such exercises in health strengthening and protection. There is deficit of students' appropriate knowledge and absence of their understanding of demand in mastering of appropriate knowledge and skills. *Conclusions:* for removal of detected drawbacks it is necessary to improve organization and content of medical colleges' students' physical education, considering the received data.
Key words: knowledge, motives, physical, education, students, medical college.

Introduction

One of important aspects of normative-legal and instructive-directive documents of national educational system is connected with health strengthening and protection of students [5, 8, 9]. It becomes still more important in case with future medical workers of primary level. It is conditioned by the fact that at the stage of education formation of students' readiness for motivation of their future patients for healthy life style is not of less importance.

In this connection it is necessary to pay attention to one of the most important its components – motor functioning with optimal parameters. This functioning is realized in different forms of physical exercises' practicing [1–3, 13]. Motor functioning is ensured in medical colleges by compulsory trainings, envisaged by curriculum. Physical trainings are conducted twice a week in the form of lessons. Besides there is an opportunity to attend extra curriculum trainings in sport circles by kinds of sports, with optional attendance. In this connection the decisive condition is students' motivation as well as students' practicing of other forms of physical trainings [4, 7, 18–20]: independent individual or group sessions. That is why formation of motivation in medical colleges' students is extremely important task of physical education theory.

The available in special literature sparse data 8, 10–12] witness about 15-17 years old youth's insufficient motor functioning. It is one of reasons of other low indicators, which characterize somatic health, organism systems' functional potentials; condition of physical abilities [14–16]. Pedagogic colleges' readiness for realization of students' health related physical culture training is at level below middle (4.7±0.01 conv.un.) at the first year. Then, there appears a tendency for reduction with every following year [10]. It was found that in 54.5% of medical colleges' students vauelogic competence is at low level [8]. Such data point at demand in increasing of their physical education effectiveness. In such case the main task is formation of firm and adequate position in respect to physical exercises' practicing for health protection and strengthening (both personal and future patients').

Thus, the received information witnesses about sparse researches in the studied direction and their fragmentary character. That is why, the researches in the mentioned direction are still important.

Purpose, tasks of the work, material and methods

The purpose of the research is to create pre-conditions for rising effectiveness of physical exercises' practicing by increasing of appropriate medical colleges students' motivation and attitude to role of such trainings in health strengthening and protection.

The tasks of the research: to substantiate demand in increase of the studied trainings' effectiveness; to determine motivation of medical colleges' students for physical exercises' practicing and their position in respect to role of such trainings in health strengthening and protection; to generalize the received data. In questioning 221 students (105 boys and 116 girls) participated; all they were 3rd year students. Selection was carried out by method of random sampling. We used the worked out by us, considering recommendations of special literature, questionnaire [17].

Results of the research

The received data witness: in issue of physical exercises' practicing for health strengthening and protection students' position does not concord with specialists' position. In particular, only 27.6% girls and 65.7% of boys allocate first place to physical exercises' practicing. Analysis of the received answers showed that in opinion of 34.5% of girls and 20% of boys physical exercises' practicing does not enter in three priority kinds. Besides, 20.7% of girls and 42.8% of boys definitely consider knowledge about means and methods of organism's state and current potentials' diagnosing to be unnecessary. Accordingly 51.7 and 28.6% – could not answer. And it is in spite of the fact that such control is rather important component of healthy life style [1–3, 5, 6, 11, 13, 14].

Such result is to large extent conditioned by students' knowledge and their motivation for realization of such functioning in every day life. The first is proved by answers to questions, connected with future professional functioning: 46.5% girls and 42.9% of boys definitely think that knowledge about physical exercises' practicing are unnecessary; accordingly only 27.6 and 28.6% – prove importance of knowledge about means and methods of organism's diagnosing; 31.7 and 28.6% – could not answer. For girl, the reason of such knowledge importance is connected with the following: control over own organism's condition (22.4%); advices of relatives and friends (20.7%). The quantity of boys' such answers was accordingly 54.2 and 20%. 8.6% of boys called consultation of future patients as the reason. Among girls such variant was absent.

The confirmation of conclusion about students' motivation are the following data: 94.3% of boys and only 32.8% of girls practiced some kinds of sports before entering college; as on the moment of questioning accordingly 94.3 and 39.7% wanted to practice sports. At the same time only 48.3% of girls and 48.6% of boys like to attend compulsory physical culture lessons.

In first case the main reason of girls' (24.2%) and boys' (17,1%) wish to practice sports means opportunity to communicate with other students. Accordingly for 13.8% and 60% it means improvement of health. For 14.3% of boys motive is improvement of physical potentials. Absence of wish 45.6% of girls is connected with absence of demand, for 5,2% deficit of free time. For boys, such absence of wish to practice physical culture exercises is connected with deficit of free time (5,7%). Concerning physical culture curriculum lessons, the obtained girls' and boys' low results are connected to large extent with their not understanding of demand in such lessons (34.5% and 14.3% accordingly). With it one of ways of such situation's overcoming is consideration of students' preferences in content of lessons. For example for 53.5% of girls and 94.3% of boys sport games are preferable. For girls – also gymnastic (20.7%), light athletic (8.6%) exercises are attractive; for other students – other exercisesупражнения.

Thus, the received data witness about noticeably higher boys' interest to physical exercises in extra-curriculum time; approximately equal quantity of those, who like physical culture lessons (<50%). Considering it, the problem of increasing of girls' interest to physical exercises' practicing in different forms is more important. Besides, the received data show that students have no formed clear position in respect of such exercises' role in health strengthening and protection and deficit of appropriate knowledge. Besides, it should be noted that there is insufficient understanding that the mentioned knowledge and skills are extremely necessary for highly qualified medical worker.

Discussion

The received results are connected with a complex of reasons. In most general form one of them is low effectiveness of formation of girls' and boys' motivation for systemic physical exercises' practicing in different forms in comprehensive educational establishment and in period of studying in medical college. The next reason is practically complete absence in academic programs of professionally oriented and general disciplines, which could give additional knowledge about physical education process's specificities. Deficit of attention to formation of students' knowledge on the regarded aspects (in college and at previous stage of learning) is of not less importance. It concerns also usage of meaningful connections with other academic disciplines.

Demand in consideration of the above delivered is noted by many scientists [3, 5, 6, 9, 13]. The authors say about importance of healthy life style practicing: knowledge of physical exercises practicing; ability to realize motor functioning with optimal parameters; systemic realization of motor functioning and control over physical condition. To some extent the received data concord with conclusions of other authors [4, 9–11, 14-16, 18] about absence of girls' and boys' belief in following healthy life style; insufficient studying of their valuelogic education in medical colleges; poor formation of theoretical knowledge and skills for application of such knowledge in every day life [8].

Concerning meaningful interdisciplinary connections of different studied disciplines and physical education in formation of valueologic knowledge their realization facilitates strengthening of motivation for such knowledge application in practice [16]. At the same time practically all specialists point at demand in re-understanding of attitude to solution of physical education tasks, connected with formation of students' theoretical knowledge on the regarded problem.

Considering the above said the received experimental data show at demand in perfection of organization and content of physical education of medical colleges' students. Realization of such approach will facilitate achieving of the required result in formation of students' clear position in respect to physical exercises' practicing for health strengthening. Finally, it will permit to strengthen students' motivation for systemic physical functioning of health related orientation and increase their professional fitness level in this aspect.

Conclusions

1. Most of medical colleges' undergraduates believe in secondary importance of physical culture exercises' practicing for health strengthening and protection in comparison with other effective means. Boys' interest to such practicing is much higher than girls'. The knowledge about methodic of organism's condition and its potentials diagnosing are definitely considered unnecessary by 56.9% of girls and 14.3% of boys.

2. To large extent such result is conditioned by low knowledge level about physical activity of health related orientation: 46.5% of girls and 42.9% of boys definitely consider such trainings unnecessary. The second reason is absence of motivation that is reflected in students' answers; unwillingness to attend curriculum physical culture trainings (51.7% of girls); absence of demand and free time (45.6%). Absence of demand and free time was marked only by 5.7% of boys. юношей. 34.5% of girls and 14.3% of boys do not understand necessity of such trainings.

3. The received result points at need in improvement of organization and content of medical colleges' students' physical education. It is necessary to consider the received data, reflecting the following wishes: of 53.5% of girls and 94.3% of boys to practice sport games; of 20.7% and 8.6% of girls to practice gymnastic and light athletic exercises.

Financing

The work has been fulfilled in compliance with governmentally financed topic "Theoretical-methodic principles of application of informational, pedagogic and medical-biological means for motor and spiritual development and healthy life style formation" (state registration number 0115U004036).

The further researches shall be directed at determination of approaches to perfection of organization and content of medical colleges' students' physical education. Their realization in appropriate program will facilitate increasing of motivation for the following: systemic use of health related physical functioning in extra curriculum time; formation and practical realization of knowledge and skills of healthy life style in personal aspect and in future professional functioning.

Conflict of interests

The author declares that there is no conflict of interests.

References:

1. Bar-Or O, Rouland T. *Zdorov'e detej i dvigatel'naia aktivnost': ot fiziologicheskikh osnov do prakticheskogo primeneniia* [Children's health and motor functioning: from physiological principles to practical application], Kiev, Olympic Literature; 2009 (in Russian)
2. Bulatova MM. Fitnes i dvigatel'naia aktivnost': problemy i puti resheniia [Fitness and motor functioning: problems and ways of their solution]. *Teoriia i metodika fizichnogo vikhovannia i sportu*, 2007;1:3–7. (in Russian)
3. Dutchak MV. *Sport dlia vsikh v Ukraini* [Sports for all in Ukraine], Kiev, Olympic Literature; 2009 (in Ukrainian)
4. Iedinak GA. Stan ta deiaki teoretichni aspekti posilennia motivacii studentiv do sistematichnoi rukhovoi aktivnosti ozdorovchogo spriamuvannia [State of students' motivation for health related systemic motor functioning and some theoretical aspects of its strengthening]. *Visnik Prikarpats'kogo nacional'nogo universitetu*, 2012;16:34–39. (in Ukrainian)
5. Iermakova TS. *Problema formuvannia zdorovogo sposobu zhittia starshoklasnikiv u vitchiznianij pedagogici (druga polovina XX stolittia).* Cand. Diss.[Problem of healthy life style formation of senior pupils in domestic pedagogic (second half of 20th century). Cand. Diss.]. Kharkiv; 2010 (in Ukrainian)
6. Ivashchenko LIa, Blagij AL, Usachev IuA. *Programmirovanie zaniatij ozdorovitel'nym fitnesom* [Programming of health related fitness trainings], Kiev, Kiev, Scientific World; 2008 (in Russian)
7. Matveev LP. *Teoriia i metodika fizicheskoj kul'tury* [Theory and methodic of physical culture], Moscow; Sportacademypress; 2008 (in Russian)
8. Ostafijchuk IaF. *Formuvannia valeologichnikh kompetencij u studentiv medichnikh koledzhiv u procesi fizichnogo vikhovannia. Cand. Diss.* [Formation of medical colleges' students' valuelogic competences in process of physical education. Cand. Diss.], Lviv; 2014 (in Ukrainian)
9. Potashniuk IV. *Shkola spriiannia zdorov'iu: teoriia, praktika, metodi doslidzhennia* [School facilitating health: theory, practice, methods of research], Luts'k, Nadstyr'ia; 2006 (in Ukrainian)
10. Romanchishin OM. *Formuvannia gotovnosti studentiv pedagogichnikh koledzhiv do fizkul'turno-ozdorovchoi roboti. Cand. Diss.* [Formation of pedagogic colleges' students' readiness for health related physical culture work], Lviv; 2013 (in Ukrainian)
11. Sainchuk MM. *Formuvannia cinnisnikh oriientacij v sferi fizichnoi kul'turi i sportu uchniv starshikh klasiv u procesi fizichnogo vikhovannia. Cand. Diss.* [Formation of senior pupils' value orientations in process of physical education. Cand. Diss.], Lviv; 2013 (in Ukrainian)
12. Semenova NV. *Obgruntuvannia rezhimu rukhovoi aktivnosti studentok 15–17 rokiv z riznim rivnem somatichnogo zdorov'ia. Cand. Diss.* [Substantiation of motor regime of 15-17 years age girl students with different level of somatic health. Cand. Diss.], Lviv; 2013 (in Ukrainian)
13. Imas EV, Dutchak MV, Trachuk SV. *Strategii i rekomendacii po zdorovomu obrazu zhizni i dvigatel'noj aktivnosti* [Strategies and recommendations on healthy life style and motor functioning], Kiev, Olympic Literature; 2013 (in Russian)
14. Tomenko OA. *Teoretiko-metodologichni osnovi nespecial'noi fizkul'turnoi osviti uchnivs'koi molodi. Doct. Diss.* [Theoretical-methodological principles of pupils' not special physical culture education. Doct. Diss.], Kiev; 2012 (in Ukrainian)

15. Topilko NIa. *Pidvishchennia rivnia somatichnogo zdorov'ia uchniv PTU zasobami fizichnogo vikhovannia. Cand. Diss.* [Rising of somatic health level of Vocational technical schools' pupils by means of physical education. Cand. Diss.] Lviv; 2011 (in Ukrainian)
16. Fedorenko IeO. *Formuvannia motivacii do special'no organizovanoi rukhovoi aktivnosti starshoklasnikiv. Cand. Diss.* [Formation of motivation for specially organized motor functioning of senior pupils. Cand. Diss.], Dnipropetrovs'k; 2012 (in Ukrainian)
17. Shiian BM, Iedinak GA, Petrishin IuV. *Naukovi doslidzhennia u fizichnomu vikhovannia ta sporti* [Scientific researches in physical education and sports]. Kamenets Podolsky, Ruta; 2013 (in Ukrainian)
18. Iurchishin IuV. *Tekhnologiia zaluchennia studentiv do rukhovoi aktivnosti ozdorovchoi spriamovanosti u procesi fizichnogo vikhovannia. Cand. Diss*. [Technology of students' involvement in health related motor functioning in process of physical education. Cand. Diss.], Kiev; 2012 (in Ukrainian)
19. Theobald MA. *Increasing student motivation: strategies for middle and high school teachers.* California: Corwin Press; 2005.
20. Yli-Piipari S, Watt A, Jaakkola T, Liukkonen J, Nurmi J-E. Relationships between physical education students motivational profiles, enjoyment, state anxiety, and self-reported physical activity. *Journ. of Sports Science and Medicine*. 2009;8:327–336.

RESILIENCE OF STUDENTS AND THEIR READINESS FOR PROFESSIONAL FUNCTIONING

Pichurin V.V.
Dnipropetrovsk National University of Railway Transport named after Academician V.Lazaryan

Abstract. *Purpose:* in structure of specialist's psychological readiness for professional functioning important place is taken by formation of the so-called professionally significant personality's features. Person's resilience shall be related to them as well. The purpose is to clear up the existing tendencies in respect to resilience and its components in students. *Material and methods:* in the research 130 students of Dnipropetrovsk National University of Railway Transport named after Academician V.Lazaryan, participated. From them 73 were boys and 57 – girls. Their age was 17-20 years old. Diagnostic of resilience level and its components (commitment, control, challenge) was conducted with the help of resilience questionnaire by S. Maddy, adapted by D. Leontyev and Ye. Rasskazova. *Results:* we determined indicators of resilience, characteristic for modern students. The received results permit to speak about psychological readiness of modern students for professional functioning by factor of resilience. *Conclusions:* 1) absolute majority of students have high indicators of resilience and indicators within standards; 2) boys and girls have statistically significant differences by factor "involvement".
Key words: resilience, commitment, control, challenge, students.

Introduction

At present, life constantly put still more difficult tasks before man. In different kinds of functioning person shall fulfill extremely complex actions, requiring maximal psychological and physical tension for successful achievement of aim. High requirements to professional functioning of modern specialist, complexity and high expenses on his (her) training with extreme conditions of labor require appropriate psychological and psych-physiological fitness.

In psychology it is considered that psychological specificities of professional functioning are conditioned by regulating influence of not separate psychic qualities and functions but by their combinations. Combination of psychological features, which is organized for fulfillment of certain functions, is called psychological system of functioning. It includes: motives, aims, programs and informational basis of functioning; taking decision, professionally important features. Insufficient formation of separate elements of functioning's psychological system; their inadequacy to peculiarities and requirements of certain professional functioning can be a reason of reduction of professional fitness. Formation of such students' features is an important task of higher school.

In formation of psychological system of functioning special place is assigned by specialists to the so-called professionally significant features of personality. They are regarded as internal psychological characteristics of a subject, in which external specific influences of labor process reflect and which exist in the form of professional requirements to a personality. In our opinion resilience shall be related to such features.

Psychology studies a number of personality's characteristics, which facilitate person's self-realization, adaptation to professional environment, ability to overcome difficulties of life (resilience, adaptive abilities, psychological stability, personal potential and so on). Resilience is regarded as system of believes about own self, about world, about correlation with the world. It includes three comparatively autonomous components: commitment, control and challenge. Development level of these components and resilience in the whole prevents from internal tension in stress situations owing to hardy coping of stresses and taking them as insignificant. Commitment is determined as confidence in the fact that involvement in what goes on gives maximal chance to find something worthy and interesting of the person. It is considered that the person with developed commitment enjoy of own functioning. In the contrast to it with absence of such confidence there appears sense of rejection, feeling of own being outside of life. Control is regarded as assurance in the fact that struggle permits to influence on result of process even in case, when this influence is not an absolute one and success is not guaranteed. The opposite is sense of own helplessness. Person with sufficiently developed component of control feels that he himself chooses own functioning and way. Challenge is regarded as human confidence in the fact that everything happening to him (her) facilitates his (her) progressing owing to knowledge, acquired from experience.

With it, it is not important, what experience is – positive or negative. Person, who regards his life as mean of acquiring experience, is ready to act even under absence of reliable guaranties of success, to his own. He considers strive for simple comfort and safety as factor, which makes life poorer. In the base of challenge there is idea of progressing through active mastering of knowledge and experience with their following usage.

Problem of resilience was the subject of scientific researches of foreign and domestic specialists D. Koshaba, S. Maddy, D. Leontyev, L. Alexandrova, L. Dikaya et al. It should be noted also such works as: [2 - 4, 9 - 20] and many other. и многие другие. Researches of resilience in psychology were conducted by such directions as connection of 5resilience and other characteristics of personality, with clinical and behavioral variables (health, effectiveness of fulfillment and etc.) Problems of development of resilience were also studied. Among the latter, domestic we can note the works by K. Mannapova [1], who regarded resilience in system of conception "vitality". Also we can mention the work by S. Babatina, who researched interconnection of resilience with temporal characteristics of student's personality [6].

The conducted analysis of all mentioned works shows that in spite of significant progress, development of modern students' resilience still is remaining and urgent problem as well as usage of physical culture and sport functioning for this purpose. One of tasks, which (in the author's opinion) can be effectively solved in the frames of psychological and psycho-physiological training at physical culture classes [5, 7], is training of students' resilience. With planning of work on resilience formation as well as its components it is necessary to clearly know existing tendencies in this sphere as well as peculiarities of boys and girls' resilience.

Purpose, tasks of the work, material and methods

The purpose of the work is to clear up the existing tendencies in respect to resilience and its components in students.

The tasks of the research:

1. Determine the level of students' resilience and such its components as commitment, control and challenge.

2. State presence or absence of statistically significant differences between boys and girls in respect to their resilience and its components.

In the research 130 students of Dnipropetrovsk National University of Railway Transport named after Academician V.Lazaryan, participated. From them 73 were boys and 57 – girls. Their age was 17-20 years old. Sample was formed with random sampling.

Diagnostic of resilience level and its components (involvement, control, taking of risk) was conducted with the help of resilience questionnaire by S. Maddy, adapted by D. Leontyev and Ye. Rasskazova. From statistical methods we used t-criterion of Student for independent samples.

Results of the research

We found the following: indicators, characterizing students by factor "commitment" are given in table 1.

Table 1.

Statistical indicators of students by factor "commitment" (N = 130)

Statistical indicators	Boys	Girls
Mean arithmetic	40.64	38.05
Median	40	39
Mode	44	40
Standard deviation	6.66	6.60

In boys' group (N = 73) low indicators by this factor was found in 4 students and was 5.5%. In girls' group (N = 57) indicators of such level were registered in 8 girl-students (14%). Indicators within standard were registered in 49 boys (67%) and 43 girls (75.5%). High indicators were diagnosed in 20 boys (27.5%) and in 6 girls (10.5%).

Indicators by factor "control" are given in table 2.

Table 2.

Statistical indicators of students by factor "control" (N = 130)

Statistical indicators	Boys	Girls
Mean arithmetic	34.11	32.56
Median	34	32
Mode	34	27
Standard deviation	6.86	6.25

By this factor low indicators were demonstrated by 2 boys (3%) and 2 girls (3.5%). Indicators within standards were registered in 50 boys (68%) and 40 girls (70%).High indicators were detected in 21 boys (29%) and in 15 girls (26.5%).

The students' indicators by factor "challenge" are presented in table 3.

Table 3.

Statistical indicators of students by factor "challenge" (N = 130)

Statistical indicators	Boys	Girls
Mean arithmetic	18.87	18.36
Median	19	19
Mode	20	23
Standard deviation	4.71	4.29

Distribution by this factor was as follows: low indicators were diagnosed in 2 girls (3.5%). In boys' group there were no indicators of such level. Indicators within standards were registered in 35 boys (48%) and in 26 girls (45.5%). High indicators by this factor were found in 38 boys (52%) and in 29 girls (51%).

Students' indicators by total mark of resilience are given in table 4.

Table 3.

Statistical indicators of students by total mark of resilience (N = 130)

Statistical indicators	Boys	Girls
Mean arithmetic	93.63	88.98
Median	93	92
Mode	98	99
Standard deviation	15.59	14.20

By this indicator low level was found in 3 boys (4%) and in 2 girls (3.5%). Indicators within standards were found in 47 boys (64.5%) and in 41 girls (72%). Indicators of high level were registered in 23 boys (31,5%) and in 14 girls (24.5%).

Secondary statistical processing of the received data was carried out with the help of Student's t0criteruion for independent samples. We compared boys' group with girls' one by indicators of commitment, control, challenge and resilience. Statistically zero hypothesis was the assumption that confidence of differences between resilience indicators (commitment, control and challenge) of boys and girls' groups does not differ significantly from zero. Alternative statistical hypothesis was assumption that confidence of differences between resilience indicators (commitment, control and challenge) of boys and girls' groups significantly differs from zero.

We have established:

a) indicators, which are in zone of insignificance ((commitment, control and challenge).

b) Statistically significant result (at level of statistical significance 0.05) by factor "commitment". Boys' indicators by this factor turned out to be statistically much higher.

On the base of the a.m.:

a) we made conclusion about validity of zero hypothesisc in respect to confidence of differences between indicators of boys' group and girls' group by such criteria as "control", "challenge" and "resilience";

б) in respect to confidence of differences between indicators of boys' group and girls' group by such criterion as "commitment" zero hypothesis was rejected.

Discussion

When planning experiment we based on the fact that modern professional activity often is accompanied by significant emotional tension. It negatively influences on specialists' workability, results in condition of their health. In psychology resilience is regarded as personal characteristic, which facilitates adaptation to professional environment, ability to overcome life difficulties; i.e. it is a professionally significant characteristic. In previous researches [8] we registered low level of students' psychological and psycho-physiological readiness for professional functioning by a number of professionally significant indicators. A question about students' psychological readiness for labor by resilience factor appeared.

Results of our research of students' resilience show that absolute majority of students have high indicators and indicators within standards. For example by factor "commitment" quantity of such students was 94.5% in group of boy students and 86% ion girls' group. By factor "control" such students were 97% in boys' group and 96.5% in girls' group. By factor "challenge" quantity of such students was 100% in group of boys and 96.5% in girls' group. By general indicator of resilience quantity of such students was 96% in boys group and 96.5% in girls' group. The received results permit to say that most of students are ready to overcome life obstacles and professional difficulties. In situations of increased emotional tension they also are bent to take reasonable decisions and continue active functioning. In our opinion the received results permit to say about psychological fitness of modern students to professional functioning by factor "resilience".

When comparing boys and girls' groups we did not find any statistically significant differences by factors "control" and "challenge" and by general indicator of resilience. At the same time we registered statistically significant differences between indicators by factor "commitment" (boys' indicators are higher). For explanation of this fact it is purposeful to carry out special psychological research.

Conclusions:

Formulating main conclusions we can note the following:

1. Absolute majority of students have high indicators of resilience and indicators within standards.

2. There are statistically significant differences between boys ands girls by factor "commitment". Indicators of boys are much higher.

The prospects of further researches we connect with studying of sport and physical culture functioning's usage for training of students' resilience.

Acknowledgement

The author acknowledges senior teacher of physical education department of Dnipropetrovsk National University of Railway Transport named after Academician V.Lazaryan Mrs. Lutayeva Nadezhda Valentinovna for her assistance in organization of girls' group testing.

The work has been fulfilled in compliance with topical plan of scientific research works of physical education department of Dnipropetrovsk National University of Railway Transport named after Academician V.Lazaryan. It is also a component of topic "Theoretical-methodological and pedagogic principles of students' psychological and psycho-physiological training in process of physical education" (state registration number 0113U006237).

Conflict of interests

The author declares that there is no conflict of interests.

References:

1. Mannapova KR. *Zhittiestijkist' v sistemi poniattia zhittiezdatnosti* [Resilience in system of conception of vitality]. Psikhologiia 2012;44(1):143–150. (in Ukrainian)
2. Aleksandrova LA. *K koncepcii zhiznestojkosti v psikhologii* [On conception of resilience in psychology]. Sibirskaia psikhologiia segodnia 2004;2:82–90. (in Russian)
3. Leont'ev DA, Rasskazova EI. *Test zhiznestojkosti* [Test of resilience], Moscow: Meaning; 2006 (in Russian)
4. Leont'ev DA. *Lichnostnyj potencial: struktura i diagnostika* [Personal potential: structure and diagnostic], Moscow: Meaning; 2011 (in Russian)
5. Pichurin VV. Osnovi organizacii psikhologichnoi i psikhofizichnoi pidgotovki studentiv zaliznichnikh vuziv v procesi fizichnogo vikhovannia [Principles of organization of psychological and psycho-physical training of railway higher educational establishments' students in process of physical education]. *Fizichne vikhovannia i sport* 2012;26:84–90. (in Ukrainian)
6. Babatina SI. Osoblivosti vzaiemozv'iazku zhittiestijkosti z temporal'nimi kharakteristikami osobistosti studenta [Peculiarities of interconnection of resilience with temporal characteristics of student's personalities]. *Aktual'ni problemi derzhavnogo upravlinnia, pedagogiki ta psikhologii* 2012;1(6):437–441. (in Ukrainian)
7. Pichurin VV. Psychological and psycho-physical training as a part of physical education of students in higher educational establishments. *Pedagogics, psychology, medical-biological problems of physical training and sports* 2014;11:44-48. http://dx.doi.org/10.15561/18189172.2014.1108
8. Pichurin VV. Psikhologichna i psikhofizichna gotovnist' studentiv-zaliznichnikiv do profesijnoi praci [Psychological and psycho-physical fitness of railway students for professional functioning]. *Fizichne vikhovannia i sport* 2013;37:95–103. (in Ukrainian)
9. Bartone PT. Resilience under military operational stress: can leaders influence hardiness? *Military psychology* 2006;18:131–148. http://dx.doi.org/10.1207/s15327876mp1803s_10.
10. Eid J, Morgan CA. Dissociation, hardiness, and performance in military cadets participating in survival training. *Military medicine* 2006;171;5:436–442.
11. Hystad SW, Eid J, Laberg JC, Johnsen B, Bartone PT. Academic stress and health: exploring the moderating role of personality hardiness. *Scandinavian journal of educational research* 2009;53(5):421–429. http://dx.doi.org/10.1080/00313830903180349.
12. Klag S, Bradley G. The role of hardiness in stress and illness: an exploration of the effect of negative affectivity and gender. *British journal of health psychology* 2004;9;2:137–161. http://dx.doi.org/10.1348/135910704773891014.
13. Kobasa SC, Maddi SR, Puccetti MC, Zola MA. Effectiveness of hardiness, exercise and social support as resources against illness. *Journal of psychosomatic research* 1985;29(5):525–533. http://dx.doi.org/10.1016/0022-3999(85)90086-8.
14. Kobasa SC, Maddi SR, Kahn S. Hardiness and health: a prospective study. *Journal of personality and social psychology* 1982;42(1):168–177. http://dx.doi.org/10.1037/0022-3514.1.168.
15. Kobasa SC, Maddi SR, Zola MA. Type A and hardiness. *Journal of behavioral medicine* 1983;6(1):41–51. http://dx.doi.org/10.1007/BF00845275.
16. Maddi SR. Hardiness: an operationalization of existential courage. *Journal of humanistic psychology* 2004;44(3):279–298. http://dx.doi.org/10.1177/0022167804266101.
17. Maddi SR. Hardiness: the courage to grow from stresses. *Journal of positive psychology* 2006;1(3):160–168. http://dx.doi.org/10.1080/17439760600619609.
18. Pengilly JW, Dowd ET. Hardiness and social support as moderators of stress. *Journal of clinical psychology*. 2000;56(6):813–820. http://dx.doi.org/10.1002/(SICI)1097-4679(200006)56:6<813::AID-JCLP10>3.0CO;2-Q
19. Sinclair RR, Tetrick LE. Implications of item wording for hardiness structure, relations with neuroticism, and stress buffering. *Journal of research in personality* 2000;34(1):1–25. http://dx.doi.org/10.1006/jrpe.1999.2265.

EFFECT OF INFORMATION PROCESSING AND DEPTH PERCEPTION UPON THROWING ACCURACY OF BASKETBALL PLAYERS

Singh Virendra Kumar[1], Agashe Chandrakant D.[2]
[1]Shri Shankaracharya Mahavidyalaya, India
[2]Pt. Ravishankar Shukla University, India

Annotation. *Purpose:* The purpose of the present study is to analyze throwing accuracy of basketball players in relation to their reasoning ability and depth perception. *Materials and Methods :* For present study, 200 intercollegiate basketball players (Ave. age = 21.34±1.87 years) were selected as sample. Johnson Basketball Throw for Accuracy (Passing Test) was the instrument which was used to assess shooting skills of selected subjects whereas reasoning ability of the selected subjects was assessed by MGTI prepared by Mehrotra (1984). To conduct the study, a 2x2 factorial design was used. Superior and inferior reasoning and perceptual abilities were ascertained by statistical method Q1 and Q3. 2x2 ANOVA results showed that the main effect of reasoning ability was not found to be statistically significant upon throwing accuracy of basketball players although it is close to .05 level of significance. *Results :* The main effect of depth perception upon throwing accuracy of basketball players turned out to be statistically significant. The two factor interaction effect of reasoning ability and depth perception upon throwing accuracy of basketball players was found to be statistically insignificant. *Conclusion :* It was concluded that reasoning ability and to some extent depth perception, are the two major variables which generate variance upon throwing accuracy of basketball players.
Keywords: information processing, depth perception, throwing accuracy, basketball.

Introduction

Player's activity during a match requires specific skills such as visual information acquisition and speed at which they process information. Researchers in the past have also showed the importance of visual skills in sports performance [1, 2, 3]. Similarly speed of information processing or reasoning ability has also been emerged as potential variable as far as performance is concerned [4, 5, 6, 7, 8]

In a sport such as basketball, good perception of depth may enables a player to accurately judge the distance between the player and other players, the role of speed of information processing or reasoning ability may also be important because of the nature of the sport which is fast paced and requires quick thinking and judgmental ability to perform fundamental ability such as throwing or passing.

Perception refers to the process of taking in, organizing, and interpreting sensory information. Perception is multimodal, with multiple sensory inputs contributing to motor responses [9]. Depth perception refers to the ability to see and understand the 3-D spatial relationship and relative distance between objects and oneself. Its primary value is to make hand-eye coordination efficient and provide for safe movement through space. Binocular depth perception is one of the most demanding visual tasks that we carry out. The horizontal separation of the eyes in the head means that each eye obtains an image of the world from a slightly different viewpoint. The differences between these images, called binocular disparities, present significant challenges that the brain's visual system must overcome in order to make use of them. Binocular vision must be highly accurate: the CNS needs to be able to register a difference between the two eyes that is smaller than the width of a single cone photo receptor. To extract these fine differences, individual features in the left eye's image must be matched with the correct partner features in the right eye.

Reasoning refers to the process of drawing conclusions or inferences from information. Reasoning always requires going beyond the information that is given [10]. In logic, an inference is called deductive if the truth of the initial information (or premises) guarantees the truth of the conclusion. The inference is called inductive if the truth of the premises makes the conclusion probable but not certain. Distinctions between deductive and inductive reasoning can be important in understanding logic; but in practice, these distinctions may exist more in the mind of the researcher developing a task than in the performance of examinees on that task. Many researchers have found that performance on deductive and inductive tests is strongly related.

When people reason, they must, in Bruner's (1957) helpful phrase, go "beyond the information given". They do this in one or both of the following ways: They attempt to infer (either automatically or deliberately) concepts, patterns, or rules that best (i.e., most uniquely) characterize the relationships or patterns they perceive among all the elements (e.g., words, symbols, figures, sounds, movements) in a stimulus set. Better reasoning is characterized by the use of concepts or rules that simultaneously satisfy the opposing needs for abstraction (or generalization) and specificity. Such concepts or rules tend to be at least moderately abstract yet precisely tuned. Put differently, a poor inference is often vague and captures only a subset of the relationships among the elements in the set. They attempt to deduce the consequences or implications of a rule, set of premises, or statements using warrants that are rendered plausible by logic or by information that is either given in the problem or assumed to be true within the community of discourse. They often seem to do this by creating and manipulating mental models of the situation. Such models tend to represent explicitly only what is assumed to be true about the situation. Better reasoning involves providing warrants that are more plausible or consistent with the rules of logic or the conditions embodied in a comprehensive mental model. More advanced deductive reasoning involves providing either multiple (possibly divergent) warrants for a single claim or an increasingly sophisticated chain of logically connected and separately warranted assertions.

John-Laird's mental models theory of deductive reasoning posits that the individual first transforms the premises of an argument into another representation that is consistent with the premises. Importantly, multiple mental models that are consistent with the premises must often be constructed and then compared in order to reach a valid conclusion. Each mental model represents a possible state of affairs that must be evaluated.[11] Bara, Bucciarelli, and Johnson-Laird (1995) identified the following factors that affect syllogistic inference in the mental models approach: (a) assembling a propositional representation of premises; (b) constructing models that integrate information from premises; (c) formulating a conclusion which integrates relationships not expressed in the premises; (d) searching for alternative models to refute conclusions; and (e) recognizing similarities between models. All these processes require working memory resources.[12]

Human reasoning occurs at different levels of awareness. Most cognitive scientists distinguish between tacit and intentional (or explicit) reasoning processes. Tacit processes that facilitate reasoning occur without conscious intervention and outside awareness; they typically do not require attention. Such thinking is sometimes described as associative, because it depends on the network of ideas and associations in memory. Tacit processes are used when we make a decision in a quick or intuitive way, often because it feels right rather than because we have a clearly articulated set of reasons. We are aware of the outcome of these tacit processes, but not of the processes themselves. Tacit processes are particularly important in focusing attention and in building an initial mental model of a problem. Effective problem solvers typically attend to different features of the problem than do less effective problem solvers. Effective problem solvers know what to seek and know what to ignore. In part, this is due to greater experience; in part, to better use of past experiences. Other researchers describe this automatic attention as the extent to which the person is attuned to certain aspects of a situation and not others.

Although researchers studied various facets of basketball [13, 14, 15, 16, 17] but while scanning through the research literature, it was observed that throwing accuracy of basketball players has not been studied so far, hence the researcher aimed to study the joint effect of depth perception and reasoning ability upon throwing accuracy of basketball players.

Materials and Methods

Ethics

The research was carried out with prior permission from Basketball Association of Chhattisgarh and the participants written consent to take part in this study.

Sample

For present study, 200 intercollegiate basketball players (Ave. age = 21.34±1.87 years) were selected as sample. The selection of subjects was done from Inter-collegiate tournaments held in the State of Chhattisgarh India. The selection of sample was based on convenience sampling technique.

Tools and Procedure

To assess throwing accuracy of selected basketball players, Johnson Basketball Throw for Accuracy (Passing Test) was used. This test is highly reliable and valid. The direction of scoring for this test is "higher the score better is the ability"[18].

Mehrotra's (1984) Mixed Type Group Test of Intelligence (MGTI) was used to assess reasoning ability of selected subjects,. It has two parts i.e. verbal and non verbal intelligence test. Both the parts have 50 statements. The test-retest reliability of the verbal test is 0.89, for non verbal test it is 0.82 while full test reliability coefficient is 0.86. The validity verbal test is .86 and for non verbal test it is 0.72 while the overall validity of the test is 0.87 when it was correlated with teacher's ratings. Only non-verbal intelligence part was used in the present investigation [19].

Depth perception of the selected subjects was recorded by a specially designed depth perception apparatus. In this test the direction is scoring is "higher the deviation, lower the binocular depth perception" [20].

Johnson Basketball Throw for Accuracy (Passing Test) was administered to selected basketball players under the supervision of investigator. Similarly experiments on depth perception apparatus was performed by the subjects under personal supervision of the investigator. The reasoning ability part of MGTI test was administered to each selected basketball player in a peaceful corner. The response pertaining to MGTI was scored off as per author's manual. Scores on Johnson basketball throw for accuracy test and depth perception was also recorded for each selected subject.

To divide cases into superior and inferior reasoning ability, Q_1 and Q_3 statistical technique was used. Subjects whose reasoning ability scores lies below Q1 was assigned to inferior reasoning ability category, and subjects whose scores lies above Q3 was assigned to superior reasoning ability category. Regarding bifurcating the scores of depth perception into superior and inferior categories, again Q_1 and Q_3 statistical technique was used. Subjects whose depth perception scores lies below Q1 was assigned to superior depth perception category, subjects whose scores lies above Q3 was assigned to inferior depth perception category.

To find out the joint action effect of depth perception (superior-Inferior) and reasoning ability (Superior-Inferior) on throwing accuracy of basketball players, 2x2 ANOVA technique was adopted. The results are presented in table 1 and 1(a) respectively.

Results

Table 1

Reasoning Ability (A) x Depth Perception (B) on Throwing Accuracy of Basketball Players (N=73)

	Depth Perception (B)		M
	b_1 Superior	b_2 Inferior	
a_1 Superior	M=17.53 N=39	M=11.40 N=05	14.46
a_2 Inferior	M=14.60 N=05	M=9.16 N=24	11.88
M	16.06	10.28	

Table 1 (a)

ANOVA Summary

Source of Variation	SS	df	MS	F
A	57.237	1	57.237	3.49(NS)
B	286.549	1	286.549	17.50**
AB	1.064	1	1.064	0.06(NS)
Within treatment (Error)	1129.426	69	16.368	

** Significant at .01 level
NS Not Significant

From the analysis of table 1 and 1 (a) following inferences were drawn:

The main effect of reasoning ability upon throwing accuracy of basketball players was not found to be statistically significant but it was close to statistical significance. The reported F=3.49(p<.06), although not statistically significant gives a clear trend that subjects with superior reasoning ability (M=14.46) have significantly better throwing accuracy as compared to subjects with inferior reasoning ability (M=11.88).

The F of 17.50, an indicator of the main effect of depth perception upon throwing accuracy of basketball players turned out to be statistically significant. It thereby reveals that subjects with subjects with superior depth perception (M=16.06) have significantly better throwing accuracy as compared to subjects with inferior depth perception (M=10.28) at .01 level of statistical significance.

The two factor interaction effect of depth perception and reasoning ability upon throwing accuracy of basketball players was not found to be statistically significant (F=0.06, p>.05).

Discussion:

In the present study, the main effect of reasoning ability upon throwing accuracy of basketball players was not found to be statistically significant F=3.49, p<.06) but it is very close to statistical significance at .05 level. This fact is also confirmed by the graphical representation of mean throwing accuracy test scores shown in Fig. (i) denotes a significant slope in the curve which is not parallel to the X axis and thus proves the partial significant main effect of reasoning ability upon throwing accuracy of basketball players. The similar results were also obtained in the past [21]. Hence, speed of information processing or in other words reasoning ability is a potential enough variable to influence basic fundamental skill in basketball i.e. field goal shooting skills.

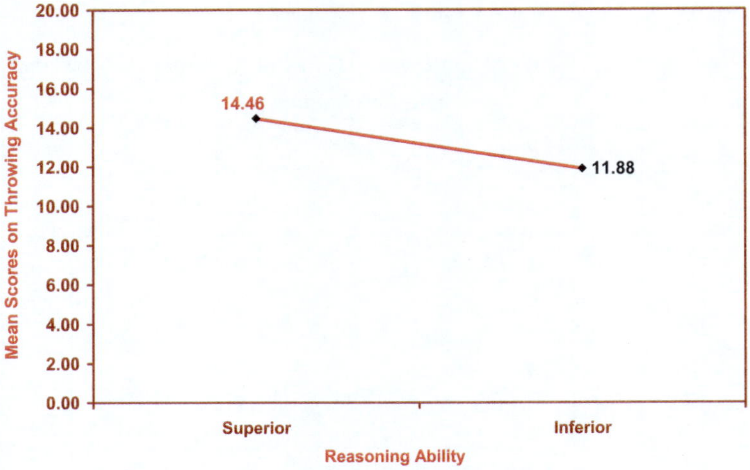

Figure (i). Line Diagram Showing Main Effect of Reasoning Ability on Throwing Accuracy of Basketball Players

In the present study, the main effect of depth perception upon throwing accuracy of basketball players was found to be statistically significant. This fact is also confirmed by the graphical representation of mean throwing accuracy scores shown in Fig. (ii) which denotes a significant slope in the curve which is not parallel to the X axis and thus proves the significant main effect of depth perception upon throwing accuracy of basketball players. Accurately throwing a ball in basketball requires a players to judge relative distance between objects and his own position in three dimensional space. Hence, a player who judgment of this distance is superior invariably throws the ball accurately. Hence the results of the present study are in expected direction.

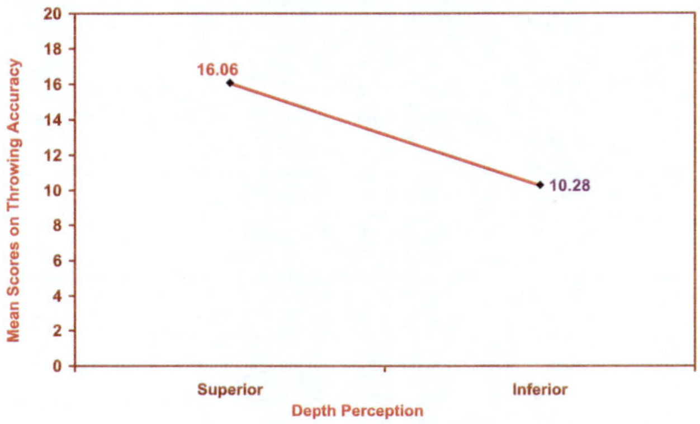

Figure (ii). Line Diagram Showing Main Effect of Depth Perception on Throwing Accuracy of Basketball Players

The two factor interaction effect of depth perception and reasoning ability was not found to be statistically significant. This fact is verified by parallel lines, which shows that each factor displayed the independence from other factor and not generating variance upon mental health jointly or in interaction with each other (Fig. iii).

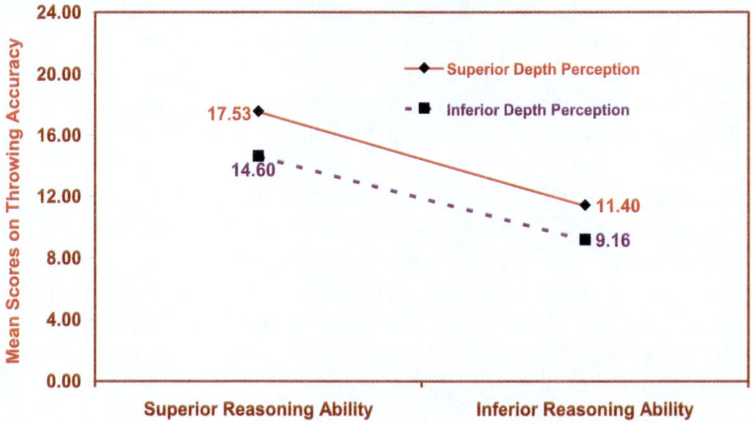

Figure (iii). Line Diagram Showing Interaction Effect of Depth Perception and Reasoning Ability on Throwing Accuracy of Basketball Players

Conclusions

Hence on the basis of results it was concluded that depth perception fully and reasoning ability partially, have a significant impact upon throwing accuracy of basketball players but same cannot be said about joint action effect of these two variables upon throwing accuracy of basketball players.

References:

1. Adolphe R.M., Vickers, J.N. and La Plante G. The effects of training visual attention on gaze behavior and accuracy. *International Journal of Sports Vision*. 1997, no.4, pp. 28-33.
2. Savelsbergh G.J.P., Williams M.A., Van der Kamp J., Ward P. Visual search, anticipation and expertise in soccer goalkeepers. *Journal of Sports Sciences*, 2002,no.20, pp. 279-287.
3. Eaves D.L, Anderton and Taylor M. *Is visual perception the key to success in young soccer players.* Perception, 36, ECVP, 2007, 240 p.
4. Vernon P. A., & Mori M. Intelligence, reaction times, and peripheral nerve conduction velocity. *Intelligence*, 1992, no.16, pp. 273–288.
5. Kioumourtzoglou E., Derri V., Tzetzis G. & Theodorakis Y. Cognitive, perceptual and motor abilities in skilled basketball performance. *Perceptual and motor skills*, 1998, no.86, pp. 771-786.
6. Planinsec J., Pisot R. Motor coordination and intelligence level in adolescents. *Adolescence*. 2006, vol.41, no.164, pp. 667-676.
7. Karalejic M. and Jakovljevic S. Cognitive abilities of young basketball players and their actual success. *Physical Culture*, 2008, vol.62, no.1-2, pp. 117-123.
8. Kamkary K., Akbari P., Shokrzadeh S. Effects of Personality Profiles and Profiles of IQ on Elite Athletes Volleyball's Performance. *European Journal of Experimental Biology*, 2012, vol.2, no. 6, pp. 2352-2359.
9. Bertenthal B. I. Origins and Early Development of Perception, Action and Representation. *Annual Review of Psychology*, 1996, vol.47, pp. 431–459.
10. Bruner J. S. *Going beyond the information given. In Contemporary approaches to cognition: A symposium held at the University of Colorado*. Cambridge, MA: Harvard University Press, 1957, pp. 41-69.
11. Johnson-Laird P. N. *Mental models and reasoning*. In J. P. Leighton, & R. J. Sternberg (Eds.), The nature of reasoning New York, NY: Cambridge University Press, 2004, pp. 169-204.
12. Bara B. G., Bucciarelli M., Johnson-Laird P. N. Development of syllogistic reasoning. *American Journal of Psychology,* 1995, no.108, pp. 157-193.
13. Pates J., Maynard I., Westbury T. An investigation into the effects of hypnosis on basketball performance. *Journal of Applied Sport Psychology*, 2001, no.13, pp. 84-102.
14. Poczwardowski A., Fisher M. *The impact of mental preparation on free throw shooting and self-efficacy with collegiate basketball players: A psychological skills training approach*. Poster presentation, European Federation of Sport Psychology Congress, Copenhagen, Denmark. 2001, pp. 100-106.
15. Pates T.; Frewan M., Beer J. Association of eye colour and sex with basketball free throws by elementary school children. *Perceptual and motor skills.* 1991, no.73, pp. 1181-1182.
16. Balcinuas M. Long term effects of different training modalities on power, speed, skill and anaerobic capacity in young male basketball players. *Journal of Sports Science and Medicine*, 2006, no.5, pp. 163-170.
17. Quintana M.S., Roman I.R., Molinuevo. Perceptual visual skills in young highly skilled basketball players. *Perceptual and motor skills*, 2007, no.104, pp. 547-561.
18. Kansal D.K. *Test and Measurement in Sports and Physical Education*. 1996, pp. 294-296.
19. Mehrotra P.N. *Manual for mixed type of group test of intelligence (Verbal and non-verbal)*, Agra National Psychological Corporation, Agra. 1984, 240 p.
20. Shahbazi, M., Taher, A. V., & Hadadi, N. Effects of Viewer-Induced Arousal on Depth Perception in Male and Female Athletes. *Procedia - Social and Behavioral Sciences*, 2011, no.15, pp. 3103–3107. http://doi.org/10.1016/j.sbspro.2011.04.253
21. Cashmore E. *Making Sense of Sports*, London, Routledge, 2005, 212 p.

PECULIARITIES OF PERFECTION OF TRAINING PROCESS OF THE QUALIFIED BODYBUILDER IN THE COMPETITIVE PERIOD

Dzhym V. Yu.
Kharkov State Academy of Physical Culture

Annotation. *Purpose:* study methods of improving the training process of skilled bodybuilders in the competitive period. *Material*: The study involved 18 athletes aged 18-25 years old. The experiment was conducted for 8 weeks. Used two variants of training techniques: large percentage weights; with smooth dynamics with emphasis on static load muscles. Efficacy was evaluated using the preparation method of expert evaluations. The method involved the use of information on the implementation of directives coach dynamics of power and endurance performance, subjective indicators (health, mood, desire to train). *Results*: comparative characteristic of the most commonly used methods of training process in bodybuilding. Developed and justified best practices, depending on the initial form of the athlete at the beginning of the competition period of training. Shows the dependence of changes in body weight of the athlete training. *Conclusions*: the proposed best practices, depending on the microcycle training in the competitive period (precompetitive and competitive mesocycles).
Keywords: training, bodybuilding, qualified, optimal, method, microcycle.

Introduction

Since 90-s, in Ukraine new for the country kinds of sports have been becoming more and more popular. In weight lifting they were, first of all, power-lifting and bodybuilding. Considering the fact that domestic theoretical and practical trainings base for such kinds of sports is only on stage of creation, the topic of this article is rather urgent for domestic sports.

One of most important problems of bodybuilders' training for competitions in Ukraine is adaptation of foreign classic methodic to domestic reality and, thus to achievement of high results.

Training system of qualified body builders is based on rationally built training process in combination with diet as factor, ensuring required material for decreasing of fat layer and growing of muscular mass.

That is why there was worked out and scientifically grounded methodic of training process of qualified bodybuilders in competition period of year training cycle [1; 2].

In domestic sports there is a little of scientifically grounded training methodic for qualified bodybuilders in preparatory period of special-training stage. Thus, coaches and sportsmen shall acquire practical experience by the method of trial and error [6; 9].

In bodybuilding competition process lasts 8 weeks. In this period qualified sportsmen of different age groups and categories try as much as possible to reduce under-skin fat layer and water with the help of trainings with optimal weights. At the end of every micro-cycle form of sportsman is estimated by coaches and anthropometric data are measured, corrections in training process and plan of diet are made [3; 15–18].

This problem was dealt with by such outstanding domestic specialists in physical culture as V.M. Platonov, L.S. Dvorkin, A.I. Stetsenko, B.I. Sheyko, V.G. Oleshko, A.I. Kamayev, D.A. Beskorovayniy, V.V. Usichenko [4-10]. Their researches based on experience of such foreign specialists as Joe Wider, Ben Wider, E. Connors, T. Kimber, M. Mc Kormic [12–14].

The present scientific research has been fulfilled as per topic of combined plan of scientific-research works in sphere of physical culture and sports for на 2011-2015. Topic 3.7 "Methodological and organizational methodic principles of determination of individual norm of human physical condition" (state registration No. 0111U000192).

Purpose, tasks of the work, material and methods

The purpose of the research: To give foundation to methodic of improvement of qualified bodybuilders' training process in competition period.

The methods of the research: Theoretical method and generalization of literature, pedagogic observation, pedagogic experiment, method of mathematical statistics.

Materials of the research: members of combined team of Kharkovska region participated in the experiment. They were 18 bodybuilder: 4 masters of sport, 14 – candidate masters of sports of 18-25 years old; mean body mass was 85±2- 100±2 kg. The participants were distributed by sport qualification into two groups": experimental (EG) and control group (CG). Control group sportsmen trained 5 times a week; experimental group trained 5-6 times a week.

Results of the research

Usage of training process of qualified bodybuilders conditioned application of two training methodic, which differed by load and scope of trainings exercises, rest periods and other components. Evaluation was conducted with the help of training diaries, in which quantity and scope of training work was noted.

Training effectiveness was evaluated with method of experts' evaluation, which envisaged application of information about fulfillment of coach's instructions, dynamic of power indicators and endurance as well as subjective qualities (self-feeling, mood, wish to train and so on).

Control group sportsmen trained during 8 weeks with great percentage loads; experimental group sportsmen trained with smooth dynamic with static exercises prevailing (see table 1,2) Before experiment we fulfilled testing measuring of sportsmen's masses, anthropological measurements for determination of better results in indicators' increment. For weighing, we used mass analyze (scales TANITA BC-545, made in Japan) and centimeter measuring tape (see table 3, 4).

Distinction of preparatory period from competition one is in more smooth transition from one training micro-cycle to other, as well as in increasing of quantity of repetitions and trials for better separation and definitions of muscles (see table 1). Increasing of trainings' quantity, shortening of breaks between trainings days is very important in preparation at this stage. Also, as it can be seen in table 1, intensity is important; time of exercises' fulfillment significantly reduced both in positive and negative phases and pauses between repetitions reduced – in preparation cycle up to 0.5 sec. and in competition micro-cycle there was no rest between repetitions at all.

Specificity of this stage is also little percent application of small weights, which was in first pre-competition meso-cycle in EG - 50%, and in CG 60 - 80%, in second competition meso-cycle - 70 - 30% in EG and 80 - 70% in CG, thus in EG greater attention was paid to work with muscles, but not to gaining mass that was most important at this stage.

Table 1

Content of training program depending on mass of load in competition period of qualified bodybuilders (experimental and control groups)

Indicators of training loads and classification of muscular groups	**Meso-cycles**			
	Pre-competition		**Competition**	
	CG	**EG**	**CG**	**EG**
Range of load in percent from maximum	60 – 80	30-60	80-70	70-30
Quantity of training days	5	6	6	6
Quantity of repetitions	10-12	12-18	12-15	15-25
Quantity of trials	5-6	5-6	5–6	6-8
Time of exercise's fulfillment, sec.				
POSITIVE PHASE (MOVEMENT UPWARD)	1	0,5	1	0,5
Negative phase (movement downward)	1,2	0,5	1	0,5
Pauses between repetitions, sec.	0,8		0,5	-
Rest between trials, min.				
In basic exercises	2-2,5	1-1,2	1,5	1
In shaping exercises	1,5	50	1	30-50
Rest time between loading of muscular groups (days)				
Hips	5	3	4	3
Back	5	3-5	4	3-5
Breast	3	4	3	4
Deltoid muscle	4	5	4	5
Biceps muscle	2	3	2	3
TRICEPS MUSCLE	3	4	3	4
Forearm	6	5	6	5
Triceps of shin	6	3	6	3
Oblique and direct abdominal muscles	3	1	3	1
Neck	0	2	0	2

The data, presented in table 2, witness that experimental group sportsmen trained with moderate weights comparing with maximal; control group trained with little quantity of repetitions but with heavy weights that is not recommended in pre-competition period, because in this period sportsmen, preparing for competitions, reduce quantity of carbon hydrates. For example, in competition period great attention is paid to muscles of hip and shin – quantity of weight bar's lifting (QWBL) is 1.797 in EG per two micro-cycles, in CG – 1.566 mainly at the account of muscles of arms, breast and back, which are practically same (650- 732 lifting of 62.500-96.400kg weight). But in this period main role is played by shaping exercises, which were different by QWBL and by calculated kilograms; that is why maximally great number of weight bar lifting was at the account of oblique and direct abdominal muscles and was in EG 9.220 QWBL and in CG 8.850 QWBL. Total scope of QWBL in basic exercises was in EG 5.254 and in CG 4.457, while in shaping exercises in EG it was 17.900 and in CG – 16.451 QWBL. Thus, CG used more powerful program of training and little quantity of QWBL with big weights. EG used more static program of training and used higher quantity of QWBL that is why scope of kilograms was higher.

Table 2

Total scope of training work, fulfilled by qualified bodybuilders of control and experimental groups in competition period

Group s of muscles	Scope of QWBL		Scope, thousands of kg.	
	CG	EG	CG	EG
Basic exercise for:				
Muscles of upper girdle	550.0	650.0	59.200	62.500
Muscles of arms	780.0	900.0	76.550	85.660
Muscles of breast	582.0	732.0	88.250	96.400
Muscles of back	979.0	1.175	166.100	182.090
Muscles of hips and shins	1.566	1.797	240.562	305.695
Total	4.457	5.254	630.662	732.345
Shaping exercises for:				
Muscles of upper girdle	1.550	1.632	110.340	139.520
Muscles of arms	820.0	965.0	58.250	65.380
Muscles of breast	520.0	630.0	63.670	65.380
Muscles of back	1.035	1.368	105.350	118.080
Muscles of hips and shins	3.676	4.105	505.250	537.740
Oblique and direct abdominal muscles	8.850	9.220	-	-
Total	16.451	17.900	842.860	926.100

Notes: QWBL – quantity of lifting of weight bar

Total scope of calculated kilograms in basic exercises is 732.345 in EG and 630.662 in CG; in shaping exercises total scope is 926.100 kg in EG and 842.860 in CG. We can make general conclusion that experimental group sportsmen trained at this stage with moderate scope of kilograms and paid more attention to abdominal muscles and muscles of legs as far as after preparatory period (28 micro-cycles) there was significant increment of subcutaneous fat layer on abdomen and hips. In their turn, CG sportsmen paid more attention to basic exercises and power indicators than to shaping exercises.

Before experiment we fulfilled anthropological measurements. As we can see in table 3, variation coefficients of all main anthropological indicators, separately for control and experimental groups, practically did not exceed general initial level.

Anthropometrical examination was fulfilled before beginning and at the end of competition period,(see tables 3, 4).

Table 3

Mean anthropological indicators of qualified bodybuilders of control and experimental groups at the beginning of competition period ($n_1 = n_2 = 9$)

Indicator	CG		EG		t	P
	$\overline{X}_1 \pm m_1$	V ,%	$\overline{X}_2 \pm m_2$	V ,%		
Body mass, kg	94.17 ± 3.74	11.91	94.00 ± 4.17	13.30	0.02	>0.05
Circumference of neck, cm	42.50 ± 1.36	9.62	42.78 ± 1.29	9.03	0.12	>0.05
Circumference of breast (inhale), cm	113.83 ± 1.88	4.95	117.88 ± 2.60	6.62	1.03	>0.05
Circumference of breast (exhale), cm	105.33 ± 1.91	5.43	107.22 ± 2.26	6.32	0.52	>0.05
Circumference of biceps, cm	43.00 ± 1.91	13.32	44.45 ± 1.59	10.72	0.48	>0.05
Circumference of waist, cm	80.33 ± 2.34	8.76	81.95 ± 2.52	9.22	0.38	>0.05
Circumference of hip, cm	79.00 ± 1.74	6.60	79.72 ± 1.84	6.93	0.23	>0.05
Circumference of shin, cm	40.33 ± 1.31	9.75	41.12 ± 1.41	10.32	0.33	>0.05
Circumference of forearm, cm	37.33 ± 1.32	10.64	39.17 ± 1.85	14.21	0.66	>0.05
Length of body, cm	168.00 ± 1.40	2.50	170.50 ± 2.25	3.96	0.77	>0.05
Length of torso, cm	77.83 ± 0.65	2.49	78.00 ± 0.63	2.43	0.15	>0.05
Length of lower limb, cm	90.17 ± 0.88	2.93	90.33 ± 0.91	3.02	0.11	>0.05
Length of upper limb, cm	83.67 ± 1.22	4.39	83.67 ± 1.22	4.39	0.001	>0.05

So, at the beginning of competition period differences are insignificant: in body mass (control group -94.17 kg and experimental group – 94.00 kg; P> 0,.05); circumference of waist (accordingly – 80.33 cm and 81.95 cm; P> 0.05); circumference of hip (accordingly – 79.00 cm, 79.72 cm; P> 0.05); circumference of neck (accordingly – 42.50 cm, 42.78 cm; P> 0.05); circumference of breast at inhale (accordingly – 113.83 cm, 117.88 cm; P> 0.05) and circumference of breast at exhale (accordingly – 105.33 cm, 107.72 cm; P> 0.05) and shin (accordingly – 40. 33 cm, 41.12 cm; P> 0.05).

Variation coefficients of all main anthropological indicators, separately for control and experimental groups, practically did not exceed general initial level. For example for control group it was V = 11.91%, and for experimental group - V = 13.30%. Accordingly for control and experimental group variation coefficients were: circumference of hips V = 6.60%, V = 6,93%; circumference of waist - V = 8.76%, V = 9.22%; circumference of biceps - V = 13.32%, V = 10.72%.

Table 4

Mean indicators of reduction of qualified bodybuilders' anthropological data of control and experimental groups at the end of competition period ($n_1 = n_2 = 9$)

Indicator	CG	EG	*t*	*P*
	$\bar{X}_1 \pm m_1$	$\bar{X}_2 \pm m_2$		
Body mass, kg	11.7±1.0	5.0±0.3	5.42	<0.01
Circumference of neck, cm	4.0±0.4	2.0±0.2	3.87	<0.01
Circumference of breast (inhale), cm	5.2±0.4	2.2±0.3	4.81	<0.01
Circumference of breast (exhale), cm	5.2±0.4	2.5±0.2	5.05	<0.01
Circumference of biceps, cm	3.3±0.5	1.8±0.3	2.18	>0.05
Circumference of waist, cm	4.8±0.4	2.7±0.2	4.15	<0.01
Circumference of hip, cm	4.3±0.3	2.5±0.2	3.84	<0.01
Circumference of shin, cm	2.5±0.2	1.5±0.2	3.16	<0.05
Circumference of forearm, cm	0.2±0.1	0.8±0.3	1.60	>0.05
Length of body, cm	168.0±1.4	170.5±1.4	0.77	>0.05
Length of torso, cm	77.8±0.6	78.0±0.6	0.15	>0.05
Length of lower limb, cm	90.2±0.9	90.3±0.9	0.10	>0.05
Length of upper limb, cm	83.7±1.2	83.6±1.2	0.0001	>0.05

For example, at the end of competition period probability of differences was proved: in body mass (control group – 11.7 kg and experimental group – 5.0 kg; P <0.01); circumference of waist (accordingly – 4.8 cm, 2.7 cm; P <0.01); circumference of hip (accordingly – 2.5 cm, 1.5 cm; P <0.05); circumference of neck (accordingly – 4.0 cm, 2.0 cm; P <0.01); circumference of breast ant inhale (accordingly – 5.2 cm, 2.2 cm; P <0.01) and exhale (accordingly – 2.5 cm, 1.5 cm; P <0.05).

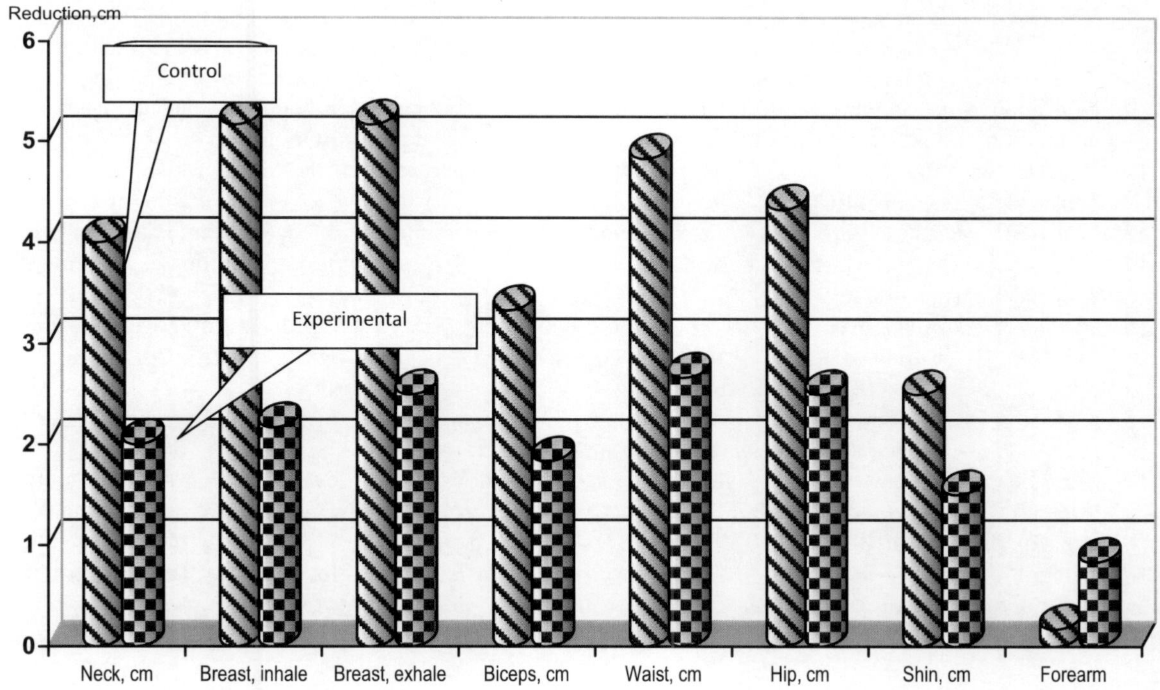

Fig.1. Comparative diagram of increment of anthropometric data of qualified bodybuilders (control and experimental groups) on competition period

Conclusions:

Thus, perfection of training process for qualified bodybuilders, permits to consider that in EG effect was more expressed and level of fitness can be estimated as optimal. Dynamic of load in this group significantly reduces probability of functional disorders (over-tension, over-training, traumas); it permits to achieve required level of sport fitness without over-tension of adaptation-compensatory mechanisms. In respect to construction of training process, in EG methodic of training more facilitates fulfillment of the set task – preservation of muscular mass during burning of subcutaneous fat and water; indicators of body mass are ($t = 5.42$; $p < 0.001$), Circumference of breast (inhale) $t = 4.81$; $p < 0.001$) and at exhale ($t = 5.05$; $p < 0.001$), waist ($t = 4.15$; $p < 0.001$), hip ($t = 3.84$; $P < 0.01$) and shin ($t = 3.16$; $p < 0.05$).

Improved methodic of training for qualified bodybuilders in competition period can be recommended for training of sportsmen with observation of sport and medical requirements, for ensuring of effective and qualitative recreation in transitive period.

Further researches shall include working out and foundation of training process of qualified bodybuilders in transitive period.

References:

1. Blauberg I. V., Iudin E. G. *Stanovlenie i sushchnost' sistemnogo podkhoda* [Formtion and essence of system approach]. Moscow, Science, 1973, 272 p. (in Russian)
2. Grishina Iu. I. *Osnovy silovoj podgotovki* [Basic strength training]. Rostov on Don, Phoenix, 2011, 280 p. (in Russian)
3. Dzhim V. Iu. Osoblivosti kharchuvannia bodibilderiv u pidgotovchomu periodi trenuvan' [Features nutrition bodybuilders in the preparatory period of training] *Slobozhans'kij naukovo-sportivnij visnik*. 2013, no. 4(37), pp. 15–19. (in Ukrainian)
4. Dvorkin L. S. *Vazhka atletika i vik* [Weightlifting and age]. Sverdlovsk, Ural University Publ., 1989, 2000 p. (in Ukrainian)
5. Shejko B. I. *Pauerlifting* [Powerlifting]. Moscow, Sports service, 2003, 532 p. (in Russian)
6. Oleshko V. G. *Silovye vidy sporta* [Strength kinds of sports]. Kiev, Olympic Literature, 1999, 287 p. (in Russian)
7. Platonov V.N. *Sistema podgotovki sportsmenov v olimpijskom sporte* [The system of preparation of sportsmen in Olympic sport], Kiev, Olympic Literature, 2004, 808 p. (in Russian)
8. Stecenko A. I. *Pauerlifting* [Powerlifting]. Cherkasy, NDITEHIMu, 2008, 459 p. (in Ukrainian)
9. Kamaiev O. I., Bezkorovajnij D. O. *Rozvitok silovikh zdibnostej 13-15- richnikh iunakiv u silovikh vidakh sportu* [Development of power abilities of 13-15-year-old boys in the power types of sport]. Kharkov, KSAPC, 2014, 106 p. (in Ukrainian)
10. Usychenko V. V. Periodizaciia godichnogo cikla podgotovki sportsmenov specializiruiushchikhsia v bodibildinge [Periodization of the annual cycle of training athletes specializing in bodybuilding]. *Pedagogics, psychology, medical-biological problems of physical training and sports*. 2006, no.7, pp. 123–125. (in Russian).
11. Zverev V. D. *Planirovanie trenirovochnoj nagruzki v podgotovitel'nom periode v bodibildinge s uchetom silovoj napravlennosti* [Planning the training load in the preparatory period in bodybuilding, taking into account power orientation]. Sankt Petersburg, SPbGAFK P.F. Lesgaft, 2003 55 p. (in Russian)
12. Dzho Uajder. *Sistema stroitel'stva tela* [The system of construction of the body]. Moscow, Physical Culture and Sport, 1991, 112 p. (in Russian)
13. Vejder B., Vejder D. *Klassicheskij bodibilding* [Classic bodybuilding]. Moscow, Exmo, 2003, 432 p. (in Russian)
14. Konnors E., Grimkovski P. , Kimber T. , Mak-Kormik M. *Bodibilding* [Bodibilding]. Moscow, FAIR PRESS, 2000, 174 p. (in Russian)
15. Djim V.Y., Comparative analysis of exercise equipment jerk in weightlifting and weight sport. *Pedagogics, psychology, medical-biological problems of physical training and sports*, 2013, no.11, pp. 10-16. http://dx.doi.org/10.6084/m9.figshare.815868
16. Kleiner S. M., Bazzarre T. L., Ainsworth B. E. Nutrional status of nationally ranked elite bodybuilders. *International Journal of Sport Nutrition*. 1994, no.4, pp. 54–69.
17. Cornelius A. E., Brewer B. W., Van Raalte J.L. Applications of multilevel modeling in sport injury rehabilitation research. *International Journal of Sport and Exercise Psychology*. 2007, vol.5, no.4, pp. 387–405. http://dx.doi.org/10.1080/1612197X.2007.9671843.
18. Visek A. J., Watson J. C., Hurst J. R., Maxwell J. P., Harris B. S. Athletic identity and aggressiveness: A cross-cultural analysis of the athletic identity maintenance model. *International Journal of Sport and Exercise Psychology*. 2010, vol.8, no.2, pp. 99–116. http://dx.doi.org/10.1080/1612 197X.2010.9671936.

CONTENT OF HEALTH RELATED SHAPING TRAINING METHODIC FOR GIRLS IN THE PROCESS OF PHYSICAL EDUCATION

Skidan A.A. [1], Sevdalev S.V. [1], Vrublewskiy E.P. [1, 2]
[1]Francisk Skorina Gomel State University, Republic of Belarus
[2]University of Zielona Góra, Poland

Abstract. *Purpose:* theoretical substantiation, working out and testing of health related trainings with girl students, practicing shaping in their physical education. *Material:* in the research 22 girl students of pedagogic specialties participated. Experiment stipulated usage of shaping methodic, based on computer program, during academic year. *Results:* experimental methodic of shaping permitted to bring physical condition indicators of experimental group's girls to patterns of computer program. Analysis of the received data of body circumferential sizes did not show statistically confident distinctions from ideal patterns ($p>0.05$) that witness about their similarity. Results of abdomen top and bottom, torso sides and bottom of back fat folds' measurements did not confidently differ from patterns ($p>0.05$). The above mentioned indicators were within normal values. With it difference for 5% of significance level was registered in the tested functional indicators of girl students, comparing with initial data. After experiment systolic and diastolic BP practically approached to normal value. Heart beats rate confidently approached to normative indicators. *Conclusions:* application of health related shaping methodic positively reflected on physical condition and functional state of girl students. We also proved that it was possible to use computer program for composing individualized training programs.
Key words: girl students, shaping, computer program, ideal patterns, physical condition, functional state.

Introduction

Recent years, students' health has been being of great concern, in spite of established opinion that youth is the healthiest category of population [2, 6, 9, and 14]. At present this group of population is socially vulnerable and do not have or do not use opportunity of its full development.

Only for recent decade the quantity of weakened students has been increased more than 2 times. Analysis of youth's health, physical condition and physical fitness shows that morbidity among students is increasing [3, 7], physical condition and physical fitness are weakening [3, 16]. The quantity of students released from practical physical culture lessons by health reasons increases as well as quantity of students – members of special health groups [2, 16]. In Belarus 70% of students do not practice physical culture. Students' physical inactivity reached 80%. Incorrect and irrational eating resulted in the fact that more than 30% of students have deficit of body mass. The same quantity of students has excessive weight [6, 15]. This problem is especially sharp for girls, having excessive fat. Such girls have increased body mass. All these influence on motor functioning and functioning of all organism's organs and systems, on psychic health [4, 18].

Researches of recent years show [11, 14, 16], that standard form of organization of physical culture lessons for HEE students is ineffective. It does not facilitate formation of sufficient motivation for physical functioning and does not ensure compensation of students' motor functioning deficit.

Involvement of students in physical trainings and formation of their conscious attitude to them is still an acute problem [4, 7]. Girl students to large extent are not satisfied with traditional forms of HEE physical education. They have increased interest to new non traditional kinds of health related physical culture activity.

In opinion of many authors [1, 4, 11, 13, 20-23], girls prefer physical functioning, containing exercises' complexes, which could influence on morphological functional indicators of woman's organism. In 18-21 years' age girls pay special attention to beauty, flexibility, mobility of their bodies. That is why girls wish to practice exercises, which would facilitate harmonious body constitution. It attracts attention of opposite sex. Girl students prefer methods, connected with music, plasticity, artistry. For them first of all positive emotions, possibility to aesthetically influence on organism by physical exercises are important.

In this connection education system in general and HEEs in particular face the task of maintenance of students' physical, psychic and moral health. That is why HEE shall be an initiator and organizer of purposeful and effective work on rehabilitation, protection and strengthening of students' health. At present this work is acquiring systemic character: new health related and diagnostic technologies are implemented; material-technical base of HEEs rises [10, 15].

In many developed countries different directions of health related physical culture are intensively developing. Great number of new body correction programs, strengthening and protection of woman's health appear [11, 17].

Recent years a number of new, modern health related physical culture systems and technologies, which are practiced mainly by girls, has appeared [11]. Among many kinds of physical functioning shaping has been taking first place during more than 20 years. With it shaping quickly develops and perfects. In opinion of many specialists modern shaping permits to effectively solve tasks of physical, mental and aesthetic perfection [5, 13, and 18].

The content of shaping trainings is determined by personalities strive for beauty and harmony. The basis of the system is idea about standard of physical perfection, which is called "model" in shaping. Such "model" has main signs of woman's beauty and attractiveness. "Shaping" system is a purposeful training of separate muscular groups, which permits for every trainee to correct defects of posture in all parts as well as to reduce weight, to improve carriage, to acquire body beauty, for which all modern girls strive. Harmonious body is one of main signs of human health, as far as defects of body hinder functioning of organism's organs and functions [5, 8, and 13].

Purpose of the research, material and methods

The purpose of the research is theoretical substantiation, working out and testing of health related trainings with girl students, practicing shaping in their physical education.

The methods and materials of the research: analysis of scientific-methodic literature was carried out in order to know existing views on the studied problems, on perfection of students' physical education.

Pedagogic observations were conducted during all period of work. The object of observation was fulfillment of the worked out methodic approaches to physical education means' application by the tested. Results were assessed by express tests and by external signs of fatigue.

Girls' testing was conducted with the help of special computer program "Shaping" [11]. The program included measurement of anthropometric indicators: a) body mass and body length; b) circumferential sizes of neck, chest, breast, waist, buttocks, hips, shins, knees, wrists; c) fat folds on forearm, front and back of shoulder, top and bottom of back, top and bottom of abdomen, front and back, inside and outside of hips; change of cardio-vascular system's indicators: blood pressure and heart beats rate (HBR). All mentioned above information was processed by computer program. By results of this processing ideal values for such contingent were received.

Besides, we used commonly accepted methods of mathematical statistic. Confidence of distinctions was determined with Student's t-criterion.

Pedagogic experiment was conducted on base of Gomel health related physical culture center during academic year. Experiment was organized ob the base of generally accepted principles. In the research 22 girl students of pedagogic specialties participated. They were trained by shaping program twice a week (60 minutes – each training session). It should be noted that experimental group of girl students was formed by selection of girls with excessive fat. The purpose of trainings was to correct their figures in general and change configuration of separate parts of their bodies. In experimental group we realized methodic of shaping training, facilitating purposeful body corrections, considering ideal values for this contingent. For this purpose we used results of special computer program "Shaping".

He offered by computer program complexes of exercises and methodic of their application are directed on correction of body parts, which deviate from standard. In process of training complexes were corrected in order to individualize approaches to every girl students. Some complexes of exercises were worked out for increasing of muscular mass (increasing of body parts' volume). Other - were directed on reducing of volumes at the account of fat decreasing. Complexes of exercises were combined by prevailing influence on different muscular groups.

Practical significance of the work was assessment of deviations from ideal values. Detection of deviations served as bench mark for targeted impact on separate body parts by shaping means. To larger extent training influence was rendered on those bode parts, which had deviations from standard. Orienting on ideal values we determined direction of correction of every part of body and selected special individual programs of appropriate training.

The structure of practical work in experimental group included execution of exercises, divided into 11 blocks (series) – fore successive work of separate muscular groups (see table 1).

Table 1. Structure of shaping trainings in experimental group

STRUCTURE OF TRAININGS			
	Block for working with muscular groups	Duration (minutes)_	Part of training
1	Warming up	10	I Introductory
2	Hip (front)	4	II Main
3	Hip (back)	4	
4	Hip (inside)	4	
5	Hip (outside)	4	
6	Buttocks	4	
7	Abdomen (top)	4	
8	Abdomen (bottom)	4	
9	Waist	4	
10	Individual block		III Additional
	– first zone	4	
	– second zone	4	
	– third zone	4	
11	Recreation	6	IV Finalizing

Results of the research

The received numerical values permitted to detect existing deviations from norm of anthropometric indicators at the beginning of pedagogic experiment.

Body mass of girls actually exceeded normal values at the beginning of experiment (by 6.71±0.23 kg). The highest deviations were detected in fat folds. For example abdomen (top and bottom) had deviations 7.37±0.17 cm; side of torso – 6.18±0.22 cm; bottom of back – 11.17±0.23 cm; hips (front, back, inside, outside) respectively – 12.2±0.23, 21.86±0.26, 11.91±0.20 and 27.36±0.22 cm.

By all tested indicators we registered confident difference ($p<0.05$) between physical condition indicators and standard indicators (SI).

By the end of pedagogic experiment, between experimental groups' physical condition data and ideal indicators we found confidential difference in measurements of the following fat folds: hip (front) (19.47±0.31 cm) deviation from SI– 4.47±0.27 cm; hip (back) – 26.45±0.13 cm, deviation from SI – 10.45±0.21cm; hip inside – 12.71±0.17 cm, deviation from SI – 3.21±0.18 cm; hip outside – 31.31±0.21 cm, deviation from SI – 11.31±0.27 cm. However, in comparison with the beginning of experiment deviations from standard indicators reduced significantly.

Analysis of circumferential sizes of body showed: waist – 63.93±0.36 cm, deviation from SI – 1.12±0.26 cm; buttocks – 91.27±0.34 cm, deviation from SI – 1.33±0.32 cm; hips – 52.29±0.23 cm, deviation from SI – 0.81±0.22 cm) and did not revealed confident distinctions from standard indicators ($p>0C5$). It witnesses about their closeness to model indicators.

Results of abdomen fat folds (top – 8.84±0.15 cm, deviation from SI – 2.32±0.14 cm, bottom – 12.84±0.21cm, deviation from SI– 2.84±0.19 cm; fat folds on side of torso - 7.75±0.24 cm, deviation from SI – 1.83±0.24 cm; fat folds on bottom of back – 19.98±0.23 cm, deviation from SI – 0.99±0.31cm also did not confidently differ from standard indicators ($p>0.05$). The delivered above indicators are within norm.

Thus, the offered by us health related shaping methodic permitted to practically approach physical condition indicators of experimental group's girls to standard indicators.

Results of research of experimental group girls' cardio-vascular system deviated from norm at the beginning of experiment. They had increased systolic BP (128.74±0.47 mm.merc.col.) and diastolic BP (87.54±0.34 mm.merc.col.).

Also, at the beginning of pedagogic experiment we registered increase of heart beats rate (73.35±0.16 with norm 60–70 b.p.m.).

After finishing of pedagogic experiment we registered confident change in the tested indicators of girl students' functional state, in comparison with initial data ($p<0.05$). Systolic and diastolic BP values were practically normal at the end of experiment (123.65±0.71 and 84.57±0.52 mm.merc.col.) Heart beats rate in rest also statistically confidently (for 5% level of significance) closed to normative indicators at the end of experiment (71.23±0.43 with norm 60–70b.p.m.).

Thus, the worked out methodic of health related shaping trainings turned out to be effective mean of formation of motor culture, physical condition , physical and functional fitness improvement for girls. Results of the research point at purposefulness of implementation of the offered health related shaping trainings methodic for girls in HEE's physical education process.

Discussion

By results of analysis of scientific-methodic literature and preliminary testing we found that girl students had low level of motor culture, of physical and theoretical fitness (that contradict to requirements of program-normative documents and scientific-methodic recommendations, regulating physical education process of girls students of not physical culture HEEs) [2, 3, 5, 8, 16]. All these are conditioned by drawbacks of HEE physical education system (orientation only on control normative indicators and body component, ignoring of motivation component of individual motor-developing impacts' application) [3, 4, 6, 7, 9, and 15]. Thus, physical education of not physical culture HEEs' girl students requires correction, considering the mentioned factors.

It should be stressed that physical education process has three vectors of impact: creation of wide circle of knowledge in field of physical culture, training of motor actions (formation of motor culture) and control of physical condition development [9, 10, 16, and 19]. All they are interconnected. Therefore wide usage of physical culture means (including non traditional) facilitates fuller physical and theoretical fitness of girl students. At the same time it is impossible to completely solve physical education tasks without positive motivation background.

As a result of "shaping" computer program every girl realized her own health related effect and could achieve more harmonious and proportional body constitution. The received results show that it is possible for girl students to influence positively on organism in process of physical education. With it perfection of external, visual status is of priority in this age. It is confirmed also by other scientists [1, 6, 8, 11, 13, and 17]. It is significant that experimental group's girl students started to actively include in independent physical exercises' practicing.

Conclusions

The conducted pedagogic experiment, health related training methodic permitted to approach every girl to indicators of shaping model. Comparing with the beginning of experiment deviations from ideal standards significantly reduced. Analysis of the received data of circumferential sizes showed that they practically correspond to ideal indicators after experiment. Sizes of fat folds are within norm.

Thus, the worked out shaping methodic permitted to substantially reduce fat component of girl students' body mass, improve functional state, rise psycho-emotional state and motivation for regular physical exercises' practicing, to form steady demand in them. All these confirmed high effectiveness of this methodic, which can be adapted to application in physical education process in conditions of other HEEs and in additional health related training of girl students.

Conflict of interests

The authors declare that there is no conflict of interests.

References:

1. Afonskaia AO. *Effektivnost' metodiki formirovaniia osnovnykh priemov ozdorovitel'noj aerobiki u studentov v processe fizicheskogo vospitaniia. Cand. Diss.* [Effectiveness of methodic of health related aerobic main techniques formation in students in process of physical education. Cand. Diss.]. Tula; 2004. (in Russian)
2. Belkina NV. Zdorov'e formiruiushchaia tekhnologiia fizicheskogo vospitaniia studentok vuza [Health-forming technology of HEE girl students' physical education]. *Teoriia i praktika fizicheskoj kul'tury* 2006;2:7–11. (in Russian)
3. Bogatyrev VS. *Fizicheskaia kul'tura v vuze* [Physical culture in HEE], Kirov: VSPU; 2001. (in Russian)

4. Volodkovich SL. *Struktura i soderzhanie ozdorovitel'no-razvivaiushchikh zaniatij po fizicheskoj kul'ture studentok podgotovitel'noj medicinskoj gruppy pedagogicheskikh special'nostej. Cand. Diss*. [Structure and content of health related- developing physical culture trainings of special health groups' girl students of pedagogic specialties. Cand. Diss.]. Moscow; 2011. (in Russian)
5. Bochenkova EV, Gubskaia NM. Vliianie fizicheskogo vospitaniia na lichnost' zanimaiushchegosia [Influence of physical education on trainee's personality]. *XXVII nauchnaia konferenciia studentov i molodykh uchenykh vuzov Iuga Rossii* [27th scientific conference of students and young scientists of the South of Russia], Krasnodar; 2000. P. 15–16. (in Russian)
6. Vrublevskij EP, Skidan AA. Metodika korrekcii teloslozheniia studentok, zanimaiushchikhsia shejpingom v processe fizicheskogo vospitaniia [Methodic of correction of girl students' practicing shaping in process of physical education, body constitution]. *II mezhdunarodnaia nauchno-prakticheskaia konferenciia "Cherez fizicheskuiu kul'turu i sport k zdorovomu obrazu zhizni", 25 maia 2014 g., Ufa* [2nd International scientific practical conference "Through physical culture and sports to healthy life style",May 25th, 2014, Ufa], 2014. P. 321–324. (in Russian)
7. Doroshenko SA. *Sportivno-vidovoj podkhod v fizicheskom vospitanii studentov v vuze. Cand. Diss.* [Sport-species approach in HEE students' physical education. Cand. Diss.], Malakhovka; 2011. (in Russian)
8. Kozlov VI. *Progressirovanie deficita dvigatel'noj aktivnosti u studentok i vybor sredstv ego kompensacii. Cand. Diss.* [Progressing of motor functioning deficit of girl students and choice of means for its compensation. Cand. Diss.], Malakhovka: MGAFK; 1995. (in Russian)
9. Kovalenko TG. *Bioinformacionnye tekhnologii pri problemno-modul'nom obuchenii v sisteme fizicheskogo vospitaniia i reabilitacii studentov s oslablennym zdorov'em. Doct. Diss.* [Bio-informational technologies with problem-module education in system of physical education and rehabilitation of students with weak health. Doct. Diss.], Volgograd; 2000. (in Russian)
10. Konikov IA. K voprosu o sushchnosti esteticheskogo [On issue of essence of aesthetic]. *Esteticheskoe soznanie lichnosti* [Aesthetic consciousness of personality], Moscow: IFRAN; 1994. (in Russian)
11. Los' EE, Glaz'ko TA. *Shejping: organizaciia samostoiatel'nykh zaniatij* [Shaping: organization of independent trainings], Minsk; 2013. (in Russian)
12. Postol OL. *Metodika ozdorovleniia studentok vuzov na zaniatiiakh po fizicheskomu vospitaniiu s primeneniem tradicionnykh i netradicionnykh sredstv. Cand. Diss*. [Methodic of HEE girl students' health improvement at physical education lessons with application of traditional and non traditional means. Cand. Diss.], Khabarovsk; 2004. (in Russian)
13. Prokhorcev IV, Maslakova E. Shejping – novyj vid ozdorovitel'noj massovoj fizicheskoj kul'tury [Shaping as new kind of health related mass physical culture], *Sport i zdorov'e* 1992;1:64–68. (in Russian)
14. Sysoev VV. *Formirovanie u studentov neprofil'nykh pedagogicheskikh special'nostej potrebnosti v fizicheskom samosovershenstvovanii. Cand. Diss*. [Formation of non profile pedagogic specialties' students' demand in physical self-perfection. Cand. Diss.], Bryansk; 2003. (in Russian)
15. Timoshenko VV. *Fizicheskoe vospitanie studentov i uchashchikhsia, imeiushchikh otklonenie v sostoianii zdorov'ia* [Physical education of students, having deviations from normal health], Minsk; 1995. (in Russian)
16. Treshcheva OL. *Formirovanie kul'tury zdorov'ia v usloviiakh sovremennogo obrazovaniia* [Formation of health culture in conditions of modern education], Omsk; 2002. (in Russian)
17. Cirkin VI, Bogatyrev VS. *Fizicheskoe zdorov'e cheloveka* [Physical health of man], Kirov: VSU; 1998. (in Russian)
18. Shchankina VV. *Novye fizkul'turno-sportivnye vidy* [New kinds of physical culture and sports],: RSU; 2006. (in Russian)
19. Iudina NM. *Metodika opredeleniia i ocenki fizicheskogo potenciala studentov vuza. Cand. Diss.* [Methodic of determination and assessment of physical potential of HEE students. Cand. Diss.], Volgograd; 2006. (in Russian)
20. Fomenko E.V., Practical recommendations for the implementation of health technologies to enhance physical fitness of students in extracurricular classes during non-traditional gymnastics. *Pedagogics, psychology, medical-biological problems of physical training and sports*, 2014, vol.7, pp. 31-36. http://dx.doi.org/10.6084/m9.figshare.1015385

21. Kurmaeva EV. Fitness - programs as mean of forming of personality physical culture of students. *Physical Education of Students* 2013;1:37-39. http://dx.doi.org/10.6084/m9.figshare.156355
22. Malenyuk TV, Kosivska AV. Training at sport circle as priority form of organization of students' physical education (on example of shaping). *Pedagogics, psychology, medical-biological problems of physical training and sports* 2015;4:38-42. http://dx.doi.org/10.15561/18189172.2015.0407
23. Martinova NP. Results of experimental testing of hee girl students' motor skills at aerobic trainings. *Physical Education of Students* 2015;5:46-53. http://dx.doi.org/10.15561/20755279.2015.0507

11

ASSESSMENT OF INDICATORS OF FACULTY MASS SPORT FUNCTIONING IN HIGHER EDUCATIONAL ESTABLISHMENT

Kirpenko V.N.
Kharkov Air Force University Kozhedub

Abstract. *Purpose:* to work out the methodic of determination of military higher educational establishment faculty's rating for improvement of organization, monitoring and control of physical education process at the faculty. *Material:* we used systemic-structural analysis; functioning of military higher educational establishment faculty was simulated; quantitative values of faculty functioning integral rating, connected with organization and conducting of sport measures, were obtained. *Results:* on the base of hierarchic model of faculty functioning we offered model of faculty rating. De-composition of its structure was carried out up to the level, at which it is possible to make objective quantitative assessments of separate kinds of functioning. *Conclusions:* the worked out rating-model of functioning results shows functional connection of faculty's integral rating with its special ratings as well as connections between different kinds of functioning at different levels of de-composition. We found clear connection of special ratings of lower level with quantitative assessments of functioning. It permits to differentially approach to comparison and assessment of faculty's functioning.
Key words: rating, model, functioning, integral, primary, assessments.

Introduction

As on to day, testing and assessment of military higher educational establishment (MHEE) faculty is a certain system, one of elements of which is assessment of physical training's organization and conduct (Methodic of complex testing (current, partial) of situation in military higher educational establishments and military educational units of higher educational establishments. Approved by Order of Ministry of defense of Ukraine, dt. 08.09.2014 № 630. Order of Ministry of defense of Ukraine, dt. 19.02.2015 № 49 "On organization of physical training in Armed Forces of Ukraine in 2015 academic year") [8–12, 13–19]. Reviews of mass sport work (RMSW) is one of those testing, which can be used as mean for assessment of faculty's functioning on organization and realization of physical trainings. However, the existing system of results' assessment strongly differs by conditions of RMSW in Armed Forces of Ukraine (AF of Ukraine) from system, which existed in period 1945 – 1990. It does not permit to completely use differentiated approach to assessment of functioning results of faculties, which prepare specialists of different military profiles [3, 7].

Analysis of recent publications witnesses that characteristic feature of modern state of Ukrainian AF reformation is transition to optimization of their structure and quantity, bringing them in compliance with economic potentials of the State. In HEEs of MD of Ukraine there appears an acute demand in searching the ways and means of comparison and assessment, activation of all kinds of faculties' functioning, including functioning, connected with organization and realization of mass sport measures [1, 3, 7]. It should be noted that assessment of faculties' mass sport functioning was always conducted. But only recent years rating system of assessment have been started to be discussed. It is explained by the fact that rating system is more perfect, comparing with earlier existing system (Report about SRW "Module" "Methodological principles of module rating system of pedagogic process organization" // МОУ НМЦ ВО. – К., 2001. – 77 с.) [4, 5].

Purpose, tasks of the work, material and methods

The purpose of the research is to determine indicators of faculty's functioning in mass sport work, to assess them and work out rating-model for mass sport and sport work at MHEE faculty.

Results of the research

It is purposeful to adopt the methodic of construction of rating model of faculty functioning results on all levels of de-composition in the form, which was developed when construction rating models of MHEEs of Ukraine (Report about SRW "Module" "Methodological principles of module rating system of pedagogic process organization" // МОУ НМЦ ВО. – К., 2001. – 77 с.). The model of mass sport and sport functioning of MHEE is shown in fig. 1.

The model of organization and realization of sport mass and sport work includes three main kinds of faculty's military officers' functioning [10, 15].

First kind "5.1. Mass sport work" stipulates training of faculty military officers and their participation in mass sport measures, conducted in HEE and out of it. They include:

- Faculty's participation in championships (full time and correspondence) among MHEEs of Ukraine;
- Faculty's participation in MHEE championship;
- Faculty's participation in regional championships among MHEEs.

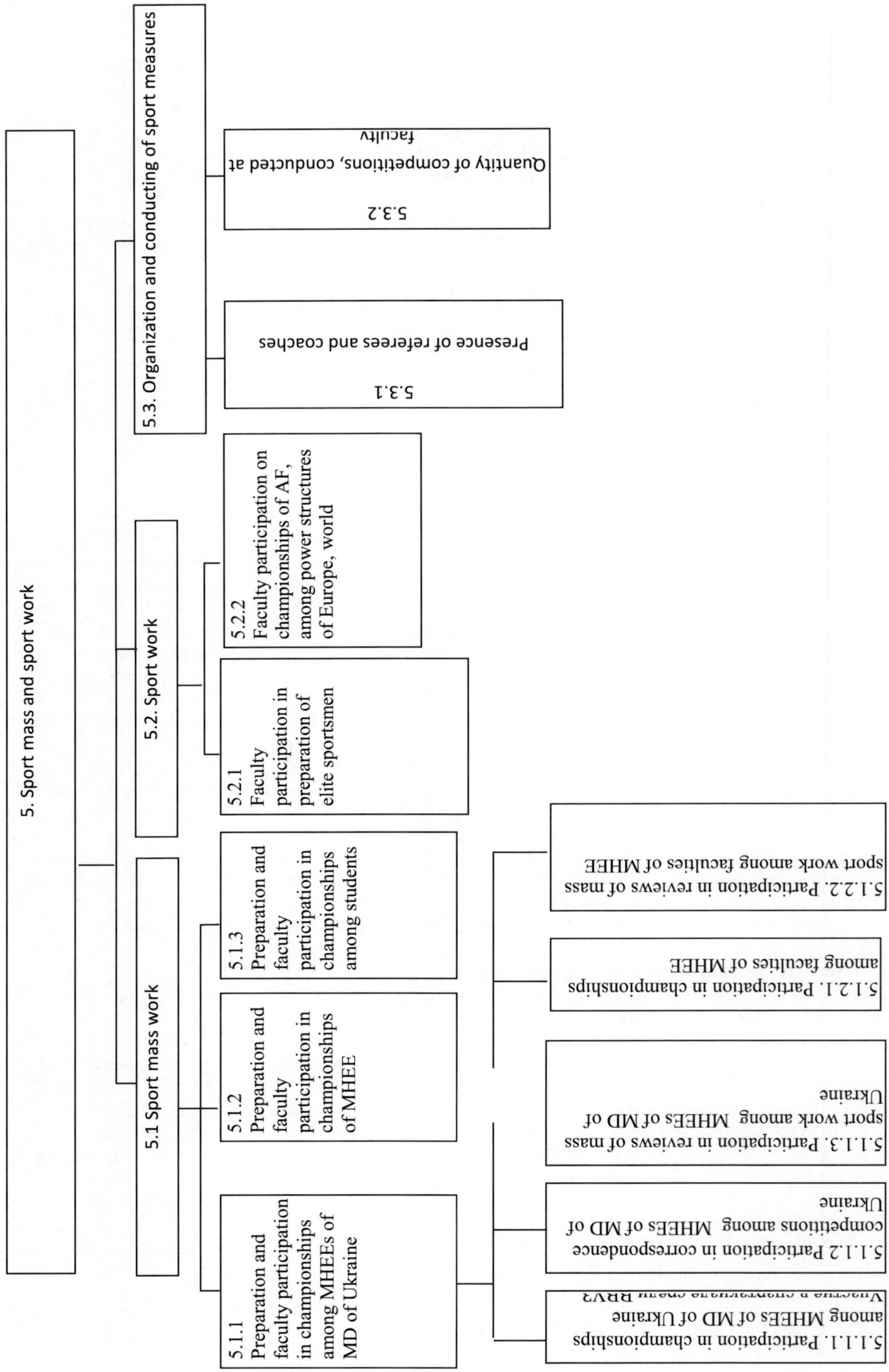

Fig.1. Model of sport mass and sport work of MHEE

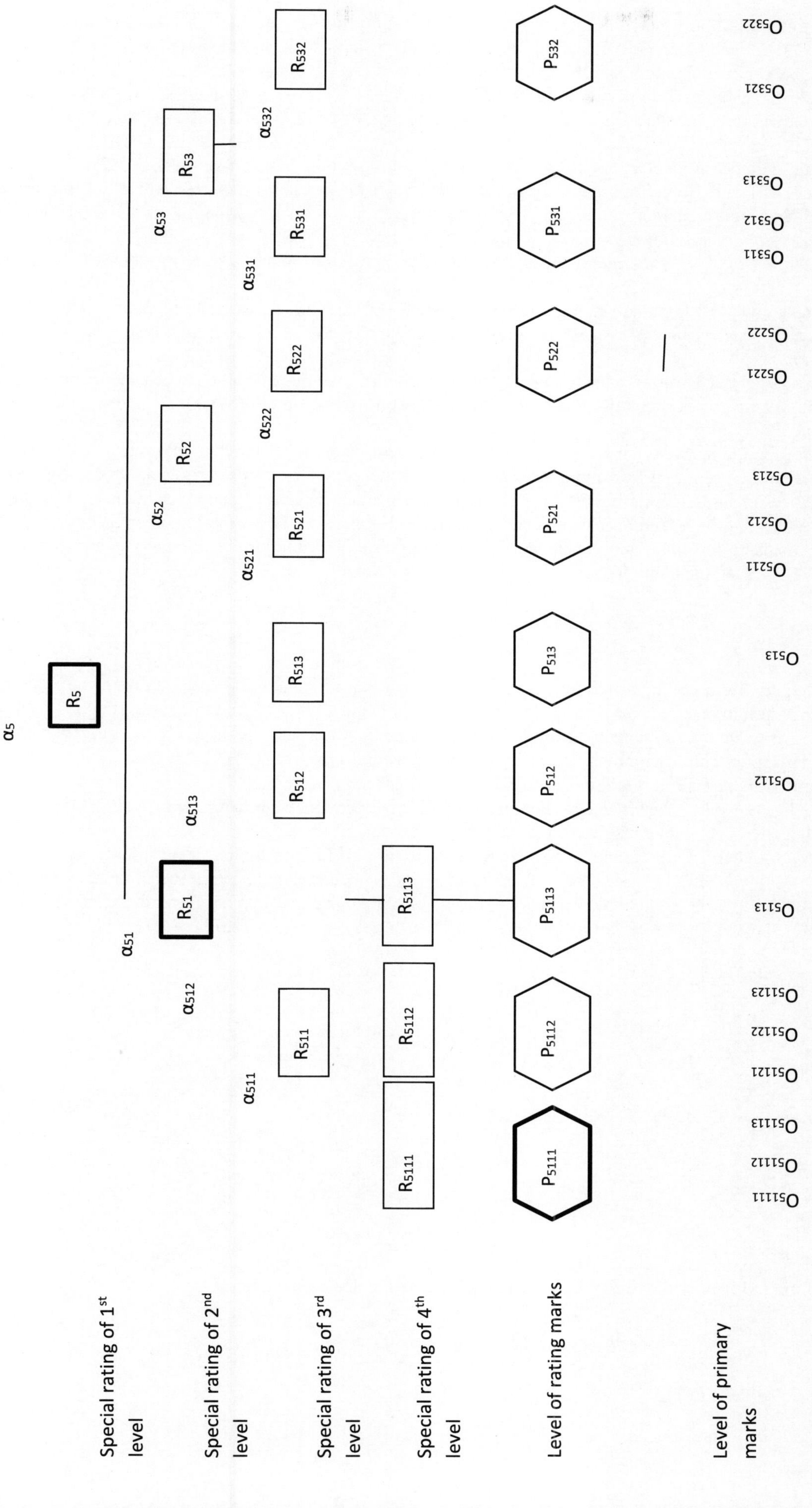

Fig.2. Rating-model of mass sport and sport work in MHEE

Second kind “5.2. Sport work” determines level of all faculty military officers’ personal readiness for passing normative, sport grades and other sport qualification requirements (candidate master of sports, master of sport and so on) as well as participation in competitions of Armed Forces of Ukraine level and higher.

Third kind “5.3. Organization and conducting of sport measures” specifies qualification level of those, who organize and conduct sport measures as well as quantitative indicators of organized and conducted sport measures on faculty.

According to model of faculty functioning adequate to it rating-model has been built (see fig.2).

As the base of faculty rating in organization and conducting of mass sport measures we applied approaches, used in military qualimetry and mathematical statistic [5, 6]. It is offered to insert some additions in them, which will permit to consider in assessment the following:

– Sport achievements of combined teams of MHEE in proportion to quantity of representatives from faculty in them;

– place, taken by MHEE team in championship among MHEEs of Ukraine as well as faculty work on preparation of qualified referees, coaches and conducting of competitions on faculty. Let us regard formation of marks by main kinds of faculty functioning.

Functioning kind 5.1.1 was assessed by faculty participation in championship and in correspondence competitions among MEEs of Ukraine, by participation in “Review for the best organization of physical training and mass sport work in AD of Ukraine”.

Kinds of functioning 5.1.1.1 и 5.1.1.2 were assessed by participation of every faculty in team of kinds of sports, which are envisaged by program of championship and correspondence competitions. By results of MHEEs’ combined teams’ performances in assessment of faculty it is necessary to consider the staff of combined team, determined by total quantity of team (K_o) and by quantity of faculty representatives in this team (K_f) as well as the place, taken by MHEE combined team in championship or at correspondence competitions (D). Primary marks of every component for kind of functioning 5.1.1.1 are calculated by formula:

$$O_{fi} = \frac{K_{fi}}{K_{oi} \times D_i}$$

K_{oi} and K_{fi}, are not constant values and can not be predicted. They depend on number (i) of MHEEs’ combined teams, which took certain place in competitions. Ordeal number of team changes within the limits $0 \le i \le N$ (where N is quantity of kinds of sports by program of championship and correspondence competitions). Rating mark shall consider achievements of all sport teams, which participate in competitions of kinds 5.1.1.1. and 5.1.1.2.

In the same way marks for other kinds of functioning 5.1.1.2 are determined.

The only difference is that D (place of our university in correspondence competitions) for all faculties will be one and the same; that is why it is not considered in the formula.

In functioning kind 5.1.1.3 results of mass sport work review within the frames of our university are considered and have only one component of primary mark. Primary mark of this component is determined by place of faculty in the university as per conditions about conduct of “Review for the best organization of physical trainings and mass sport work in AF of Ukraine”. Then, rating mark will coincide with primary mark, i.e. $P_{5113} = O_{5113}$.

$$P_{5113} = \frac{D_f}{\sum_{i=1}^{N} D_i}$$

$$R_{5111} = \frac{P_{5111}}{\sum_{i=1}^{N} (P_{5111})_i}$$

$$P_{5111} = \sum_{i=1}^{N} \frac{K_{fi}}{K_{oi} \times D_i}$$

$$R_{5113} = \frac{P_{5113}}{\sum_{i=1}^{N} (P_{5113})_i}$$

Special rating of faculty by kind of functioning 5.1.1 is calculated by formula:

$$R_{511} = \alpha_{111} R_{5111} + \alpha_{112} R_{5112} + \alpha_{113} R_{5113}$$

Primary mark O_{5121} of functioning kind 5.1.2 is determined by results of faculty participation in every kind of sports, envisaged by MHEEs' championship program. For calculation of the mentioned primary marks the following expression is used:

$$O_{5121} = 1 - \frac{n}{N}$$

Where n is the place, taken by faculty in certain kind of sports at championship;
N is the sum of faculties places in this kind of sports (faculties, participating in championship).
Rating mark is calculated by formula:

$$P_{5121} = \sum_{i=1}^{N} (O_{5121})_i$$

In functioning kind 5.1.2.2 results of mass sport work review within the frames of our university are considered and have only one component of primary mark. In functioning kind 5.1.1.3 results of mass sport work review within the frames of our university are considered and have only one component of primary mark. Primary mark of this component is determined by place of faculty in the university as per conditions about conduct of "Review for the best organization of physical trainings and mass sport work in KhUAF".

Faculty sport work (kind of functioning 5.2) is assessed by quantity of faculty military officers, who confirmed or passed sport normative and qualification requirements during academic year as well as took proper places at competitions of Armed Forces and MHEEs. The procedure of scoring for fulfillment of sport normative (international master of sports, master of sports, candidate master of sports, first, second, third grades) and for places, won at competitions was determined by appropriated rules.

Faculty work on organization and conducting of sport measures was assessed by place of faculty by quantity of faculty military officers, having qualification of referee of International, National, first and second categories, coaches. The procedure of scoring for qualification level was determined by appropriated rules.

Total faculty rating is calculated by formula:

$$R_5 = \alpha_1 R_{51} + \alpha_2 R_{52} + \alpha_3 R_{53}$$

Finally, it would be purposeful to render the values of weight coefficients α (see table 1), which are recommended to be used when determining faculty rating on mass sport and sport work. They were received on the base of generalization of many years' experience of physical education, special physical training and sport department as well as experience of sport committee of Kharkov university of Air Forces in assessment of mass sport and sport work at the university. The rendered data are not final; they can be specified.

Table 1. Recommended numerical values of weight coefficients α

Description	α_{51}	α_{52}	α_{53}	α_{511}	α_{512}	α_{513}	α_{521}	α_{522}
Numerical value	0,6	0,3	0,1	0,25	0,3	0,45	0,45	0,55
Description	α_{531}	α_{532}	α_{5111}	α_{5112}	α_{5113}	α_{5121}	α_{5122}	–
Numerical value	0,7	0,3	0,25	0,3	0,45	0,4	0,6	–

Discussion

The content of functions and kinds of faculty activities, methods of their accounting and assessment are determined by normative documents, regulating separate directions of armed forces' functioning [9–12].

For improvement of military officers' physical fitness, development of mass sport, organization of meaningful leisure of personnel at faculty mass sport and sport work are organized [Order of Minister of defense, dt. 19.02.2015 № 49 "On organization of physical training in Armed Forces of Ukraine in 2015 academic year"]. It is known that organization level and content of mass sport and sport work on faculty directly influence on effectiveness of cadets' functioning and quality of graduates. That is why traditional approach to assessment of results of this work can not permit to objectively assess and compare faculties, which prepare specialists of different profiles. In earlier offered assessment methods quantity of indicators for objective assessment of MSW* is not sufficient. For example, in work [7] it is noted that MSW results are assessed by data, rendered by units' commanders. Methods of conducting and assessment of MSW do not differ noticeably. Difference in results is explained by authors by different approaches to planning.

*MSW – mass sport work *(note of translator)*.

However, the results, received by us, show that rating system of assessment plays rather important role. This system has been worked out and substantiated on the base of model of faculty functioning. De-composition of its structure is carried out up to the level, at which it is possible to realize objective quantitative assessment of separate kinds of functioning. We determined required mathematical correlations, permitting to express integral rating of faculty though special ratings by separate kinds of functioning as well as to express special ratings through assessment of these kinds of functioning. List of initial data and mechanism of their re-calculation in primary marks of faculty kinds of functioning do not require additional researches of rating object.

Conclusions

On the base of the worked out model of functioning we have offered rating-model, permitting to objectively assess and compare functioning of faculties in MSW.

We have found the list of initial data and mechanism of their re-calculation in primary marks of faculty functioning. These data can be inserted in data base of automatic system of faculty rating's determination.

The offered in this work model of MHEE mass sport and sport work can be regarded as variant. The model undoubtedly requires discussion and specifying by physical training and sports departments of all MHEEs of Ukraine.

Conflict of interests

The authors declare that there is no conflict of interests.

References:

1. Barybina LN, Semashko SA, Krivencova EV. Osobennosti organizacii sportivno-massovoj raboty v tekhnicheskom vuze [Specific features of porganization of mass sport work in technical HEE]. *Physical education of students,* 2011;1:18–21.
2. Kirpenko VM, Piddubnij OG, Bozhko SA. Ocinka efektivnosti iakosti pidgotovki kursantiv z disciplini «Fizichne vikhovannia, special'na fizichna pidgotovka i sport» [Assessment of effectiveness of cadets' training in discipline" physical education, special physical training and sports"]. *Pedagogics, psychology, medical-biological problems of physical training and sports*, 2008;12:14–18. (in Ukrainian)
3. Kirpenko VM. Pidvishchennia efektivnosti pedagogichnogo procesu special'noi fizichnoi pidgotovki kursantiv VVNZ povitrianikh sil na osnovi idei optimizacii [Increase of effectiveness of pedagogic process of special physical training of Air Forces' MHEEs cadets, considering optimization]. *Slobozhans'kij naukovo-sportivnij visnik*, 2013;2:169–174. (in Ukrainian)
4. Liamec VI, Teviashev AD. *Sistemnyj analiz* [Systemic analysis]. Kharkov: KhTURE; 1998. (in Russian)
5. Oleksiienko BM. *Teoretichni osnovi vijs'kovoi kvalimetrii* [Teoretichni osnovi vijs'kovoi kvalimetrii]. Hmelnitsky; 2000. (in Ukrainian)
6. Sidorenko EV. *Metody matematicheskoj obrabotki v psikhologii* [Methods of mathematical processing in psychology]. Sankt Petersburg: Socio-Psychological Center; 1996. (in Russian)
7. Sukhorada GI. *Sportivno-masova robota u vishchikh vijs'kovikh navchal'nikh zakladakh. Cand. Diss*. [Mass sport work in military higher educational establishments. Cand. Diss.]. Kiev; 2003. (in Ukrainian)
8. *Army Regulation 350-1, Army Training and Leader Development.* Washington, DC: Headquarters, Department of the Army, 18 December 2009; Section VI, "Army Training Programs", 1–24. "Army physical fitness training"; 2009.
9. *Army Regulation 40–501 Standards of Medical Fitness*. Washington, DC: Headquarters, Department of the Army, 14 December; 2007.
10. *Canadian Forces, Expres Operations Manual* (4-th Edition); 2010.
11. *Field Manual FM 7–22 Army Physical Readiness Training with Change 13 May 2013 Paperback*. by United States Government US Army; 2013.
12. Joseph E. *Raycroft Mass Physical Training*: For Use in the Army and the Reserve Officers Training Corps Forgotten Books; 2015.
13. McGraw LK, Out D, Hammermeister JJ, Ohlson CJ, Pickering MA, Granger DA. Nature, correlates, and consequences of stress-related biological reactivity and regulation in Army nurses during combat casualty simulation. *Psychoneuroendocrinology*. 2013;38(1):135–144.
14. McGeachan C. Needles, picks and an intern named Laing: exploring the psychiatric spaces of Army life. *Journal of Historical Geography*. 2013;40:67–78.
15. Lewandowski-Romps L, Peterson C, Berglund PA, Collins S, Cox K, Hauret K, et al. Risk Factors for Accident Death in the U.S. Army, 2004–2009. *American Journal of Preventive Medicine.* 2014;47(6):745–753.
16. Walker D, Neighbors C, Walton T, Pierce A, Mbilinyi L, Kaysen D, et al. Spicing up the military: Use and effects of synthetic cannabis in substance abusing army personnel. *Addictive Behaviors*. 2014;39(7):1139–44.
17. Portman N, Šlapeta J. The flagellar contribution to the apical complex: a new tool for the eukaryotic Swiss Army knife? *Trends in Parasitology*. 2014;30(2):58–64.
18. Raiha NK, Soma DJ. Victims of child abuse and neglect in the U.S. army. *Child Abuse & Neglect*. 1997;21(8):759–768.

12

CHARACTERISTIC OF BIO-GEOMETRIC PROFILE OF STUDENTS' POSTURE AND PHYSICAL FITNESS IN PROCESS OF PHYSICAL EDUCATION

Dudko M.V.
Kyiv National Economic University named after Vadym Hetman

Abstract. _Purpose:_ to determine specific features of bio-geometric profile of posture and physical fitness of students in process of physical education. _Material:_ 250 students were tested. Video-recording and analysis of bio-geometric profile of human posture were fulfilled. Program Torso was used for this purpose. _Results:_ it was found out that only 15.2% of students had correct posture. The most quantity of posture abnormalities was detected in 36.4% of the tested. In sagittal plane we observed the following types of abnormalities: round back – in 24.4% of students, slouching back – in 24% of students. We found that 63.3% of students with normal posture are in zone of risk. Low backbone flexibility, mobility of hip joints and elasticity of hamstrings was detected on students. _Conclusions:_ students with unsatisfactory bio-geometric profile of posture (scoliosis posture – 43.33%; round back – 23. 33%; slouching back – 22. 73%) are in the called pre-morbid state of muscular-skeletal apparatus.
Key words: students, physical education, posture, visual screening.

Introduction

In modern conditions, educational process in higher educational establishments is connected with continuously increasing informational flow and with significant psychological loads. It sets high requirements to students' health condition and physical fitness that is important condition of ensuring of students' harmonious development. [13, 20, 23].

Most of specialists [1, 3, 7, 8] connect it with unfavorable social economic conditions of life and ecology, with substantial reduction of students' interest to physical culture and sports, weakening of physical education system in higher educational establishments.

Numerous researches [2, 4, 10, 17-19, 22] witness that mass character of posture abnormalities – is one of the most pressing problems of modern society. Functional abnormalities of posture are one of the most wide-spread deviations in muscular skeletal system of modern students [8, 9, 24]. Postures disorders negatively influence on function of internal organs, cardio-vascular, respiratory and digestive systems. They negatively impact on human mental; and physical workability [1, 3, 8, 9, 25-30].

At present time there is great number of scientific publications [4, 5, 6, 7, 13, 21] on studying of posture abnormalities of students and approaches to their correction by physical education means. However, some problems have still been remaining unsolved.

In our opinion, for effective planning of health related work it is purposeful to use "screening" [10]. Its purpose is to detect students with "risk zones" of posture's bio-geometric abnormalities as well as determination of pre-morbid states of muscular-skeletal apparatus (MSA).

Generalizing specialists' views we can state the fact that correction of posture's bio-geometrical profile abnormalities of students is reflected in many publications. At the same time some questions, concerning prophylaxis of such abnormalities have not been profoundly worked out yet.

Purpose, tasks of the work, material and methods

The purpose of the work is to determine specific features of bio-geometric profile of posture and physical fitness of students in process of physical education.

The tasks of he work:

1. To generalize scientific data on prophylaxis and correction of students postures' abnormalities by means of physical education, by data of special literature.
2. To determine the most frequent abnormalities of posture's bio-geometrical profile, level of its state and specificities of students' physical fitness.

The methods of the research: we used the following methods: theoretical analysis and generalization of special scientific-methodic literature, pedagogic observations, pedagogic testing, anthropometry, video recording and analysis of human posture's bio-geometrical profile with the help of program "Torso", visual screening", methods of mathematical statistic. In the research 250 first year students of Kyiv National Economic University named after Vadym Hetman participated.

Results of the research

Collection of data from students' medical records was conducted with direct participation of vertebra-neurology specialist. Visual screening and application of "Torso" program [9] permitted to detect that only 15.2% of students have normal posture. Types of posture's abnormalities were distributed in the following way: scoliosis posture 36.4% of the tested, slouching back 24%, round back – 24.4% of students.

To receive urgent information about bio-geometrical profile of students' postures it is necessary to have simple informative indicators. These indicators shall be easily accessible to physical culture teacher; not require diagnostic apparatuses and great time losses. In our case we used improved record of control over posture's bio-geometric profile [7].

For assessment of posture's bio-geometric profile we used the following indicators:

- In respect to sagittal plane – position of head and torso in respect to vertical axis, chest kyphosis and lumbar lordosis, shape of abdomen, angle between hip and shin;
- In respect to frontal plane – position of head in respect to horizontal axis, location of shoulders, of blades lower angles and pelvis bones, triangles of waist, position of feet.

Every indicator was assessed by three points' scale. We used method of comparison of individual posture on photograph and graphic pictures of variants on sample. "Point" 1 corresponded to mark "bad", "2" – "satisfactory, "3" – "good".

All 250 students were tested by map of visual screening of posture's bio-geometrical profile. It permitted to distribute students by levels, separately for every kind of posture: "low", "middle", "high" (see table 1).

Table 1

Distribution of students by state of posture's bio-geometrical profile, %

Type of posture	Level of bio geometrical profile state		
	low	middle	high
Normal posture	0	63.33	36.67
Scoliosis posture	43.33	56.33	0
Round back	23.33	76.67	0
Slouching back	22.73	77.27	0

For determination of "risk zones" of functional disorders in muscular skeletal apparatus (MSA) orthopedist assessed students' posture in frontal and sagittal planes. We used map of express control of posture's bio-geometrical profile (norm – 2 points, pathologies – 1 point). All students were divided into two groups: with normal posture and with posture abnormalities. For determination of "risk zones" of MSA functional disorders we constructed graphs of normal distribution of generalized summarized points of students with normal postures and students with posture abnormalities. Sections of graphs overlapping were classified as "risk zones" (see table 2).

Table 2

Determination of level of bio-geometrical profile's state and "risk zones" by integral mark of 17-18 years' age students, points

Age, years	Level			Risk zone
	Low	Middle	High	
17	11—17	18—23	24—33	18—20
18	11—16	17—23	24—33	17—20

Analyzing the received data we can conclude that 63.33% of students with normal posture are in "risk zone". It means that these tested require deepened control of bio-geometric profile of posture. They need in prevention prophylaxis of MSA disorders.

Students with different kinds of posture abnormalities and low bio-geometrical profile level are in the so-called pre-morbid state of MSA. Pre-morbid state (from Latin prae – pre and morbus disease) is an initial human state before disease. This state is characterized by reduction of organism's adaptation potential. It has 2 stages of progressing: with prevailing of non-specific changes and preservation of homeostatic characteristics; with prevailing of specific changes in organs and systems (pathology is still not expressed and changes are of compensatory character).

Thus, slouching and round back – are types of posture, which are favorable ground for progressing of pathological kyphosis, while scoliosis posture can result in scoliosis.

At the next stage of our researches we studied physical fitness of students with different types of posture (see table 3).

It was found that students with normal posture have middle level of general endurance 2567.11 m (S= 317.99 m). It should also be noted that students with scoliosis posture and slouching back also have middle level of general endurance– 2467.58 m (S=357.18 m) and 2440.83 m (S=283.51 m). But these indicators have statistically significant distinctions ($p<0.05$). At the same time students with round back demonstrated the worst result 2359.02 m (S= 361.42 m). It corresponds to the lowest level of general endurance ($p<0.05$), comparing with students with normal posture.

Testing resulted in statistically significant distinctions in indicators of students with normal posture (9.58 s., S=0.59) and students with round back (10.05 s., S=0.48) ($p<0.05$). At the same time students with scoliosis back showed middle level of dexterity (9.77 s., S=0.63 and 9.71 s., S=0.63). It should also be noted that these values did not statistically confidently differ from indicators of students with normal posture ($p>0.05$).

Table 3

Physical fitness indicators of students with different posture abnormalities (n=250)

Description of test	Posture type							
	Normal posture (n=38)		Scoliosis posture (n=91)		Round back (n=61)		Slouching back (n=60)	
	$\bar{x}$	S	$\bar{x}$	S	$\bar{x}$	S	$\bar{x}$	S
12 minutes Cooper's test of walk and run, m	256711	317.99	2467.58*	357.18	2359.02*	361.42	2440.83*	283.51
Shuttle run «4 x 9», multiple passing of one and the same distance, sec.	9.58	0.59	10.01	0.59	10.05*	0.48	10.0	0.72

Initial position (i.p.): hanging with seizing from above, legs are closed; chin ups above bar, quantity of times	15.11	2.26	13.35*	2.00	10.30*	1.54	12.18*	1.82
I.p.: lying on back with legs bent in knees and arms behind head. Rising in sitting position, quantity of times per 1 minute.	50.08	5.46	45.03*	7.23	37.92*	3.02	41.32*	6.09
I.p. – sitting position. Maximally bend forward with arms stretched also forward, cm	3.53	0.67	3.31	0.56	2.21*	0.33	3.32	0.41
I.p. lying on abdomen with arms behind head. Rising and keeping of shoulder girdle, sec.	90.08	9.04	60.71*	10.88	50.80*	3.45	58.77*	11.16

Notes: * – $p<0.05$ in comparison with indicators of students with normal postures.

Discussion

Results of our researches supplemented the data of other specialists [7, 13, 21, 24]. Besides, they confirmed the conception of V.A. Kashuba et al. [4-6] about prophylaxis approaches to students' physical education.

The received data witness that indicators of dynamic power endurance of shoulder girdle and back muscles of students with normal posture correspond to level above middle (15.11 times, S=2.26). It is statistically confidently higher than in students with round back (10.30 times, S=1.54; level below middle) and students with scoliosis posture (13.35 times, S=2). Power endurance of shoulder girdle and back muscles of students with round back and scoliosis posture corresponded to middle level ($p<0.05$).

Statistically confident differences between static power endurance of students with normal posture (90.08 s., S=9.04), scoliosis posture (60.71 s., S=10.88), round back (50.80 s., S=3.45) and slouching back (58.77 s.., S=11.16) ($p<0.05$) are rather substantial.

For assessment of backbone flexibility, hip joints' mobility and elasticity of hamstrings we used test "bending of torso from sitting position". Analysis of this test's results showed low level of this indicator in students with all types of posture. For example in students with normal posture this indicator was, in average, 3.53 cm (S=0.67), with scoliosis posture – 3.31 cm (S=0.56), with slouching back – 3.32 cm (S=0.41). With it, it should be noted that these indicators had no statistically significant distinctions ($p>0.05$). At the same time students with round back showed the lowest result 2.21 cm (S=0.33 cm) ($p<0.05$).

Conclusions:

1. Recent decade in Ukraine there have been observed reduction of students' health that is conditioned by a number of objective and subjective reasons: low social-economical level of life of most of students; conditions of educational functioning; deficit of students motor functioning. As a result – increase of students with functional disorders of muscular skeletal apparatus.

2. We have determined the types of posture abnormalities of students: scoliosis posture was registered in 36.4% of the tested; slouching back - 24% of students; round back - 24.4%. Also attracts attention the fact that only 15.2% of students have normal posture. Increasing of quantity of students with functional disorders of muscular skeletal apparatus creates a problem situation. This potentially unfavorable state earlier or later inevitably results in weakening of organism's functional potentials.

3. Express control of bio-geometric profile of students (5 indicators in frontal and 6 indicators in sagittal planes) points at the fact that 63.33% of the tested with normal posture have middle level of posture state. They are in the so-called "risk zone". In the future they can have functional disorders of muscular skeletal apparatus. It should also be noted that students with low level of posture's bio-geometrical profile (scoliosis posture – 43.33%; round back– 23. 33%; slouching back– 22. 73%) are in the so-called pre-morbid state of MSA.

4. We detected low flexibility of backbone, mobility of hip joints and elasticity of hamstrings. Students with normal posture had this indicator, equal, in average, to 3.61 cm (S=4.18), students with slouching back – 2.77 cm (S=2.81), with round back – 2.21 cm (S=1.43); students with scoliosis posture had 2.19 cm (S=2.55). With it, it should be noted that the above mentioned indicators had no statistically significant distinctions ($p>0.05$).

5. Indicators of dynamic power endurance of shoulder girdle and back muscles of students with normal posture correspond to above middle level and are 15.11 times, (S=3.94). It is statistically confidently higher than indicators of students with round back (10.30 times, S=2.40; - level below middle); students with scoliosis posture (13.35 times, S=4.49) and round back (12.18 times, S=3.82). It is very important that with registration of static power endurance statistically confident distinctions were found in students with scoliosis posture (60.71 sec., S=10.88), round back (50.80 sec., S=3.45), slouching back (58.77 sec., S=11.16) in comparison with students with normal posture (90.08 sec., S=9.04) ($p<0.05$).

The prospects of further researches are connected with working out of technology of not fixed MSA disorders' prophylaxis in students, in process of their physical education.

Conflict of interests

The author declares that there is no conflict of interests.

References:

1. Belikova ZhA. *Uprazhneniia khatkha-jogi kak sredstvo korrekcii deformacii pozvonochnika studentov special'nykh medicinskikh grupp s narusheniiami osanki. Cand. Diss*. [Hatha yoga exercises as mean of backbone deformation's correction of special health groups' students with posture abnormalities. Cand. Diss.], Belgorod, 2012. (in Russian)
2. Zabalueva TV. Pedagogicheskie aspekty formirovaniia vozrastnoj osanki cheloveka [Pedagogic aspects of formation of human age posture]. *Uchenye zapiski universiteta imeni P.F. Lesgafta*, 2009;5:27 – 31. (in Russian)
3. Isaeva OV. *Differencirovannye podkhody k ozdorovleniiu studentov 16-17 let s narusheniiami osanki v processe fizicheskogo vospitaniia. Cand. Diss.* [Differentiated approaches to health improvement of 16-17 years' age students with posture abnormalities in process of physical education. Cand. Diss.], Ivanovo, 2015. (in Russian)
4. Kashuba VA, Bibik R, Nosova N. Kontrol' sostoianiia prostranstvennoj organizacii tela cheloveka v processe fizicheskogo vospitaniia [Control of human body space organization in process of physical education]. *Molodizhnij naukovij visnik Volins'kogo nacional'nogo universitetu imeni Lesi Ukrainki*. 2012;7:10-19. (in Russian)
5. Kashuba VA, Dudko MV. Sovremennye podkhody, metodiki i tekhnologii k formirovaniiu zdorovogo obraza zhizni studentov v processe fizicheskogo vospitaniia [Modern approaches to, methodic and technologies of students' healthy life style formation in process of physical education]. *Fizichne vikhovannia, sport i kul'tura zdorov'ia u suchasnomu suspil'stvi.* 2015;1:52 - 57. (in Russian)
6. Kashuba VA, Martyniuk OA. K voprosu ispol'zovaniia korekcionno-profilakticheskikh programm v processe fizicheskogo vospitaniia studentok s razlichnymi narusheniiami prostranstvennoj organizacii tela [On the question of usage of correction-prevention programs in physical education of girl students with different disorders of body space organization]. *Naukovij chasopis NPU im. M.P. Dragomanova*, 2013;1(27):28-35. (in Russian)
7. Kashuba VA, Ivchatova T, Sergienko K. K voprosu izmeneniia prostranstvennoj organizacii tela cheloveka v processe fizicheskogo vospitaniia s ispol'zovaniem komp'iuternykh tekhnologij [On the question of change of human body space organization in physical education with the help of computer technologies]. *Sportivnij visnik Pridniprov'ia.* 2014;1:42-45. (in Russian)
8. Kolos MA. *Korekciia funkcional'nikh porushen' oporno-rukhovogo aparatu studentov v procesi fizichnogo*

vikhovannia. Cand. Diss. [Correction of functional disorders of students' muscular skeletal apparatus in process of physical education. Cand. Diss.], Dnipropenrovsk, 2010. (in Ukrainian)

9. Martyniuk OA. *Korrekciia narushenij prostranstvennoj organizacii tela studentok v processe fizicheskogo vospitaniia. Cand. Diss*. [Correction of disorders of girl students' body space organization in process of physical education. Cand. Diss.], Kiev, 2011. (in Russian)
10. Nosova NL. *Kontrol' prostorovoi organizacii tila shkoliariv u procesi fizichnogo vikhovannia. Cand. Diss*. [Control of schoolchildren's body space organization in process of physical education. Cand. Diss.], Kiev, 2008. (in Ukrainian)
11. Retivykh IuI. *Metodika korrekcii narushenij osanki studentov sredstvami ozdorovitel'noj fizicheskoj kul'tury na osnove ucheta vidov i stepeni deformacij pozvonochnika. Cand. Diss*. [Methodic of correction of students' postures by means of health related physical culture on the base of registration of kinds and degree of backbone deformation. Cand. Diss.], Volgograd, 2009. (in Russian)
12. Temchenko VA, Burko VL, Konik GA. Organizaciia upravleniia fizicheskoj kul'turoj i sportom v vysshem uchebnom zavedenii [Organization of management of physical culture and sports in higher educational establishment]. *II regional'na naukova konferenciia "Strategichne upravlinnia rozvitkom galuzi Fizichna kul'tura i sport", 14 grudnia 2013 r., Kharkiv* [II regional scientific conference "Strategic management of development of Physical culture and sports' branch". December 14th, 2013, Kharkiv], Kharkiv, HDAFK; 2014. p. 16—18. (in Russian)
13. Futornyj SM. *Zdorov'esberegaiushchie tekhnologii v processe fizicheskogo vospitaniia studencheskoj molodezhi* [Health related technologies in process of physical education of students], Kiev: Poligrafservis, 2014. (in Russian)
14. Erdenko DV. *Metodika ispol'zovaniia vostochnoj gimnastiki pri narusheniiakh osanki studentok gumanitarnykh vuzov. Cand. Diss*. [Methodic of application of oriental gymnastic with posture's abnormalities of humanitarian HEEs' girl students. Cand. Diss], Moscow, 2009. (in Russian)
15. Iumasheva LI. *Korekciia porushen' postavi studentiv muzichnogo vishchogo navchal'nogo zakladu u procesi fizichnogo vikhovannia. Cand. Diss*. [Posture's corrections of musical higher educational establishment's students in process of physical education. Cand. Diss], Kiev, 2007. (in Ukrainian)
16. Iakovenko DV. *Ozdorovitel'naia fizicheskaia kul'tura studentov s osteokhondrozom pozvonochnika na osnove kompleksnykh korrigiruiushchikh vozdejstvij. Cand. Diss*. [Health related physical culture of students with backbone osteochondrosis on the base of complex correcting impacts. Cand. Diss.], Sankt Petersburg, 2009. (in Russian)
17. AbouHassan J, Milosavljevic S, Carman A. Can postural modification reduce kinetic and kinematic loading during the bowing postures of Islamic prayer? *Ergonomics*. 2010;53(12):1446–1454.
18. Andrejeva Julija, Mockiene Asta, Zukauskiene Milda. Fatigue and faulty posture connection among children, diagnosed with dysarthria. *Pedagogics, psychology, medical-biological problems of physical training and sports*. 2015;8:75-81. http://dx.doi.org/10.15561/18189172.2015.0810
19. Andrews DM, Fiedler KM, Weir PL, Callaghan JP. The effect of posture category salience on decision times and errors when using observation-based posture assessment methods. *Ergonomics*. 2012;55(12):1548–58.
20. Boak A, Hamilton HA, Adlaf EM, Beitchman JH, Wolfe D, Mann RE. The mental health and well-being of Ontario students. *CAMH Research Document*. 2014;38:213—244.
21. Bothmer M, Fridlund B. Gender differences in health habits and in motivation for a healthy lifestyle among Swedish university students. *Nursing and Health Sciences*. 2005;7:107—110.
22. Cavalheri V, Camillo CA, Brunetto AF, Probst VS, Cipulo Ramos EM, Pitta F. Effects of arm bracing posture on respiratory muscle strength and pulmonary function in patients with chronic obstructive pulmonary disease. *Revista Portuguesa de Pneumologia* (English Edition). 2010;16(6):887–91.
23. Futornyi S. Actual issues of improving the process of student`s physical education through the application of modern health-saving technologies. *Molodizhnij naukovij visnik nacional'nogo universitetu imeni Lesi Ukrainki*. 2014;14:26–30.

24. Gorelov A.A., Kondakov V.L., Belikova Zh.A. About necessity of use of Hatha Yoga exercises for correction of deformation of students' spine of special medical groups with violations of posture. *Physical education of students*, 2013, vol.2, pp. 35-44. http://dx.doi.org/10.6084/m9.figshare.156378
25. Hong Y, Fong DT-P, Li JX. The effect of school bag design and load on spinal posture during stair use by children. *Ergonomics*. 2011;54(12):1207–13.
26. Kalinichenko IO, Dyachenko YL. State changes in posture and arch of the foot in children aged 4 - 6 years with hypermobility of the joints under the influence of rehabilitation activities in schools. *Pedagogics, psychology, medical-biological problems of physical training and sports,* 2013;8:26-30. http://dx.doi.org/10.6084/m9.figshare.745781
27. Litvinenko Y.V., Niznikowski Tomasz, Boloban V.N. Evaluation of the kinematic structure of indicators key elements of sports equipment exercise by postural orientation movements. *Physical education of students*, 2014;6:29-36. http://dx.doi.org/10.15561/20755279.2014.0606
28. Mani R, Milosavljevic S, Sullivan SJ. Control of posture during tasks representing common work-related postures – a reliability study. *Ergonomics*. 2015;3;58(6):980–989.
29. Torlakovic A, Muftic M, Radjo I, Talovic M, Mahmutovic I. Evolution of Sports-medical Team Management in the Program of Posture Correction in Children. *Materia Socio Medica*. 2014;26(2):104.
30. Żukowska Hanna, Szark-Eckardt Mirosława, Muszkieta Radosław, Iermakova TS. Characteristics of body posture in the sagittal plane and fitness of first-form pupils from rural areas. *Pedagogics, psychology, medical-biological problems of physical training and sports*, 2014;7:50-60. http://dx.doi.org/10.6084/m9.figshare.1015583

13

STUDYING OF INTERCONNECTIONS OF MORPHOLOGICAL FUNCTIONAL INDICATORS OF STUDENTS, WHO PRACTICE MARTIAL ARTS

Podrigalo L.V., Iermakov S.S., Alekseev A.F., Rovnaya O.A.
Kharkov State Academy of Physical Culture

Abstract. *Purpose:* to study interconnections of students' morphological functional indicators and their influence on level of sportsmanship. *Material:* in the research 17 students, practicing martial arts, participated. 62 indicators were determined: anthropometrical, goniometrical criteria of arms joints' status; tapping test and maximal frequency of grabs in impulse mode. *Results:* we found that maximal contribution in system is made by hand dynamometry of right and left hands, body length and mass, chest circumference, width of shoulders; maximal frequency of grabs by right and left hands. It was confirmed that there are correlations between students' morphological functional indicators. The highest contribution to formation of functional system is characteristic for anthropometric indicators. Results of maximal grabs in impulse mode made rather sufficient contribution in system's formation that is confirmed by great quantity of correlations. Analysis of character, strength and orientation of correlations witnesses about informative potential of this test and permits to recommend it as screening for control of sportsmen's state. *Conclusions:* we determined that indicators of hand dynamometry system formation illustrate that for martial arts wrestlers strong grab was very important. It is ensured by strength of hand muscles.
Key words: martial arts, morphological functional, indicators, correlations, students.

Introduction

Achievement of high sportsmanship depends on the whole complex of indicators, among which important places are taken by peculiarities of physical condition and level of fitness. Besides their absolute values, when analyzing sportsmen's status, interconnections between them shall be considered. It permits to reflect the state of homeostasis and is an illustration of prognosis of sportsmen's success.

As on to day there has been sufficient quantity of works, devoted to this problem in different kinds of sports. For example, Baláš, J. et al. [7], who studied body composition, muscular strength and endurance of sport mountaineers, determined presence of correlations between these components. Authors outlined the most informative indicators, which included strength of grab, hanging on bent arms and fingers, content of fat, rock climbing experience (dispersion 97%).

Studying men's body composition (members of baseball combined team of Poland), Yagello V. et al. [6] determined characteristic features of their somatic condition. The authors connect it with tactic and technical peculiarities of this kind of sports.

Kocharian T.N. et al. [2], analyzed specific features of morphological development of elite basketball players of different game roles. The authors determined regularities of decreasing of absolute sizes of body (longitudinal, transverse and perimeter) from central players to forwards and backs. They confirmed dependence of proportion types on basketball players' game roles.

Comparative analysis of power kind of sports' sportsmen' physical condition confirmed correlation between anthropometrical indicators and sportsmanship. Besides, the most informative indicators and physical condition indices were found [3, 11–13, 15-20].

The available results permit to conclude that studying of sportsmen's physical condition shall consider peculiarities of kind of sports. It permits to optimize the procedure of selection and substantially increase effectiveness of control and prognosis of sportsmen's success.

Coming from the above mentioned, *the purpose of the research* was to study morphological functional indicators of students (practicing martial arts) as factors of influence on level of sportsmanship.

Material and methods

In the research 17 students, practicing martial arts, participated. Mean age was (17.53±0.15) years. Level of sportsmanship varied from sportsmen-beginners' to candidate masters of sports and masters of sports. The participants were representatives of strike kinds (karate, hand-to-hand fighting, thae-quan-do) and throw kinds of martial arts (Judo,

Greco-Rome wrestling). Design of the research implied determination of 62 morphological and functional indicators. They included anthropometrical indicators (somatic-metric and physical-metric), reflecting general physical condition, status of upper and lower limbs. We conducted goniometric researches of amplitude of movements in upper limbs' joints. Results of tapping test were used as illustration of nervous system's liability. Peculiarities of martial arts conditioned interest to study of maximal frequency of hand's grab in impulse mode. For assessment of this quality we used electronic device "Kepai" (made in China). The methodic implied registration of maximal quantity of device's pressing during 10 seconds.

Statistical analysis of the received data was conducted with the help of licensed electronic tables Excel. On the base of the received results we built correlation matrix, which included coefficients by Pirson. For analysis we chose only confident dependences ($r>0.482$). Contribution of each indicator in system was assessed by indicator of system formation. This criterion was offered by Zosimov A.N. [21] for analysis of correlation matrixes. It reflects quantity of connections, formed by the tested indicator and their strength. The indicator is expressed in conventional units and calculated by formula:

$$PS = \sum rj \cdot n,$$

where, $\sum rj$ – sum of values of significant correlation coefficients, formed by given indicator,
n – quantity of significant correlations of given indicator of structure.

Results of the research

For comparative analysis we determined indicators of system formation for values, which are traditionally used in analysis of physical conditions: bode length and mass, chest circumference, width of shoulders, hand dynamometry by both hands, tapping test results and maximal frequency of grabs by both hands. The received results are shown in fig.1.

Indicator of system formation,
Conventional units

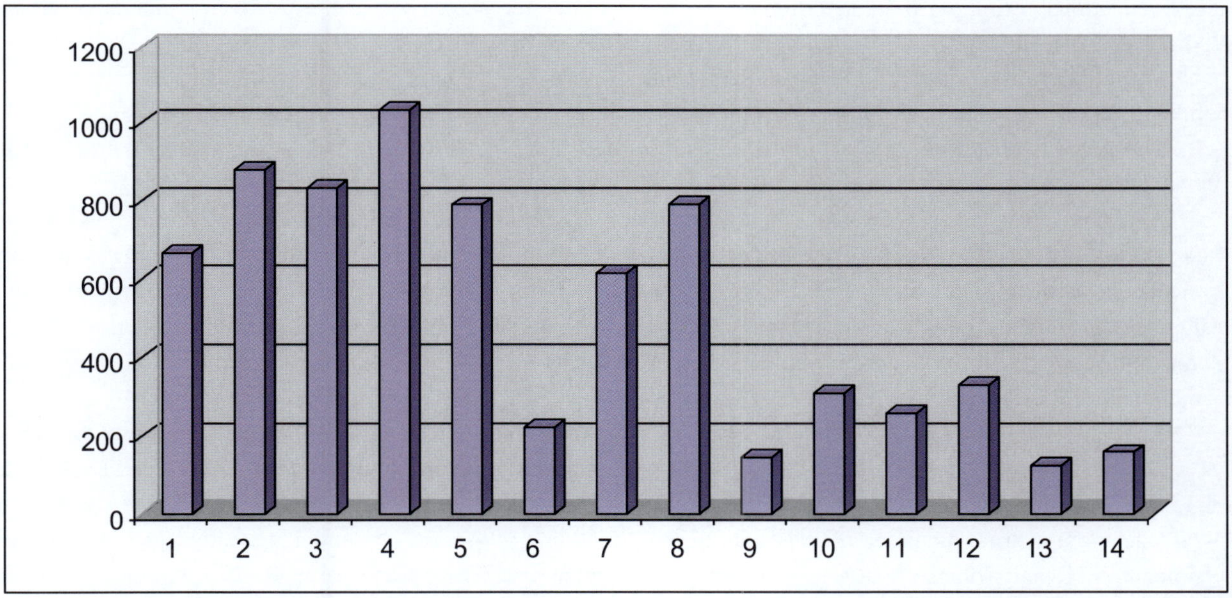

Criteria

Fig. 1. Value of system formation indicator of the tested criteria: 1 –body length; 2 –body mass; 3 – chest circumference; 4 – right hand dynamometry; 5 – left hand dynamometry; 6 – maximal frequency of grab by right hand; 7 – maximal frequency of grab by left hand; 8 – width of shoulders; 9–14 – tapping test results – in every sub-test accordingly.

We have determined that right hand dynamometry is characterized by maximal value (1036.48), second place is taken by body mass (878.18), then go chest circumference (832.28), width of shoulders (791.34), left hand dynamometry

(789.10); body length (669.06). The seventh rank place is taken by maximal frequency of left hand grab (616.78). Results of this test's fulfillment by right hand are at 11th place (221.11). Results of tapping test take 8–10 and 12–14rank places. Their values are within 330–124.

Contribution of anthropometric indicators in system illustrates importance of physical condition for success in martial arts. It is witnessed by closeness of system formation indicator of main physical condition values: body length, body mass, chest circumference and width of shoulders. The used indicators are integral criteria of physical condition, reflecting condition of muscular system. With it, in this context especially noticeable is the fact that system formation indicators decrease in the following order: body mass- chest circumference- width of shoulders- body length. The least value for body length is especially expressed because this indicator reflects genetically conditioned peculiarities of growth and development. The rest criteria are more informative as reflecting development of just muscular mass. At the same time values of system formation indicator of hand dynamometry substantially exceed values of main anthropometric indicators. They can be a proof of importance of just arms' strength in martial arts.

It is rather difficult to explain substantial difference between contribution of maximal grab's frequency by right and left hands due to little scope of available information. Such situation justifies detail analysis of available correlation dependences.

Analysis of tapping test results' contribution (see fig.1) permits to speak about different significance of this test's components for functional state. It is confirmed by wave-like character of dynamic of system formation indicator. Coming from quantity of significant correlations, results can be divided into two groups: marginal (1,5, and 6) and middle (2–4). With it, first group is characterized by less value. It is connected with adaptation to conditions of test and with complexity of maintaining of high temp of its fulfillment. At the same results of second group can be interpreted as proof of high lability of nervous system of martial art sportsmen, which ensure rather high success in sports.

Considering the purpose of the research it was interesting to analyze the character of dependences between maximal frequency of left and right hands' grabs and other indicators. We determined confident interconnections ($p<0.05$) between maximal frequency of right hand grab with circumference of right and left wrist ($r=0.483$). It reflects direct dependence between development of forearm muscles and ability for maximal quantity of pressing for short times. The presence of these connections permits to offer determination of wrist circumference as screening test, which can be of prognostic importance in martial arts.

Sufficiently high correlation between fulfillment of maximal frequency of right and left hands' grabs ($r=0.695$) shall be interpreted as witness of harmonious physical condition and functional state of the tested sportsmen.

The found dependence on heart beats rate is also interesting ($r=-0.529$). The inverse nature of connection in our context can be assessed as witness of stress and time consuming character of the applied methodic.

Analysis of results of test for maximal quantity of left hand pressing in impulse mode showed much higher quantity of correlations. First of all there were more confident correlations with anthropometric indicators, illustrating general physical condition and status of upper limbs. For example, we confirmed confident ($p<0.05$) correlations with body mass ($r=0.648$), chest circumference (in pause, $r=0.657$; at inhale $r=0.646$; at exhale $r=0.652$) and width of shoulders ($r=0,644$). It confirms again the made earlier assumptions about direct dependence of maximal grab' frequency results on development of muscles.

Analysis of correlations of maximal frequency of left hand grab showed confident correlations with length of right ($r=0.553$) and left ($r=0.529$) forearms. It illustrates higher importance in comparison with results of right hand test. In our opinion it witnesses about validity of earlier assumption about importance of upper limbs' training for test's efficiency.

One more witness in favor of it is confident correlations with circumferential indicators and results of hand dynamometry. Results of maximal frequency of grab correlated with right arm parameters: circumference of biceps ($r=0.716$), forearm ($r=0.687$) and wrist ($r=0.67$). Correlations with left arm were accordingly: ($r=0.658$), ($r=0.61$) and ($r=0.75$). Value of correlation of grab's maximal frequency with hand dynamometry was at the right ($r=0.639$) and at the left ($r=0.76$). Thus, validity of assumption about importance of arm' muscles' development for maximally quick and strong grabs, is confirmed again.

Correlation with systolic blood pressure was higher than with results of maximal frequency of right hand grab ($r=0.504$). It must also be interpreted as witness of physical loads stresses' progressing in fulfillment of this test.

Fulfillment of maximal frequency of right hand grabs did not have confident correlations with goniometric indicators. For maximal frequency of left hand grabs we found dependence with bending in right elbow joint ($r=-0.566$)

and moving aside in left wrist joint (r=0.562). The latter dependence was the most important: it illustrates connection of muscles, realizing grab and movement.

Assessment of sportsmanship level's correlations with the tested indicators was also of certain interest. We found confident correlations with body mass (r=-0.55), length of right (r=-0.526) and left (r=-0.49) forearms; results of last sub-test in tapping test (r=-0.503), amplitude of moving inside in right wrist joint (r=-0.764), moving aside in right (r=0.573) and moving inside in left (r=0.508) shoulder joints. The presented dependences reflect importance of morphological and functional indicators for success in martial arts.

Discussion

Comparative analysis of morphological functional characteristics is widely used for analyzing of martial art sportsmen's state. For example Jesu' et al. [9] offered to use mass of free fat, maximal strength in absolute and relative expression, muscular strength, average and peak power in test Wingate, strength of direct and reverse grab as prognostic indictors.

Jagiello et al [5], regarded interconnection of anthropometric indicators with sportsmanship level of elite Polish Judo wrestlers. The authors noted tendency to increase of skeleton mass (width of pelvis, shoulder and elbows) and muscles (diameter of forearm) with rising of sportsmanship. The found correlations of anthropometric indicators with sport rating confirm its objectivity as criterion of wrestlers' skillfulness.

Erkan Demirkan et al. [8] used complex of anthropometrical and functional indicators for comparison of free style and Greco-Rome wrestlers. They determined that arms' peak power, dexterity and flexibility were selective factors of distinctions in these kinds of wrestling.

Researches of Parola F., Musso E. [10] witness about existence of problem of effective criteria's determination in assessment of physical fitness. To large extent this problem is conditioned by specific character of physical qualities' manifestation in competition functioning.

A.V. Voronkov et al. [1] studied the problem of control of power fitness in arm-wrestling. The authors noted authenticity of traditional tests. The received by them results prove demand in accounting of correlation dependences between level of sportsmanship, competition success and fulfillment of tests and control exercises.

Effectiveness of muscular strength's determination in separate movements in wrist joint for prognosis of sportsmen's success in arm-wrestling has been confirmed. Besides, there was established presence of correlation dependences, permitting to assess and prognosticate sportsmen's state [13].

Analyzing morphological predictors of sport talents in female free style wrestling, V.V. Semenov [4] outlines the most informative indicators, which differ, depending on weight categories. They include longitudinal, transversal and circumferential indicators of hip, shin, shoulder and forearm. On the base of them discriminant equations, permitting to prognosticate success, were built.

In this context and on the base of received results we can conclude that maximal frequency of grab is rather important for success of martial art sportsmen. The value of system formation indicator of these criteria (especially for left hand) is comparable with value of important anthropometric indicators (body length). It significantly exceeds contribution to formation of system of tapping test's results. The found indicators of hand dynamometry system formation illustrate that strong grab is very important for martial art wrestlers. This ability is ensured by strength of hand muscles. With it right hand (as stronger one) is characterized by much higher contribution. At the same time system formation indicators has opposite character: value of indicator for right hand is practically three times less than indicator for left hand. May be it is connected with different character of movements in determination of hand dynamometry and maximal frequency of grab. In the first case there takes place maximal static single load, fulfilled during 1-2 second. In the second case mean, multiple dynamic loads take place. It takes much more time. Different values of hand dynamometry pre-condition different maximal frequencies of grab. With it, the higher static force is, the less dynamic manifestations are. Just it is reflected by opposite values of system formation indicators.

Conclusions

The conducted researches confirmed presence of correlation dependences between morphological functional indicators of students, who practice martial arts. It has been found that the highest contribution to formation of functional system of sportsmanship growth is made by anthropometrical indicators (body length and mass, chest circumference, hand dynamometry, width of shoulders). At the same time results of test for maximal grab in impulse mode also made substantial contribution to system formation. It is confirmed by presence of great number of correlations. Analysis of character, strength and orientation of correlations witnesses about high informative potential of this test. It permits to recommend it as screening in control of sportsmen's, practicing martial arts, state.

References:

1. Voronkov AV, Nikulin IN, Sobyanin FI. On the improvement of the control force readiness of students engaged arm sport. *Physical Education of Students*, 2014;2:3–7. http://dx.doi.org/10.6084/m9.figshare.917169
2. Kocharian TN, Krikun EN, Martirosova EG. Osobennosti morfologicheskogo razvitiia vysokokvalificirovannykh basketbolistok razlichnykh igrovykh amplua [Specific features of morphological development of elite female basketball players of different game roles]. *VII Mizhnarodnij kongres integrativnoi antropologii, 17–18 zhovtnia 2013 roku* [7th International congress of integrative anthropology, October 17-18, 2013], Vinnitsa; 2013. (in Ukrainian)
3. Podrigalo LV, Galashko AI, Lozovoj AD. Sravnitel'naia ocenka antropometricheskogo razvitiia sportsmenov silovykh vidov sporta [Comparative assessment of anthropometrical development of sportsmen of power kinds of sports]. *Pedagogics, psychology, medical-biological problems of physical training and sports* 2007;3:107 – 111.
4. Semenov VV. Morfologicheskie prediktory sportivnoj odarennosti v zhenskoj vol'noj bor'be [Morphological predictors of sport talents in female free style wrestling]. *Mizhnarodnij kongres integrativnoi antropologii, 17–18 zhovtnia 2013 roku* [7th International congress of integrative anthropology, October 17th-18th, 2013], Vinnitsa; 2013. (in Ukrainian)
5. Iagello Vladislav, Tkachuk Vladimir, Blakh Veslav. Vzaimosviaz' antropometricheskikh pokazatelej s urovnem sportivnogo masterstva vysokokvalificirovannykh dziudoistov Pol'shi [Interconnection of anthropometrical indicators with sportsmanship level of elite Polish Judo wrestlers]. *Fizicheskoe vospitanie studentov tvorcheskikh special'nostej* 2004;2:36–45. (in Russian)
6. Iagello Vladislav, Iagello Marina, Kozina ZhL. Profil' stroeniia tela muzhchin, zanimaiushchikhsia bejsbolom [Profile of body composition of men, practicing baseball]. *Physical education of students* 2012;6:140–143. http://dx.doi.org/10.6084/m9.figshare.96607
7. Baláš J, Pecha O, Martin AJ, & Cochrane D. Hand–arm strength and endurance as predictors of climbing performance. *European Journal of Sport Science*, 2011;12(1):16–25. http://dx.doi.org/10.1080/17461391.2010.546431
8. Erkan Demirkan, Mehmet Kutlu, Mitat Koz. Physical Fitness Differences between Freestyle and Greco-Roman Junior Wrestlers *Journal of Human Kinetics* 2014;41:245–251. http://dx.doi.org/10.2478/hukin-2014-0052.
9. Jesu's Garcı'a-Pallare's, Jose' Marı´a Lo'pez-Gullo'n, Xabier Muriel. Physical fitness factors to predict male Olympic wrestling performance *Eur J Appl Physiol* 2011;111:1747–1758 http://dx.doi.org/10.1007/s00421-010-1809-8.
10. Parola F, Musso E. Market structures and competitive strategies: the carrier–stevedore arm-wrestling in northern European ports. *Maritime Policy & Management*. 2007;34(3):259–278. http://dx.doi.org/10.1080/03088830701343369
11. Podrigalo LV, Galashko MN, Galashko NI. Study of specificities of arm wrestlers' psychological status in competition period. *Physical Education of Students*, 2015;3:44–51. http://dx.doi.org/10.15561/20755279.2015.0306
12. Podrigalo LV, Galashko MN, Galashko NI, Prusik Krzysztof, Cieslicka Miroslawa. Research of hands' strength and endurance indications of arm sport athletes having different levels of skills. *Physical Education of Students* 2014;2:37–40. http://dx.doi.org/10.6084/m9.figshare.907140.
13. Podrigalo LV, Iermakov SS, Nosko MO, Galashko MN, Galashko NI. Study and analysis of armwrestlers' forearm muscles' strength. *Journal of Physical Education and Sport*, 2015;15(3):531–537. http://dx.doi.org/10.7752/jpes.2015.03080
14. Podrigalo LV, Istomin AG, Galashko NI. *Monitoring of the functional state of the athletes in arm sport.* Kharkov: KNMU Publ.; 2010. (in Russian)
15. Tamborini R, Chory RM, Lachlan K, Westerman D, Skalski P. Talking Smack: Verbal Aggression in Professional Wrestling. *Communication Studies*. 2008;59(3):242–258. http://dx.doi.org/10.1080/10510970802257689
16. Xiong J. The Functions and Methods of Mental Training on Competitive Sports. *Physics Procedia.* 2012;33(0):2011–4.

17. Zaccagni L. Anthropometric characteristics and body composition of Italian national wrestlers. *European Journal of Sport Science*. 2011;12(2):145–151. http://dx.doi.org/10.1080/17461391.2010.545838
18. Zaporozhanov VA. About reliable indicator of proprioception in agility control. *Pedagogics, psychology, medical-biological problems of physical training and sports* 2013;4:21-25. http://dx.doi.org/10.6084/m9.figshare.693023
19. Zaporozhanov VA, Borachinski T. On the transfer of skills skill in different conditions of motor activity. *Pedagogics, psychology, medical-biological problems of physical training and sports* 2013;9:25-28. http://dx.doi.org/10.6084/m9.figshare.749693
20. Zaporozhanov VA, Boraczynski Tomasz. Discussion on the concepts of "coordination" and "agility" in terms of physical education. *Pedagogics, psychology, medical-biological problems of physical training and sports* 2015;3:15-19. http://dx.doi.org/10.15561/18189172.2015.0303
21. Zosimov AN. *Analysis of the systems in medicine*. Kharkov: Tornado; 2000. (in Russian)

QUICKNESS AND ENDURANCE FITNESS OF PEDAGOGIC COLLEGE GIRL STUDENTS UNDER INFLUENCE OF CHEER-LEADING

Masliak I.P.
Kharkiv State Academy of Physical Culture

Abstract. *Purpose:* to determine dynamic of quickness and endurance indicators of pedagogic college girl students under influence of cheer-leading. *Material:* in the research 385 girl students participated, who composed 3 control and 3 experimental groups. Quickness fitness was registered by indicators of 60 meters' run (sec.); latent time of motor response (msec.); run on the sport during 5 sec (quantity of steps); tapping test (quantity of points). Level of endurance fitness was registered by results of 2000 meters' run (min). *Results:* the most effective cheer-leading exercises, which positively influence on girl students' endurance, have been determined. The most favorable age periods for training of quickness and endurance under influence of cheer-leading exercises have been found. The higher increment in quickness indicators was registered in 15 years old girls. The most substantial increment of endurance was registered in 16 years old girls. *Conclusions:* it is recommended to include cheer-leading exercises: basic movements, jump elements, constants, in variable components of girl students' academic training program.
Key words: physical education, students, quickness, endurance, cheer-leading.

Introduction

Physical education is an integral component of teaching, education and vocational training at higher educational establishments [10]. In process of future specialists' training significant attention shall be paid to mastering of professional knowledge and skills, development of physical qualities and formation of healthy life style [15]. Modern students endure much less physical and much higher emotional-psychological loads, stress states, hypodynamia. It results in reduction of adaptation potentials of young people's organisms and increase of morbidity. That is why the problem of increasing of students' physical education effectiveness at the account of introduction of new and non traditional motor functioning's kinds is rather topical.

A number of authors note improvement of students' health and motor fitness at the account of priority usage of volleyball [19, 23], light athletic [1], football [8], body-flex and pilates [20], swimming [17], aqua-fitness [6], futsal [22] in academic training program.

Cheer-leading is one of innovative kinds of motor functioning. Cheer-leading, as a kind of sports, has appeared comparatively not long age and has acquired wide acclaim among USA youth, in European countries and in Ukraine. It has show character, renders different impacts; it is dynamic and can be practiced by wide age range of people [4, 16, 18]. With it cheer-leading does not require special equipment and apparatuses. It is especially important in conditions of social-economical crisis.

A number of authors note in their works positive influence of cheer-leading of pre school age children's physical condition [12]; on physical health, motor fitness and interest to physical culture of secondary schools' pupils [2, 3, 13, 14]; physical condition and physical workability of first years girl students of technical university [11]; on formation of wide arsenal of motor skills of higher educational establishments' students [5]; on development of specific physical qualities of college girl students [7, 21].

With it influence of cheer-leading exercises on complex manifestation of college girl students' motor abilities has still been studied insufficiently.

Purpose, tasks of the work, material and methods

The purpose of the research is to determine dynamic of quickness and endurance indicators of pedagogic college girl students under influence of cheer-leading.

The methods of the research: theoretical analysis and generalization of scientific-methodic literature; pedagogic experiment; pedagogic testing;; methods of mathematical statistic.

Quickness fitness was registered by indicators of 60 meters' run (sec.); latent time of motor response (msec.); run on the sport during 5 sec (quantity of steps); tapping test (quantity of points). Level of endurance fitness was registered by results of 2000 meters' run (min).

The researches were conducted on the base of pedagogic college of Kharkov humanitarian-pedagogic institute. 385 first - third years girls students of physical culture profile participated in the researches. They composed 3 control and 3 experimental groups: 1st group – 1st year girl students; 2nd group – 2nd year girl students and 3rd group – 3rd year girl students. All girl students were the members of main and preparatory health group. The research was approved by ethic committee of Kharkov humanitarian pedagogic institute.

In the course of experiment control groups' girl students were trained by traditional physical education program. In variable component of experimental groups' training process cheer-leading exercises were introduced (basic movements, jump elements, constants and so on).

Results of the researches

Analysis of the received results of quickness testing (see table 1) showed absence of confident distinctions between indicators of girl students of experimental and control groups (p>0.05). Analysis of initial data permitted to detect the absence of definite system of distinctions in results (p>0.05). The exclusion were indicators of motor response and run on the spot, where distinctions in results of 1st and 2nd as well as between 2nd and 3rd groups were confident (p <0.05 – 0.001).

Table 1

Quickness indicators of experimental and control groups girl students before experiment

Groups	I	II	III
	Indicators $\overline{X} \pm m$		
	60 meters' run (sec.)		
n	*75*	*108*	*95*
Experimental	10.75±0.08	10.70±0.07	10.84±0.05
n	*23*	*34*	*50*
Control	10.81±0.13	10.73±0.10	10.91±0.08
t	0.38	0.24	0.71
p	>0.05	>0.05	>0.05
	Latent time of motor response (msec.)		
Experimental	0.29±0.00	0.27±0.00	0.28±0.00
Control	0.29±0.01	0.27±0.00	0.28±0.00
t	0.62	0.30	0.73
p	>0.05	>0.05	>0.05
	Run on the spot (quantity of steps)		
Experimental	18.25±0.35	17.95±0.18	17.59±0.19
Control	18.74±0.38	17.74±0.28	17.22±0.27
t	0.94	0.65	1.10
p	>0.05	>0.05	>0.05
	Tapping test (quantity of points)		
Experimental	68.67±0.62	66.34±1.05	67.36±0.87
Control	67.39±1.63	66.74±1.29	66.54±1.34
t	0.73	0.24	0.51
p	>0.05	>0.05	>0.05

Analysis of the received data and normative [9] showed that indicators of 60 meters' run, latent period of motor response and run on the spot correspond to marl 2 points in all tested groups; tapping test corresponded to 4 points. Thus, level of quickness of 1st – 3rd year girl students in average corresponds to mark "unsatisfactory".

Analysis of data after experiment (see fig.1) showed that all quickness indicators of experimental groups' girl students significantly and confidently improved (p <0.05 – 0.001).

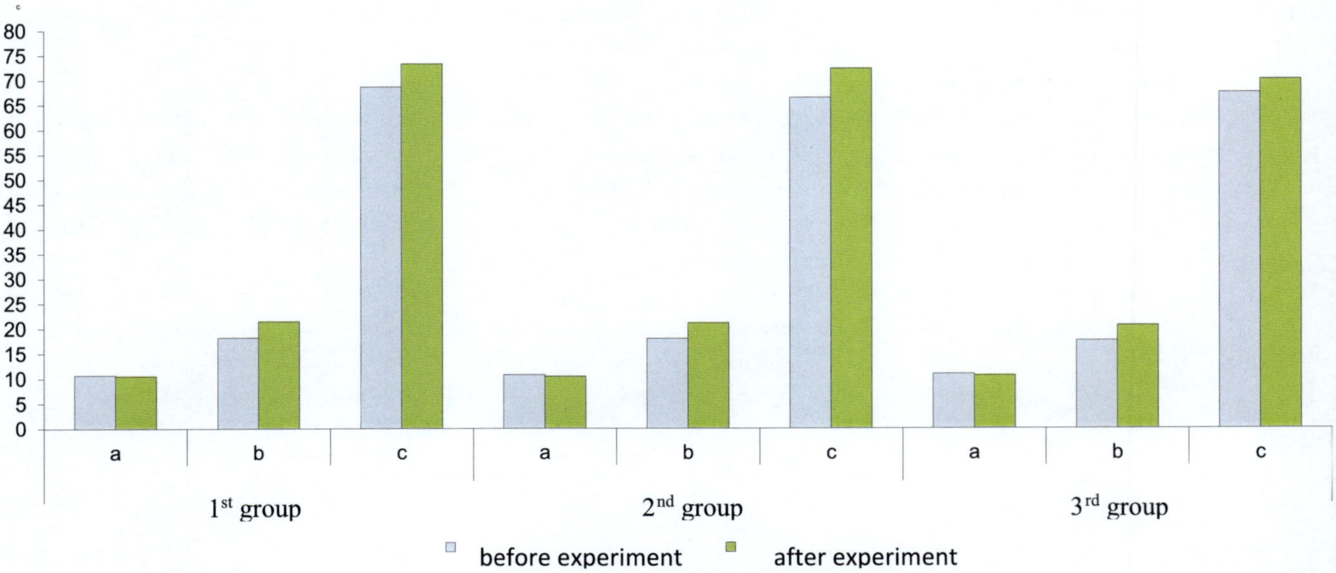

Fig 1. Indicators of quickness level in experimental groups before and after experiment:
a – 30 meters' run (sec.), b – run on the spot (quantity of steps), c – tapping test (quantity of points).

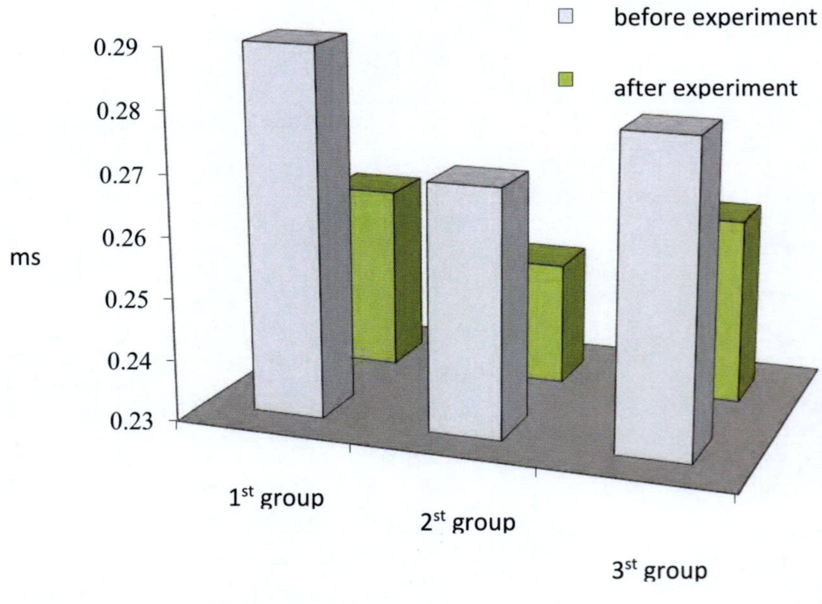

Fig. 2. Indicators of motor response in experimental groups before and after experiment

Analysis of experimental data showed that in 60 meters' run results of 1st year girl students improved by 2.32%, 2nd year girl students – by 2.33%, 3rd – by 2.39%; latent period of motor response improved by 10.34%; 7.40%; 7.14% accordingly; run on the spot – by 17.26%; 17.32%; 1.,99% accordingly; tapping test – by 6.61%; 8.90%; 3.88% accordingly. Thus, substantial changes took place in frequency of legs' movements. The highest increment in quickness was observed in girls of 15 years old age.

Analysis of control groups' data after experiment showed that their results also improved to some extent. But these changes were less significant than in experimental groups and were not confident ($p>0.05$). Results of tests were as follows: 60 meters' run of 1st group girl students – improved by 1.48%, 2nd group – by 2.05%; 3rd group – by 1.83%); latent period of motor response – by 3.44%; 3.70%; 3.57% accordingly; run on the spot – by 6.24%; 4.79%; 4.52% accordingly; tapping test – by 2.83%; 2.68%; 4.68% accordingly.

Analysis of repeated data in age aspect revealed confident difference in indicators of tapping test between 1st and 2nd as well as between 2nd and 3rd experimental groups ($p<0.05$-0.001). The rest indicators do not significantly differ in comparison with initial data.

Comparison of repeated data of experimental groups with normative [9] showed increasing of results by 1 point of assessment scale in the following indicators: 60 meters' run and tapping test (1st group's girl students) and latent period of motor response (1st and 2nd groups' girl students). As for the other indicators we observed their significant and confident improvement. But there were no changes by assessment scale. In our opinion it is explained by imperfectness of available assessment criteria.

Comparison of control groups' results showed analogous to experimental groups' character of changes by assessment scale in the following indicators: 60 meters' run and latent period of motor response.

Thus, application of specially selected cheer-leading exercises in process of girl students' physical education rendered positive influence on quickness level. The most substantial increment of results was noted in girls of 15 years old age.

Analysis of endurance data revealed absence of confident differences between indicators of control and experimental groups ($p>0.05$) (see table 2). In age aspect we observed worsening of results with age (but statistically not confident $p>0.05$). Exclusion were the data of 1st and 2nd experimental groups' girl students, whose data were statistically different ($p<0.001$).

Table 2

Endurance indicators of experimental and control groups' girl students before experiment

Groups	I	II	III
	Indicators $\overline{X} \pm m$		
	2000 meters' run (min.)		
n	*75*	*108*	*95*
Experimental	16.69±0.12	17.69±0.93	17.41±0.14
n	*23*	*34*	*50*
Control	16.89±0.21	16.70±0.17	17.03±0.19
t	0.81	1.04	1.59
p	>0.05	>0.05	>0.05

Comparison of 2000 meters' run results with normative (governmental physical education program) showed that in all tested groups they are significantly lower than standards and are far from reaching the lowest limit. That is why their mark was 0 points.

Analysis of results after application of cheer-leading (see fig.3) showed that endurance indicators in experimental groups significantly and confidently improved ($p<0.001$). For example, results of 1st year girl students improved by 6.59%, 2nd years – by 16.05%, 3rd year – by 11.37%. The highest increment in results of endurance training was observed in 16 years' old girls.

Analysis of analogous data of control groups' girl students showed confident improvement of results in 2nd and 3rd groups ($p<0.05$ – 0.01). For example, 1st group girl students' results improved by 2.13%; 2nd group – by 2.93%; 3rd group – by 4.46%. Percent increment of indicators in control groups was significantly lower than in experimental groups. It should be noted that in repeated results of control and experimental groups' girl students we observed significant and confident domination of experimental groups' results ($p<0.001$).

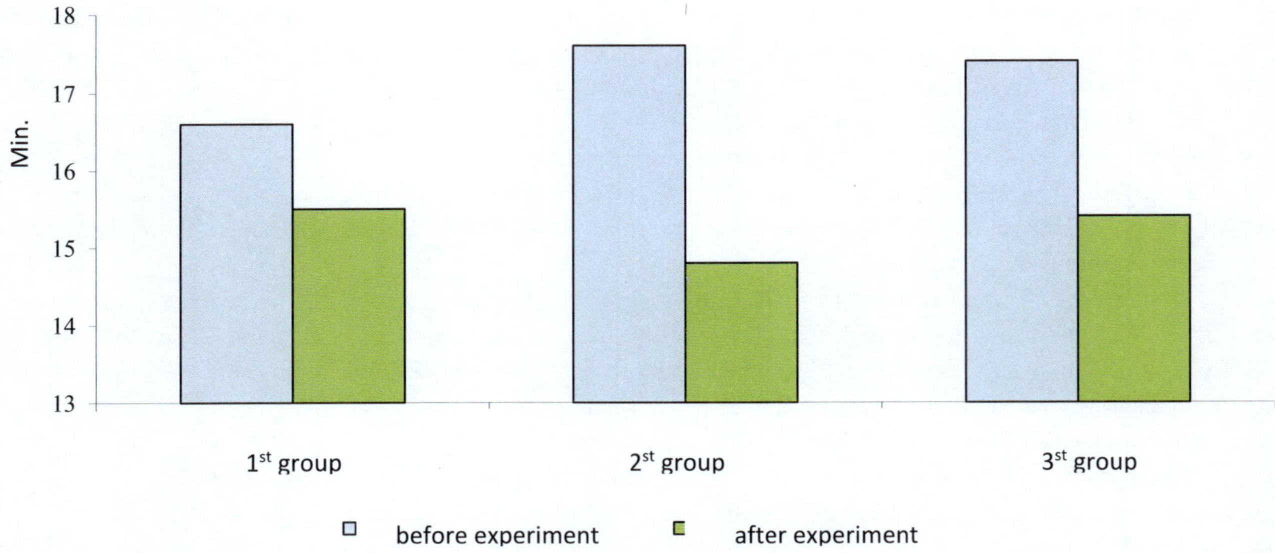

Fig.3. Indicators of endurance fitness of experimental groups' girl students before and after experiment

Analysis of repeated results in age aspect showed that character of differences changed significantly in experimental groups. For example, indicators of 1st and 3rd groups became much better and it was statistically confident ($p < 0.001$). Analysis of analogous indicators of control groups did not reveal significant changes in comparison with initial data.

Comparison of repeated results of endurances testing with normative showed absence of changes by assessment scale: they equal to zero in all tested groups.

Thus, application of specially selected cheer-leading exercises in physical training of girl students positively influenced on endurance fitness. The highest increment of results was observed in 16 years' old girl students.

Discussion

Analysis of scientific-methodic literature showed that there is quite few works, devoted to cheer-leading implementation in physical education process in different educational establishments. Also quite a few works on problems of cheer-leading's influence on different aspect of training and formation of students' motor competence was found. In available works influence of cheer-leading exercises on pre school age children's physical condition was analyzed [12];on physical health and motor qualities' condition of secondary schools pupils [2, 3, 13, 14]; on level of physical condition and physical workability of technical university girl students [11]; on power and coordination training of college students [7, 21].

On the base of analysis and generalization of the conducted research's results we supplement the data of T.M. Bala [13] about positive influence of cheer-leading exercises on motor skills' training; expanded the data of N.V. Kryvoruchko, I.P. Masliak [7, 21] about influence of cheer-leading on students' motor abilities.

For the first time we determined: the most suitable for training by cheer-leading exercises forms of girl students' quickness; the most favorable age periods for training of quickness and endurance under influence of cheer-leading exercises.

Conclusions:

1. As a result of initial testing we detected "low" level of quickness and endurance of pedagogic college girl students.

2. Application of cheer-leading exercises in physical education influenced positively on quickness and endurance of the tested contingent.

The further researches in this direction can be realized by means of determination of cheer-leading influence on physical abilities of higher educational establishments' girl students.

Acknowledgement

The researches have been fulfilled in compliance with topical plan of scientific-research works of Kharkov State Academy of Physical Culture for 2013 - 2015 by topic 3.5.29. "Theoretical and applied principles of organization of physical training, physical fitness and physical condition of different population strata monitoring".

Conflict of interests
The author declares that there is no conflict of interests.

References:

1. Andres A, Serbo E, Festriga S. Sportivno-orientovane fizichne vikhovannia studentiv [Sport oriented physical education of students]. *Moloda sportivna nauka Ukraini*, 2015;19:6-12. (in Ukrainian)
2. Bala TM, Maslyak IP. Zmina rivnia fizichnogo zdorov'ia shkoliariv 5-6-kh klasiv pid vplivom vprav cherlidinga [Change of physical health of 5-6 forms' pupils under influence of cheer-leading exercises]. *Moloda sportivna nauka Ukraini*, 2011;15:10-15. (in Ukrainian)
3. Bala TM, Maslyak IP. Zmina rivnia fizichnogo zdorov'ia shkoliariv 7-9-kh klasiv pid vplivom vprav cherlidinga [Change of physical health of 7-9 forms' pupils under influence of cheer-leading exercises]. *Sportivnij visnik Pridniprov'ia*, 2011;2:21-23. (in Ukrainian)
4. Bala TM, Maslyak IP. *Chirliding u fizichnomu vikhovanni shkoliariv* [Cheer-leading in physical education of schoolchildren], Kharkov; 2014 (in Ukrainian)
5. Zinchenko IA. *Pobudova trenuval'nogo procesu sportsmeniv u cherlidingu na etapi specializovanoi bazovoi pidgotovki. Cand. Diss*. [Building of sportsmen's training process in cheer-leading at stage of specialized basic training. Cand. Diss.], Kharkov; 2013 (in Ukrainian)
6. Kozina ZhL, Iermakov SS, Bazylyuk TA, Voloshina EV. Innovacionnye tekhnologii akvafitnesa igrovoj napravlennosti s primeneniem tekhnicheskikh ustrojstv v fizicheskom vospitanii studentok [Aqua-fitness innovative technologies of game orientation with application of technical devices in girl students' physical education]. *Physical education of students*, 2012;1:42-46. (in Ukrainian)
7. Krivoruchko N, Maslyak I. Dinamika pokaznikiv rozvitku koordinacijnikh zdibnostej studentiv VNZ pid vplivom vprav chirlidingu [Dynamic of coordination indicators of HEE students under influence of cheer-leading exercises]. *Moloda sportivna nauka Ukraini*, 2013; 7: 87-91. (in Ukrainian)
8. Malyar EI. *Rozvitok profesijno vazhlivikh iakostej studentiv special'nosti «Opodatkuvannia» zasobami futbolu. Cand. Diss*. [Training of professionally significant qualities of students (specialization "Taxation") by means of football. Cand. Diss.], Lviv; 2008 (in Ukrainian)
9. Romanenko VA. *Diagnostika dvigatel'nykh sposobnostej* [Diagnostic of motor abilities], Donetsk: Don NU; 2005 (in Ukrainian)
10. Terenteva NM, Mameshina MA, Maslyak IP. *Teoriia ta metodika fizichnogo vikhovannia* [Theory and methodic of physical education], Kharkov, KSAPC; 2010. (in Ukrainian)
11. Timofeeva OV. Chirliding v sisteme fizicheskogo vospitaniia studentok [Cheer-leading in system of girl students' physical education]. *Teoriia i praktika fizicheskoj kul'tury*, 2008;11:36-38. (in Russian)
12. Timofeeva TN,. Tatarinova OO, Vladimirova SM. Cherliding dlia doshkol'nikov [Cheer-leading for pre school age children]. *Detskij sad: teoriia i praktika*, 2011;10:68-75. (in Russian)
13. Bala T. Change in the level of strength and endurance development of 5-6 grades pupils under cheerleading exercises influence. *Slobozhanskyi herald of science and sport* , 2015; 3: 14-18.
14. Bala TM. The influence of cheerleading exercises on the schoolchildren's physical health of 5-9th forms. *Pedagogics, psychology, medical-biological problems of physical training and sports*, 2012; 4: 12-16.
15. Belykh S. I. Health, physical education and physical development of students in historically and personally developing paradigm. *Pedagogics, psychology, medical-biological problems of physical training and sports*, 2013; 5: 7-12. http://dx.doi:10.6084/m9.figshare.707091
16. Carrier Justin, McKay Donna. Complete cheerleading. Human Kinetics: USA, 2006: 240.
17. Cieślicka M. Swimming lessons in improving the health of students. *Pedagogics, psychology, medical-biological problems of physical training and sports*, 2013; 12: 101–104. http://dx.doi:10.6084/m9.figshare.880636
18. Chappell Linda Rae. Coaching cheerleading successfully (second edition). Human Kinetics: In Canada, 2005: 206.
19. Grutsyak N. Volleyball in unsportsmanlike university : development trends. *Slobozhanskyi herald of science and sport*, 2015; № 2(46): 59-62.
20. Ilnitskaya AS, Kozina ZhL, Korobejnik VA, Ilnickiy SV, Cieślicka Mirosława, Stankiewicz Błażej, Pilewska Wiesława. The method of application of health systems Bodyflex and Pilates in physical education of

students. *Pedagogics, psychology, medical-biological problems of physical training and sports,* 2014; 2: 25-32. http://dx.doi:10.6084/m9.figshare.923510

21. Kryvoruchko NV, Masljak IP, Zhuravlyova IN. Impact on the display of power cheerleading ability of university students I-II levels of accreditation. *Pedagogics, psychology, medical-biological problems of physical training and sports,* 2013; 9: 38-42. http://dx.doi:10.6084/m9.figshare.749696.
22. Temchenko V. Influence of informational technologies on physical background of students engaged futsal in sport-oriented physical education. *Slobozhanskyi herald of science and sport*, 2015; 3(47): 93-96.
23. Salatenko IA. Direction improvements professionally-applied physical preparation of students of economic specialties. *Pedagogics, psychology, medical biological problems of physical training and sports*, 2012; 11: 90-93. http://dx.doi:10.6084/ m9.figshare.97369.

STABILITY OF EQUILIBRIUM IN UPRIGHT STANCE AND VOLUNTARY MOTION CONTROL IN ATHLETES-SHOOTERS IN THE PROCESS OF READY POSITION AND TARGET SHOOTING

Pryimakov A.A.[1], Eider E. [1], Omelchuk E.V. [2]
Szczecin University, Poland[1]
M.P. Dragomanov National Pedagogical University[2]

Annotation. *Purpose:* consists in studying the relationships between the system of equilibrium regulation in upright stance and voluntary motion control in athletes-shooters during ready position and target shooting. *Material:* 19 highly skilled athletes specialized in pistol shooting were studied. Physiological and biomechanical characteristics of posture and voluntary motions were assessed by methods of stabilography, electromyography and tremorometry; besides, accuracy of target shooting was registered. *Results:* high degree of shooting accuracy dependence on posture somatic parameters has been revealed, of which the greatest impact upon the result is exerted by low-frequency vibrations of the body general centre of mass, subjected to voluntary control. Prognostic models of shooting accuracy dependence upon the character of posture regulation during ready position and the shot have been developed. *Conclusions:* obtained results reveal the mechanisms of functioning and interacting of two systems of management – posture and voluntary motion. Elaborated regression models permit to model and predict posture stability and shooting accuracy during ready position and the shot.

Key words: orthograde posture, equilibrium, accuracy, relationships, athletes-shooters.

Introduction

It is known that in the process of long-term adaptation to physical loads (PL) mechanisms of upright posture regulation are improved in athletes, and provide not only the high quality and reliability of equilibrium maintenance under extreme conditions of athletic activity but determine the quality and reliability of voluntary motion control to a great extent as well [8, 14, 16, 19, 20].

System approach in biological studies has demonstrated that both posture regulation and voluntary motion control are realized by hierarchically organized functional systems (FS) with clearly defined final adaptive outcome of the activity of each system [1, 2, 8, 10]. Interaction of FS may be realized at different levels of each system [8]. It depends on the structural and functional organization of both the voluntary motion and assumed posture, which preceds it and interacts with it both at the stage of “afferent synthesis” and “decision making” [1, 9] and in the process of formation and realization of voluntary motion program [2, 3, 18]. However, interaction mechanisms of functional systems of upright posture regulation and voluntary motion control are rather insufficiently highlighted in the literature from system positions: that is, from position of their hierarchically organized component interactions and final adaptive results of each system [5, 10, 11]. Peculiarities of improvement of these interactions in the process of long-term adaptation to physical loads are insufficiently covered in the literature as well.

The objective of this work consists in studying the relationships between the system of equilibrium regulation in upright stance and that of voluntary motion control in athletes-shooters during ready position and target shooting.

Purpose, tasks of the work, material and methods

Methods of combined multiparameter registration of physiological and biomechanical characteristics of posture and voluntary motions including stabilography, electromyography, tremorometry, pulsometry, target shooting accuracy were used [8, 9, 12].

Eighting highly skilled pistol shooterts participated in studies.

Mechanisms of posture regulation were studied during equilibrium maintenance in three upright stances: the Romberg stance (posture 1), the common stance (posture 2) and complicated upright stances (postures 3-4) during ready position, just before and during target shooting.

In one case the posture was complicated by four-time pistol lifting and holding in outstretched arm until fatigue (posture 3), whereas in the other – by upright stance maintenance with knee joint angle equal to 110° (posture 4). In both cases testing ended in apparent signs of fatigue due to isometric activity of the upper and the lower extremity muscles.

During ready position and shot somatic and vegetative parameters of the posture and formed motion were synchronously registered along with calculation of energy expenditures. Accuracy of target shooting was recorded.

Shifts of the body general centre of mass (GCM) while maintaining equilibrium in upright stance, tremor of the hand holding the pistol and accuracy of target shooting were considered as the parameters of the “final adaptive results”.

Synchronous registration of somatic, vegetative and biomechanical indices followed by respective mathematical processing allowed to examine physiological mechanisms underlying interrelated activity of two systems of control, integrating for realization of the program of accuracy motion under various conditions. Methods of variance statistics including correlation, regression, dispersion, etc. methods of statistical analysis in *STATISTICA* system of Windows were applied for experimental material processing [4].

Results of the research

The results of studies have demonstrated that pistol holding in outstretched arm in shooter's *specific stance* insignificantly influences equilibrium stability: high equilibrium stability was observed in athletes both during convenient and specific posture of the shooter. Amplitude of high-frequency shifts of the body GCM varied from 0,6 ± 0,09 to 0,8 ± 0.03 mm, whereas that of low-frequency – from 0,9 ± 0,1 to 1,6 ± 0,16 mm. Some somatic characteristics of the posture, activity of muscular and cardiovascular (CV) system showed significant changes both during ready position assumption and just before the shot.

For instance, standing with pistol in outstretched arm in shooter's specific posture while aiming was accompanied with significant increase of hand tremor amplitude relative to that in initial posture, and electric activity of brachioradial muscle (BRM), tendency to increase of electric activity of deltoid muscle (DM), enhancement of CV system activity and increased energy expenditures.

Just before the shot the character of posture regulation and hand voluntary motion control during aiming appeared to change: decrease of the amplitude of slow high-amplitude shifts of the body GCM was observed in frontal and sagittal planes, whereas fast ones – in frontal plane; besides, an increase of the frequency of fast vibrations of the body GCM and decrease of slow ones in sagittal plane, tendency to reduction of heart rate (HR), tremor amplitude (TA) of hand holding the pistol and amplitude of electromyograms (EMG) of BRM and DM were noted.

Coefficients of correlation (r) between somatic parameters of the posture varied during ready position from –0,44 ± 0,03 to 0,738 ± 0,0002, reflecting different interdependence of the upper extremity muscle functioning, vibrations of the body GCM and tremor of hand holding the pistol. It is noteworthy, that in this case the dependence of CV system functioning and energy expenditure on somatic parameters of posture stability was also manifested.

Just before the shot interrelation between somatic parameters of the posture and their correlation with HR tended to enhance.

Sustained static tension of the upper and the lower extremity muscles while holding pistol in outstretched arm in complicated stance (with knee joint angle equal to 110°) induces more expressed shifts of the parameters of posture stability, muscular and cardiac activity, accelerates fatigue development and activates mechanisms of equilibrium correction in orthograde posture. The above is accompanied with synchronization of arm and the lower extremity vibrations, appearance of spike discharges of motoneurons on EMG and increase of energy expenditures, which finds its manifestation in high degree of correlations between parameters.

Improvement of the mechanisms of posture stability regulation and voluntary motion control in top level shooters is characterized by short-term decrease of EMG amplitude of deltoid and brachioradial muscles, tremor amplitude of hand holding the pistol and the main vibrations of the body GCM just before the shot.

Insignificant decrease of HR may be observed in some shooters in specific posture at the moment preceding the shot. Despite the fact that direct voluntary control for discrete involuntary vibrations of the body GCM is not possible (as according to N.A.Bernstein (2) their regulation is realized with participation of rubrospinal level of motion control), mechanisms of tremor amplitude, the body GCM vibrations and HR decrease are indirectly activated by top level athletes.

An artificial introduction of confounding factors (change of habitual posture, additional vestibular irritants, prolonged isometric regime of muscular activity) impairs the quality of posture regulation and is accompanied with increased energy expenditures and deterioration of shooting accuracy (Table 1).

Table 1

Somatovegetative indices and accuracy of shooting under different conditions of upright posture maintenance

Indices	**Initial posture of shooter**		**Pistol holding until fatigue**		**Low stance maintenance until fatigue**	
	X	±M	X	±M	X	±M
Tremor amplitude, mm	7,5	0,9	8,0	0,27	10,9	1,6
Sagittal stabilogram ampl., mm	1,6	0,1	1,78	0,14	4,76	0,57
EMG of DM, mkV	321	20,0	382,9	25,0	513,0	53,3
EMG of BRM, mkV	232	17,6	219,6	19,9	295,3	17,9
EMG of QMT, mkV*	74.6	1,4	16,7	3,0	221,1	9,2
EMG of GM, mkV	74.6	3,4	107,4	8,4	184,2	14,4
HR, bt·min^{-1}	92.8	1,7	102,4	2,5	111,2	3,2

Indices	Initial posture of shooter		Pistol holding until fatigue		Low stance maintenance until fatigue	
	X	±M	X	±M	X	±M
Energy expenditure, kcal	4.2	0,2	4,45	0,12	5,15	0,12
Shooting result (5 shots)	49.4	0,29	48,45	0,53	46,74	0,91

*EMG of QMT = electromyogram of quadriceps muscle of thigh; EMG of GM = electromyogram of gastrocnemius muscle.

Despite the fact that confounding factors (prolonged pistol holding in outstretched arm and low stance until fatigue) decrease posture stability, increase and synchronize various vibrations of standing person, more fit athletes damp down these vibrations before the shot, preventing their "spreading" on the arm holding the pistol. Unfit athletes do not possess this capacity, therefore the shot is made in the face of decreased equilibrium stability, increased TA of arm, EMG of DM and BRM, HR and energy expenditures, which leads to impaired shooting accuracy.

Correlation analysis has demonstrated that under complicated standing conditions (while holding pistol in outstretched arm until fatigue or keeping knee joint angle equal to 110°), interaction of functional systems of posture stability control and accuracy of voluntary motion tends to increase.

Analysis of interactions at the moment of ready position and just before the shot shows that control for posture stability, tremor vibrations of arm holding the pistol and HR at the moment preceding the shot, is dependent on the character of posture regulation during ready position (15-10 sec before the shot). This is evidenced by revealed high positive correlations, reflecting dependence of amplitude of the body GCM shifts, arm tremor, and EMG at the moment preceding the shot on respective indices registered during assuming ready position (Table 2).

Table 2

Interactions of somatic indices and HR of athletes-shooters, recorded just before the shot with analogous indices registered while assuming ready position

Position	Indices:		Before the shot:						
			tremor	stabilogram			EMG		HR
			amplitude	sag.A_1*	fr.F_2	fr.A_2	DM	BRM	
R	tremor	frequency	-0,725		-		-	-	-0,770
e		amplitude	0,966		-		-	-	0,921
a	stabilogram	sag.A_1	-	0,605	-	-0,617	-	-	0,654
d		sag.A_2	-	0,685	-	0,630	-	-	-
y		sag.F_1	-	0,751	-	-	-	-	-
		fr. F_2	-	-	-0,778	-			-
p	EMG	DM	-	-		-	0,878	0,898	
o		BRM		-		-	0,898	0,918	0,748
s.	HR					-		0,748	0,789

* **Notes**: **sag.** – sagittal, **fr.** – frontal, $\mathbf{A_1}$ – amplitude of high-frequency vibrations, $\mathbf{A_2}$ – amplitude of low-frequency vibrations, $\mathbf{F_1}$ – frequency of low-amplitude vibrations, $\mathbf{F_2}$ – frequency of high-amplitude vibrations.

Correlation analysis results indicate that the greater are the arm TA while assuming ready position, the body GCM vibrations, muscle electric activity and HR (10-15 sec before the shot), the higher are their meanings just before the shot and vice versa. Fit athletes tend to manifest more expressed capacity for reduction of these vibration amplitude and HR decrease before the shot.

The less is the posture stability at the beginning of ready position, the more expressed are correctional reorganizations of posture just before the shot in athletes: high correlation interactions have been observed between amplitude of the body GCM and tremor while assuming ready position and the degree of their decrease just before the shot ($r=0,913<0,01$ and $r=0,717<0,01$, respectively), which is indicative of control on the basis of signals of negative feedback (2).

At the same time, deterioration of equilibrium stability in sagittal plane while assuming ready position activates compensatory responses aimed at decrease of amplitude (r=-0,677 ± 0,008) and increase of frequency (r=0,736 ± 0,003) of tremor, rise in frequency of the main vibrations of frontal stabilogram (r=0,623±0,02) just before the shot. Increase of amplitude of the main vibrations of the body GCM in frontal plane while assuming ready position leads to decrease of amplitude of deltoid muscle EMG (r=-0,669 ±0,009) just before the shot.

Analysis of regulation mechanisms of posture stability during ready position shows that programing of responses, which provide maximal accuracy of shooting in case of regular hindrances to posture maintenance, includes the development of efficient program anticipating posture reorganization, consisting in activation of motor units, stabilization of equilibrium and joint angle during ready position assumption and just before the shot, between the parameters of which and voluntary motion accuracy there exist high correlations.

The findings demonstrate that arm tremor depending on EMG activity of DM during ready position exerts the greatest influence on accuracy of shooting: there exist strong negative linear dependences between arm TA, electric activity of DM and shooting accuracy – the higher are arm TA and electric activity of DM, the lower is the result of shooting.

Presented in Fig.1 coefficients of correlation and determination, regression models reflect high dependence of the result of accuracy motion on posture somatic parameters recorded during ready position and just before the shot under ordinary and complicated conditions of standing: the higher is the amplitude of tremor, body GCM vibrations and electric activity of DM and BRM, the lower is the result of shooting, and vice versa.

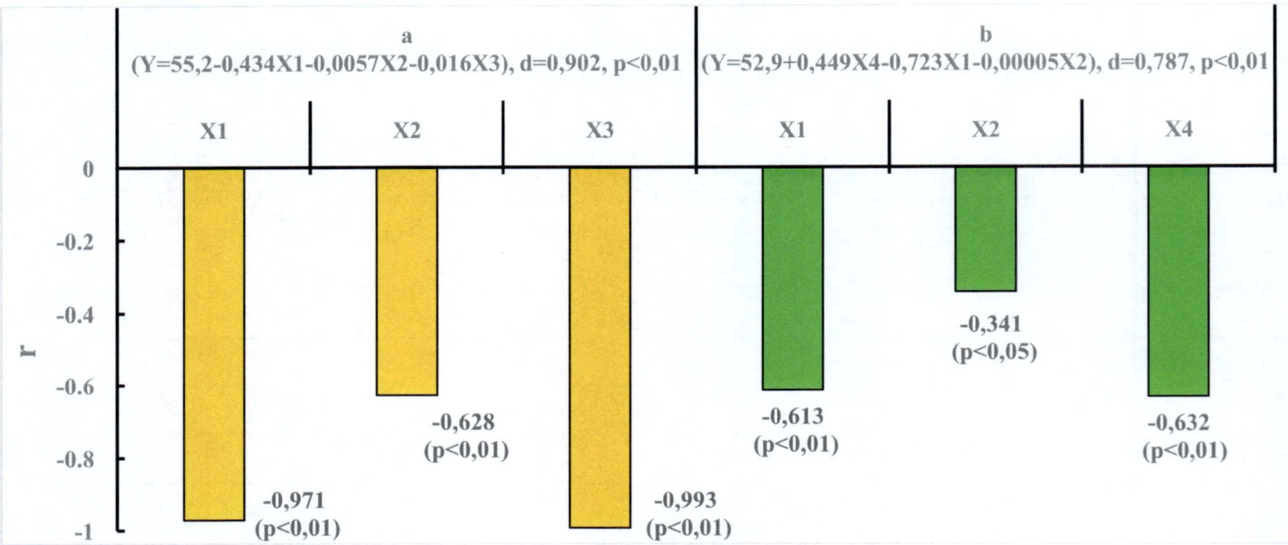

Fig.1. Coefficients of correlations and regression models reflecting association between accuracy of target shooting and posture somatic parameters, recorded during ready position (a) and just before the shot (b): r – coefficients of correlation; Y – result of shooting, points; X1 – tremor amplitude, mm; X2 – EMG of DM, mkV; X3 – EMG of BRM, mkV; X4 – amplitude of sagittal stabilogram, mm.

Coefficients of pair and multiple correlations, determination and regression equations indicate that accuracy of voluntary motion is determined not only by partial contribution of individual parameters of examined system but their interaction as well, as a result of which there occurs dependence, different in the degree and the form from pair correlations, which is approximated rather precisely by means of multiple regression equations presented in the Figure.

Discussion.

Carried out studies have confirmed the findings of several authors indicating close association between the parameters of shooter's upright posture stability and accuracy of target shooting [6, 7, 14-16]. Dependence of shooting accuracy on the peculiarities of cardiac activity has been also revealed, which corresponds to the results reported by several authors [6, 13].

At the same time, conducted studies have specificated the mechanisms of posture regulation while assuming ready position and just before the shot as well as their associations providing optimum background conditions for realization of voluntary accurate motion – target shooting.

For instance, it has been revealed that at the beginning of aiming the character of deviating posture regulation is manifested providing alteration of equilibrium stability control during the shot, depending on stability in ready position.

Statistical processing of findings has revealed rather strong influence of individual somatic characteristics of posture and their interactions upon the mechanisms of accurate volitional motion control during ready position and target shooting. This is also indicative of close interrelation of regulation mechanisms of two systems of control: the system of upright posture stabilization and that of voluntary motion.

Analysis of coefficients of correlation, determination and regression equations, presented in Fig.1, demonstrates high degree of dependence of shooting accuracy on simultaneous interrelated impact of posture somatic parameters, of which the greatest influence on the result is exerted by relatively slow, low-frequency vibrations of the body GCM, sequacious to voluntary control. Top level athletes have a knack for damping them down, manifesting higher quality of posture stability control at the moment of accurate motion realization.

On the basis of obtained results it is safe to conclude that formed program of realization of forthcoming accurate motion includes both standard parameters of posture and voluntary motion and the mechanisms of correcting their interaction when confounding factors and hindrances are acting, thus providing control of perturbation and deviation.

As a result of the above, high accuracy during the shot is achieved in adapted athletes at well-timed (in accordance with created standard and the character of correctional inverse afference) preliminary posture reorganization – its stability and biomechanical parameters.

During fatigue in less adapted to physical load athletes, one may observe increase of amplitude and synchronism of vibrations of different body links in upright posture, loss of ability to damp down these vibrations, which are propagating to the barrel, thus deteriorating shooting quality the more, the higher are their amplitude and the degree of synchronization.

The worse posture stability at the beginning of ready position, the more expressed are its correctional reorganizations just before the shot: the more decreased are the arm TA, the body GCM vibrations; besides the tendency to HR reduction is observed. The above reflects deviation control on the basis of negative feedback.

Hence important tasks follow: a) elaboration of means and methods of posture stabilization during ready position, aimed at improvement of stability within equilibrium zone, decrease of amplitude of tremor, muscle electric activity, HR just before the shot; b) usage of prognostic models allowing to predict the system state, the character of posture control just before the shot and accuracy of voluntary motion realization on the basis of initial data.

Conclusions.

1.Obtained results reveal the mechanisms of functioning and interacting of two control systems – posture and voluntary motion.

2.High degree of shooting accuracy dependence on simultaneous interacting impact of posture somatic parameters has been revealed, of which the greatest influence on the result is exerted by relatively slow, low-frequency vibrations of the body GCM, sequacious to voluntary control.

3. Elaborated regression models permit to model and predict: 1) posture stability, the character of its regulation just before the shot depending on analogous parameters during ready position; 2) change of CV system activity at the moment of shot depending on posture stability, activity of muscles, tremor of arm holding the pistol during ready position and just before the shot; 3) accuracy of shooting depending on the character of posture regulation during ready position and the shot.

References:

1. Anokhin P.K. *Ocherki po fiziologii funkcional'nykh sistem* [Essays on the physiology of functional systems], Moscow, Medicine, 1975, 448 p. (in Russian)
2. Bernshtejn N. A. *O postroenii dvizhenij* [On the construction of movements], Moscow, Medicine, 1947, 255 p. (in Russian)
3. Bernshtejn N.A. *O lovkosti i ee razvitii* [About dexterity and its development], Moscow, Physical Culture and Sport, 1991, 288 p. (in Russian)
4. Borovikov V.P., Ivchenko G.I. *Prognozirovanie v sisteme STATISTICA v srede Windows* [Forecasting in the STATISTICA for Windows], Moscow, Finance and Statistics, 2006, 275 p. (in Russian)
5. Bozerzhan Zh. *Spravochnik po sportivnoj strel'be* [Handbook of sports shooting], Rostov on Don, Phoenix, 2006, 192 p. (in Russian)
6. Ivanov K.O., Kubriak O.V. Vliianie oshchushchenij ot serdca i stabil'nosti pozy na tochnost' strel'by v predstavlenii elitnykh strelkov [Influence of feelings from the heart and stability pose on accuracy in the representation of elite shooters]. *Vestnik sportivnoj nauki*, 2011, no.5, pp. 13-22. (in Russian)
7. Kudelin A. Kak povysit' ustojchivost'? [How to improve stability?]. *Oruzhie*. 2005, no.2, pp. 64–66. (in Russian)
8. Prijmakov O.O. Vzaiemozv'iazok mekhanizmiv reguliuvannia stijkisti postavi ta svavil'nogo tochnist'n'ogo rukhu u sportsmeniv [Relationship resistance mechanisms regulating posture and arbitrary precision motion in athletes]. *Fiziologichnij zhurnal*. 1995, vol.41, no.3-4, pp. 23-28. (in Ukrainian)
9. Prijmakov A.A. Vzaimosviazi sistem regulirovaniia ravnovesiia v vertikal'noj stojke i upravleniia proizvol'nymi dvizheniiami u sportsmenov-strelkov [Relationship management systems of equilibrium in the vertical rack and control voluntary movements in athletes-riflemen]. *Fizicheskoe vospitanie studentov*. 2010, no.3, pp. 75-77. (in Russian)
10. Sudakov K.V. *Funkcional'nye sistemy organizma* [Body functional systems], Moscow, Medicine, 1987, 432 p. (in Russian)
11. Tarasova L.V. Faktory ustojchivosti sistemy «strelok-oruzhie» v trenirovke vysokokvalificirovannykh strelkov [Resistance factors of the "shooter-weapon" in the training of highly skilled riflemen]. *Vestnik sportivnoj nauki*, 2009, no.3, pp. 25-27. (in Russian)

12. Boloban V. Systemic stabilography: methodology of measuring, estimating and controling sportsman body balance and the system of bodies. *Coordination motor abilities in scientific research.* Biala Podlaska, 2005, pp. 102-109.
13. Christodonlou V.X., Dinas P.C., Baliamis N.G., Felouris A.D. *Changes in heart rate variability during an archery competition. 15th annual congress of the European College of Sport Science*: book of abstracts. 2010, no.15, pp. 339.
14. Era P., Konttinen N., Mehto P., Saarela P., Lyytinen H. Postural stability and skilled performance – a study on top-level and naive rifle shooters. *Journal of Biomechanics*, 1996, vol.29, no.3, pp. 301–306.
15. Herpin G., Gauchard G.C., Lion A., Collet P., Keller D., Perrin P.P. Sensorimotor specificities in balance control of expert fencers and pistol shooters. *Journal of Electromyography and Kinesiology.* 2010, vol.20, no.1, pp. 162-169.
16. Lakie M. The influence of muscle tremor on shooting performance. *Exp. Physiol.* 2010, vol.95, no.3, pp. 441–450.
17. Matthias E., Schandry R., Duschek S., Pollatos O. On relationship between interoceptive signal information and the process of visual stimulus processing. *Int. J. Psychophysiol.* 2009, vol.72, no.2, pp. 154–159.
18. Perrot C., Deviterne D., Perrin P. Influence of training on postural and motor control in a combative sport. *J. Hum. Mov. Studies.* 1998, no.35, pp. 119-135.
19. Terekhov A.V. *Concerning the nature of slow component in postural sway. European Workshop on Movement Science. 2005,* Vienna, 2005, 123 p.
20. Terekhov A.V., Levik Yu.S. The forming of the reference vertical in the orthograde posture stabilization task. *Progress in motor control*. 2006, no.5, pp. 4-20.

PROFESSIONAL PORTRAIT OF FUTURE INSTRUCTORS FOR PHYSICAL EDUCATION OF PRESCHOOL

Semanychyn T.M., Popel' S.L.
Prikarpatskiy National University

Annotation. *Purpose:* identify the degree of readiness of students to conduct valeological activity in preschool educational institutions. The objective of the study was to identify the relationship between educational level and health education and readiness of students to valeological activities. *Material*: in the experiment took part 550 students. *Results*: the survey allowed to establish pedagogical assumptions that characterize the training of students. This will include valeological activity for the formation of their own culture valeological children. It is shown that students' valeological culture is a prerequisite for the effective functioning of the system in pre-secondary institutions. It is noted that the training of students of the Faculty of Physical Education and Sports to valeological activity is low. *Conclusions*: studies have shown that only 11.7% of the students have been trained and have the necessary knowledge and practical skills.

Keywords: physical education, valeology, culture, children, instructor.

Introduction

After I.I. Brekhman's [9] introducing of term "valueology as science about health" many specialists try to carry out valueology activity among wide strata of population [5, 10, 12]. With it they pay special attention to children. Recent time valueology knowledge has become integral part of training of highly qualified specialists in system of physical education [8]. Cultivation of students' valueology culture is a core and , at the same time, a determining condition of effective functioning of such system in children educational establishments (CEE).

Valueology orientation of modern education in Ukraine, oriented on a person as the highest value of social being regards him (her) as a subject of cognition, communication and creativity. That is why it is so important to create conditions, in which person would take position of "creator" of own personality in constantly varying modern social environment [11].

The problems connected with formation of valueology culture were elucidated in works of many scientists [1, 3, 6]. Considering their results we can say that training of students at physical culture and sports faculty to valueology functioning corresponds to realization of their own creative potential.

Nowadays term "valueology culture" is interpreted in different ways. It is often is understood as:

– system of knowledge and ideas, on the base of which health related human functioning is constructed and regulated [7];

– high level of ecological thinking, its orientation on HLS, ability to quickly change manner of actions in compliance with new conditions of environment[8];

– special quality, which characterizes measure of certain social role for correspondence of individual's qualities to social standards, which id required for self determination of valueology activity's subject [1];

– one of aspects and, at the same time, axiological potential of personality, who takes position of "creator" of own somatic health in condition of modern social environment [3, 7];

– humanistic orientation of modern valueology education in Ukraine with its orientation on a person as the highest value of social being and regards him (her) as a subject of cognition, communication and creativity [11];

– social-psychological setting for non-traditional solution of contradictions of objective reality, connected with practicing of HLS [13];

– integrating and synthetic quality, characterizing the measure of personality's potentials for creative valueology functioning [2, 4];

– integral personality's quality, expressed in relation (position, orientation) of a person to own health [15-17];

– combination of real potentials, skills for practicing of HLS, which determine level of valueology education [5, 18-21].

From medical point of view valueology culture or culture of health is a part of general culture and is a reasonable system of actions and relations to own health and health of other people, i.e. ability to live not injuring own organism but benefiting it [14]. With it scientists mention that health culture implies not simple "collecting" of useful recommendations but active application of them in everyday practice.

Valueology culture implies also ability to propagate valueology knowledge. Pedagogues shall cultivate firm motivation for health and healthy life style (HLS) starting from pre school age (with the help of academic programs, pedagogic work with parents, with own example in everyday communication).

Thus, it is evident that it is necessary to have interconnection between educational and health related directions in pre school educational establishments. Such interconnection can be ensured by readiness of modern student and future instructor of physical culture in CEE for valueology functioning on the base of system of valueology knowledge, which forms certain level of valueology culture.

Purpose, tasks of the work, material and methods

The purpose of the work is to determine the level of readiness of physical culture and sports faculty for valueology functioning.

The main tasks of the research were analysis of scientific literature on theoretical principles of physical culture instructors' training and carry out questioning of students, devoted their readiness for valueology functioning.

The methods and organization of the research. Modern status of training of future physical culture instructors of pre school children for valueology functioning was studied by us with the help of empiric methods, i.e. questioning of 550 HEE students of Ukraine.

The questionnaire had several parts, concerning presence and development of own resources, facilitating formation of valueology culture, strategy and skills in prevention from HLS violation, knowledge of professional valueology culture's structure, its cognitive development, acquiring of personal professional knowledge and creation of functional behavior's strategy. Such construction of questionnaire permits to more completely evaluate problems and disadvantages in theoretical and methodic valueology preparation of future physical culture instructors of pre school educational establishments.

Evaluation was fulfilled by 5-points' scale. All results were processed by methods of parametrical statistics with the help of "Statistika 5" programs.

Results of the research. Discussion.

Characteristics of valueology knowledge are given in table 1. Results of analysis showed that most of the questioned students (86.7%) have no oriented understanding of own resources, which would facilitate formation of pre school children's HLS.

Table 1

Characteristics of knowledge and skills of 3rd -0 5th year students of physical education and sports faculty in sphere of valueology culture (n=550, %)

Characteristics of knowledge and skills in sphere of valueology culture	+2	+1	0	–1	–2
Available personal resources, facilitating formation of valueology culture	2.1	6.8	72.3	10.9	7.9
Development of personal resources facilitating formation of valueology culture	6.9	12.1	69.3	5.7	6.0
Development of strategy and behavior for prevention of HLS violations	2.0	16.5	36.8	19.3	25,4
Structure of professional valueology culture.					
1. Cognitive development	3.0	8.1	60.5	12.0	16.9
2. Development of personal professional resources	4.6	10,3	20.1	40.4	2.6
3. Development of strategy of functional behavior and skills	10.2	12.5	30.3	30.6	1..4

Question "Do you have own ready system of values, targets and settings in sphere of HLS?" positive answer was given only by 14.2 % of the questioned; "cannot answer" – by 53.4 %: "don't have" – by 32.4%. With it, it was determined that 66.9% students are not able to communicate with children professionally; 43.2% do not know how to solve their life problems; 77.9% – cannot evaluate situations in children collective and cannot use own professional potentials to control such situations. In our opinion this can be explained by quantity of negative points (92.3%), received by students for their answer to question: "Do you understand behavior of children, render them psychological and social support?"

Low level of valueology fitness of future specialists in pre school physical education is also proved by data about development of personal resources, facilitating formation of valueology culture. More than half (56.1%) of respondents have no personal resources, facilitating determination of own mistakes in HLS practicing; 45.6% points at inability to adequately evaluate problem situations and solve life problems; 68.8% cannot change themselves and their life; nearly one third (32.3%) cannot control own behavior and 55.2% are not able to listen to children.

The latter is explained by the fact that more than 2/3 of students are not able to express own feelings and take decisions on psychological-social children's support.

Such status of students' valueology training reflects in certain way on their ability to work out strategy and behavioral skills for prevention of HLS violations. It was determined that 72.3% cannot take decisions on overcoming of harmful habits, while 45.3% do not take such habits as harmful at all. With it only 30.2% of students can evaluate social situation and feel responsibility for own behavior; 34.7% can defend own rights and personal space. Insignificant part of students (24.2%) can defend own "Self", are able for self-support and support. Most students (76.3%) cannot avoid situations, connected with taking harmful substances and other forms of destructive behavior. However 98.6% of respondent mentioned about ability for non conflict effective communication, including with pedagogues.

Thus, we received answers to three blocks of questions, which touched on characteristics of knowledge and skills in sphere of valueology culture and these answers point at insufficient students' knowledge, at demand in acquiring of such knowledge for successful future professional functioning.

Correction of situation, which exists in this problem, can imply correction of evaluation points with answering on cognitive structure of students' professional valueology education. It was found that holistic idea about processes and phenomena, which occur in nature, only 46.8% of students have. From them 91.2% understand potentials of modern scientific methods of cognition of nature. However, only 12.4% know these methods and are able to apply them in professional functioning. Only 30.1% have some knowledge about main mental functions of a child, but 78.9% have knowledge about main human mental functions. So, knowledge of children's psychology requires more attention from the side of pedagogues to students, who are taught to practice valueology activity in pre school educational establishments. Data, concerning development of personal professional resources, were also interesting: 41.1% of students have skills in analysis of educational situations. Only 23.4% of them know general philosophical laws of culture of thinking; 26.9% can express results of educational, scientific and pedagogic functioning both in oral and written forms. Only 37.2 of respondents know national specificities of everyday life, family and family education and can use their knowledge in work. Only one third (33.1%) of students think that they have high level of personal health and only 11.7% can feel responsibility for health and life of other people. All these, undoubtedly influence on development of strategy of students' functional behavior and skills in mastering of own valueology culture. Positive answer to question: "Do you know and apply modern methods of scientific cognition?" was given only by 25.3% from them, while only 10.4% of respondents know the principles of organizational-sociological researches. Nearly half (48.7%) of positive answers were received to question: "Do you have means and methods of pedagogic influence on personality?", with it only 24.6% from them have knowledge of general and individual features of child's mentality; 22.1% – use in pedagogic process knowledge of main biological processes, mechanisms, phenomena and etc.

It should be noted that only 25.3% of respondents consider themselves to be ready for re-evaluation of experience, accumulated by science and social practice in sphere of children's physical education in pre school educational establishments. The most troublesome are students' answers to such challenges of modern system of pre-school education as usage of modern informational educational technologies (only 12.3% of positive answers), knowledge of modern psychological methodic of correction of child's psycho-emotional state (8.9%), ability to diagnose temper and character of a child (3.4%), ability to compose psychological characteristic of a child (6.6%), to personally determine the nearest prospects of a child (5.9%), determination of psychological climate of children's group (9.2%) and sociological; status of a child in group (7.1%). Not less troublesome is inability in 63.2% of cases to determine type of family relations and type of family education. Only 18.6% of students can carry out work on prevention from family conflicts. With it, it is no surprising that very little part (3.1%) of students can compose programs for correction of children's behavior in family. However, rather significant percentage (47.2%) of students can practically apply knowledge and skills in pedagogic influence on older sociological strata of people. Such status of valueology problem requires integrated program of continuous valueology education for receiving by students both general and basic valueology competences.

Formation of modern strategy of students' functional behavior and skills for formation of own valueology culture is called for also by very low percentage of positive answers to question about ability to create safe and friendly atmosphere in children's collective (9.5 %), to bring knowledge "between lines", i.e. use non-verbal component of communication (14.2 %), have knowledge of children's styles and methods of material's mastering and great stock of different forms of teaching functioning (4.7 %), are satisfied with work with children and enjoy with it (16.5 %).

Analysis of answers to questions, touching on employment and competence in valueology functioning in CEE is shown in fig. 1 and 2.

It was found that staff positions in CEE are engaged by workers from other branches, who passed brief course of retraining as instructors in pre school children physical culture. Answers to first question "Do you agree that owing to deficit of specialists in valueology the appropriate positions are engaged by workers from other branches – coaches, physical culture school teachers, after brief retraining course?" distributed in the following way: from 550 of respondents 48.2% agreed with our opinion, 32.8% – agreed partially, 11,7% – did not agree, for 7.3% it was difficult to answer.

The second question: "To what extent do you have knowledge about valueology functioning in CEE?" results distributed in the following way: from 550 of respondents only 11.1% of students have knowledge in this field, 39.2% – have partial knowledge, 36.8% – have no knowledge and for 12.9% of students it was difficult to answer.

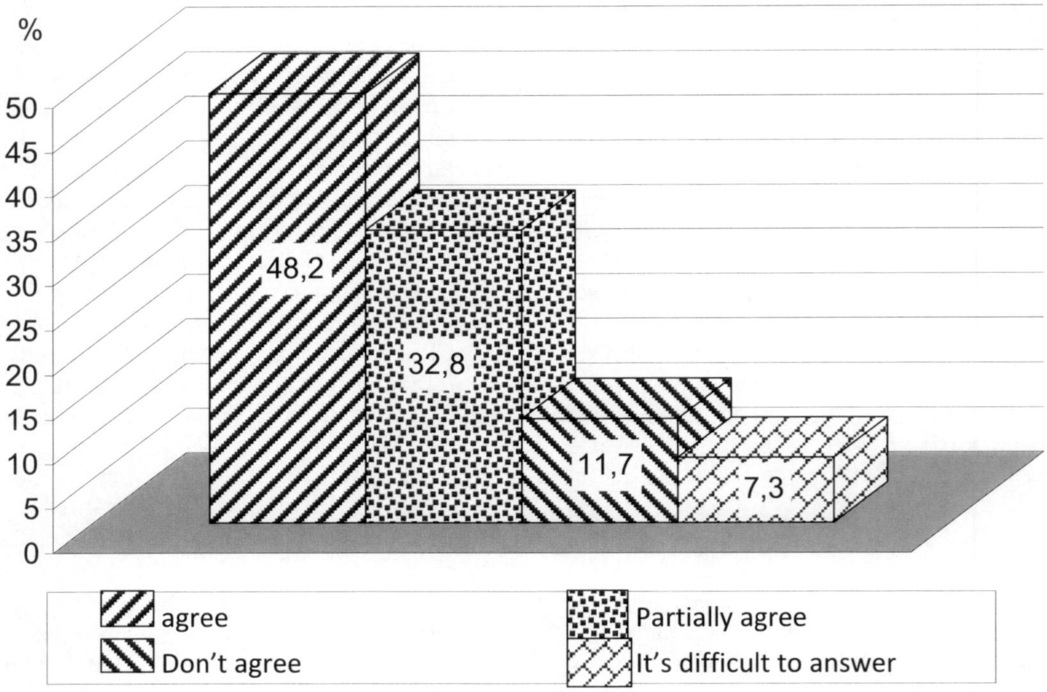

Fig.1. Quantity of students, questioned about staff provisioning for valueology functioning in CEE.

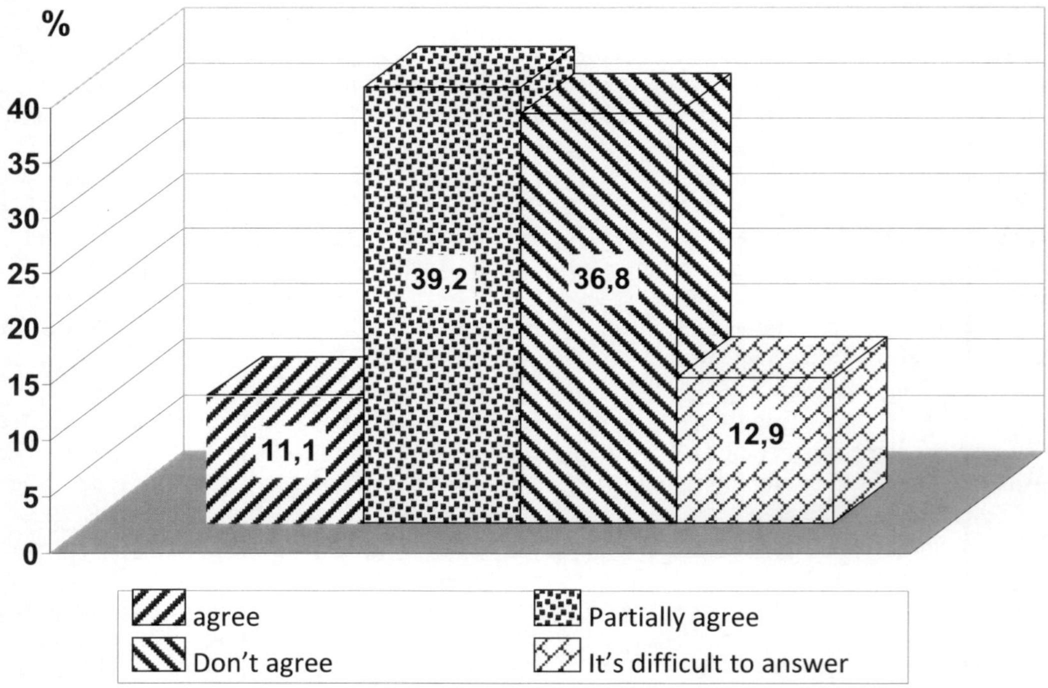

Fig.2. Quantity of students, questioned about knowledge of valueology functioning technologies in CEE (%).

Therefore, very little quantity of students, videlicet 11.1%, have sufficient level of valuelogy culture and knowledge about valueology functioning in CEE that witness about urgency and purposefulness of this problem.

Conclusions:

1. On the base of analysis of pedagogic literature and research of theoretical principles of professional training of future physical education instructors for valueology functioning in CEE we showed that only 11.7% of the questioned students have proper fitness and required knowledge and skills.

2. Formation of future physical education instructor's readiness for valueology functioning is oriented on opening of higher educational establishment student's potentials to successfully respond to new requirements of social environment.

3. Future physical education instructor in CEE shall be professionally competent creative, humanistic personality with prevailing spiritual-moral qualities and brightly expressed subjective position, individual style of functioning and significant creative potential.

The prospects of further researches in this direction are working out of scientific-methodic complexes for effective training of CEE future physical education instructor for practicing of valueology activity.

References:

1. Aliev M.N., Gusejnov A.G. Vospitanie nravstvenno-volevykh kachestv u detej sredstvami fizicheskoj kul'tury [Education of moral and volitional qualities in children by means of physical culture]. *Pedagogika*, 2008, no.1, pp. 67–73. (In Russian)
2. Kovtun R.F. *Podgotovka molodykh specialistov vysshikh uchebnykh zavedenij k vospitatel'noj rabote so studentami. Kand.diss.* [Training of graduates of higher educational institutions for educational work with students. Cand. Diss.], Chelyabinsk, 2005, 327 p. (In Russian)
3. Korotaeva E.V. Kachestvo podgotovki budushchego pedagoga [The quality of training of future teachers]. *Pedagogika* [Pedagogy], 2006, no.9, pp. 61–66. (In Russian)
4. Krucevich T.Iu. *Teoriia i metodika fizicheskogo vospitaniia* [Theory and methodology of physical education], Kiev, 2003, 423 p. (In Russian)
5. Kutek T. [Features of the learning process of future industry professionals "Physical Culture and Sports"]. *Molodaia sportivnaia nauka Ukrainy* [Young sports science in Ukraine], 2009, no.4, pp. 90 – 94. (In Russian)
6. Kuc A., Tret'iakov M., Lapichak I. Integraciia cennostej fizicheskoj kul'tury v professional'noj podgotovke pedagoga po fizicheskomu vospitaniiu [Integration of the values of physical culture in teacher training in physical education]. *Pedagogika, psihologia ta mediko-biologicni problemi fizicnogo vihovanna i sportu*, 2003, no.1 pp. 119–124. (In Russian)
7. Martishina N.V. Cennostnyj komponent tvorcheskogo potenciala lichnosti pedagoga [Value component of creative potential of the teacher]. *Pedagogika*, 2006, no.3, pp. 48–57. (In Russian)
8. Matveev L.P. *Teoriia i metodika fizicheskoj kul'tury* [Theory and methods of physical culture]. Sankt Petersburg, Lan, Omega, 2004, 159 p. (In Russian)
9. Moskalenko N.V. Innovacionnaia programma razvitiia fizkul'turno-ozdorovitel'noj raboty v obshcheobrazovatel'nykh shkolakh [Innovative program of development sports and recreation activities in secondary schools]. *Sportivnij visnik Pridniprov'ia*, 2005 no.2, pp. 37–40. (In Russian)
10. Nikolaev Iu.M. Obshchaia teoriia i metodologiia fizicheskoj kul'tury [General theory and methodology of physical education]. *Teoriia i praktika fizicheskoj kul'tury*, 2005, no.11, pp. 9–14. (In Russian)
11. About the state and prospects of development of adult education: college decision MES from 27.11.2008, vol. 14 / 3-3. Information Collection MES of Ukraine, 2009, no.1, pp. 31–45. (In Russian)
12. Skarednova I.V. [Development and implementation of modular routines aimed at creating culture of healthy and safe lifestyle of younger students]. *Opyt vnedreniia federal'nykh gosudarstvennykh obrazovatel'nykh standartov nachal'nogo obshchego obrazovaniia v Tiumenskoj oblasti* [Experience of implementing the federal state educational standards of primary education in the Tyumen region], Tyumen, 2012, pp. 33–36. (In Russian)
13. Solov'ev G.M. Genezis stanovleniia sovremennogo celepolaganiia po fizicheskoj kul'ture v sisteme obrazovaniia [The genesis of the emergence of modern goal setting in physical culture in the education system]. *Teoriia i praktika fizicheskoj kul'tury*, 2003, no.8, pp. 10–14. (In Russian)
14. Usol'ceva L.A. [Creating the conditions for a healthy lifestyle in a GEF implementing children]. *Opyt vnedreniia federal'nykh gosudarstvennykh obrazovatel'nykh standartov nachal'nogo obshchego obrazovaniia v Tiumenskoj oblasti* [Experience of implementing the federal state educational standards of primary education in the Tyumen region], Tyumen, 2012, pp. 32–33. (In Russian)
15. Iakovleva I.V. [Actual issues of culture of a healthy and safe lifestyle during the implementation of the GEF]. *Opyt vnedreniia federal'nykh gosudarstvennykh obrazovatel'nykh standartov nachal'nogo obshchego obrazovaniia v Tiumenskoj oblasti* [Experience of implementing the federal state educational standards of primary education in the Tyumen region], Tyumen, 2012 pp. 30–32. (In Russian)
16. Jang S-J., Tsai M-F., Chen H-Y. Development of PCK for novice and experienced university physics instructors: a case study. *Teaching in Higher Education*. 2013, vol.18, no.1, pp. 27-39. http://dx.doi.org/10.1080/13562517.2012.678329.

17. Osova O.O. contribution of native teachers of the second half of the XIX-th century to the working out of the teacher`s problem. *Pedagogics, Psychology, Medical-Biological Problems of Physical Training and Sports.* 2009, no.1, pp. 103 - 105.
18. Sá M.M., Azevedo R., Martins C., Machado O. Portuguese Physical Education Instructors' Exposure to Noise and Perception of Associated Risk. *Human and Ecological Risk Assessment: An International Journal.* 2014, vol.20, no.2, pp. 448-460. http://dx.doi.org/10.1080/10807039.2013.786922.
19. Semanyshyn T.M., Popel S.L. The professional valeological portrait of instructor of physical culture. *Pedagogics, psychology, medical-biological problems of physical training and sports*, 2014, no.10, pp. 41-44. http://dx.doi.org/10.5281/zenodo.10489
20. Whitehead K., Thorpe S. The problematic place of a woman physical education instructor: an historical case study. *Gender and Education.* 2004, vol.16, no.1, pp. 77-95. http://dx.doi.org/10.1080/0954025032000170354.

17

RESULTS OF EXPERIMENTAL TESTING OF HEE GIRL STUDENTS' MOTOR SKILLS AT AEROBIC TRAININGS

Martinova N. P.
Luhansk Taras Shevchenko National University

Abstract. *Purpose:* to analyze dynamic of motor skills' formation in girl students, who practice aerobic by experimental program. *Material:* in the research 40 girl students participated. Motor skills level was tested with the help of state and additional tests. *Results:* it was found that for training quickness it is necessary to use rope skipping in mode, corresponding to development of this quality. For training maximal strength it is purposeful to use more complex power exercises in ground part of the complex. *Conclusions:* implementation of rope skipping means in dance aerobic trainings increases training influence on practically all motor skills. Rope skipping permits to doze and regulate training load. The same under musical accompaniment develop sense of rhythm. In some modes such jumps facilitate training of speed power qualities and power endurance.
Key words: motor skills, aerobic, rope skipping, methodic, girl students, education.

Introduction

Training and perfection of students' motor skills in HEE is one of important and necessary component of discipline "Physical education". But recent years there have been observed weakening of students' motor skills, especially in girls [19, 21, 22].

Health related aerobic is a part of girl students' physical education practically in all HEEs. Interest to aerobics is conditioned by its high effectiveness, accessibility, bright emotional character and attractiveness [3, 20, 23].

Modern specialists worked out different approaches to development of motor skills at health related aerobic trainings. Methodic of motor skills' training on the base of graphic analytic models and bio-mechanical motor skills' indicators has been implemented [13]. Module technology of motor coordination training has also been implemented [16], and it permits to individualize training process on the base of girl students' potentials. Effectiveness of rhythm qualities simulation of girl students, who train health related aerobic has been experimentally substantiated [4].

Application of attractive kinds of training, considering girl students' individual features, is of the same importance for physical qualities' training [6–8, 10]. Specialists recommend not to limited to only one kind of aerobic. It is possible to vary them periodically [5]. Our attention was attracted by rope skipping aerobic. Specialists say that rope skipping is one of the best trainings by covering of muscular system and by its variety [9, 17]. The first rope skipping program was worked out by K. Cooper [5]. N.M. Amosov and I.V. Muravov think that it can not ensure versatile training of youth [1]. Analysis of scientific-methodic literature witnesses about absence of reliable aerobic rope skipping methodic for training of HEE girl students' motor skills. In this aspect the urgency of the topic of our research is rather evident.

Purpose, tasks of the work, material and methods

The purpose of the article is to analyze dynamic of motor skills' formation in girl students, who practice aerobic by experimental program and prove effectiveness of this program.

The methods and organization of the research: the research was conducted on the base of East-Ukrainian National university, named after Vladimir Dal. In experiment 40 girl students, who practice health related aerobic, participated. They were divided into two groups: experimental (EG) – 20 girls and control (CG) – 20 girls. CG girl students were trained by traditional program; EG girl students – by experimental methodic.

Level of motor skills was tested with state tests, envisaged by academic program for discipline "Physical education in HEE" and with additional tests.

Results of the researches

For training of girl students' motor skills at aerobic classes we offered experimental methodic. In dance aerobic program we introduced rope skipping. Such approach stipulates strengthening of aerobic influence on girl students' motor skills. For the period of experiment in both groups we registered confident improvement of results by all tested indicators (see table 1).

At the end of experiment we registered confident improvement of test results "2000meters' run" in EG – 11.03 ± 0.62 min ($p < 0.001$). It was 8.24% of increment in comparison with initial indicators. In CG we did not register any significant changes – 11.77 ± 0.52 min ($p < 0.001$), increment was 1.92%. Analysis of test "Long jump from the spot" showed significant difference in final CG indicators (1.69 ± 0.07 m) and in EG (1,77 ± 0,11 m) at level $p < 0.05$. Increment of CG results was 0.01 m ($p < 0.001$), and in EG – 0.11 m ($p < 0.001$). Increment of results in test "High jump from the spot" was in EG – 12.74% and in CG there were no significant changes (2.48%). Final result was, accordingly, the following: 38.05 ± 2.11 cm ($p < 0.001$) and 35.10 ± 2.20 cm ($p < 0.001$).

As we can see, in test "Torso risings in sitting position from lying position during 1 minute) confident increment of results was in both groups ($p < 0.001$). But in EG rate of increment was higher – 21.61%. It was very good result. In CG increment rate was only 4.31%. In test "100 meters' run" there were significant differences ($p < 0.001$) in both groups (EG – 17.09 ± 0.59 (2.57%), CG – 17.30 ± 0.67 (1.31%). Differences between final values between two groups were not significant ($p > 0.05$). In test "Shuttle run 4x9 m" we registered significant increment of indicators in EG – 6%. At the end of experiment result was 10.81 ± 0.35 sec. ($p < 0.001$). Control group indicators nearly did not change: 0.26%, 11.40 ± 0.48 sec. ($p < 0.001$). Increment of test "Pressing ups from the floor" did not have significant differences ($p > 0.05$) between EG (18.20 ± 7.06) and CG (15.55 ± 7.07). In test "Forward torso bending in sitting position" we registered confident changes in EG – 18.50 ± 3.79 cm, CG – 15.60 ± 4.65 cm ($p < 0.05$). Increment rates were accordingly: EG – 31.21%, CG – 12.23% .

To receive more information about effectiveness of experimental methodic we used additional tests (see table 2).

Changes in test "Rope skipping during 30 sec." were confident in every group and between groups ($p < 0.001$). At the end of experiment in EG (73.35 ± 3.56) there was much better result than CG 59.45 ± 6.92). Percentage of increment rates was in EG – 34.71% and in – 7.6%. Analysis of "Romberg's test" showed that EG girl students' balance indicators increased up to 13.35 ± 3.07 ($p < 0.001$). In CG they increased only to 6.45 ± 2.54 ($p < 0.001$). The registered differences were statistically confident at level $p < 0{,}001$.

Test "Integral coordination indicators" (ICI) [2] showed significant difference between results of both groups at level $p < 0.001$. Increment rate of ICI in EG was 84.32%. It witnesses about high level of jump coordination (0.72 ± 0.09, $p < 0.001$). CG girl students improved their results by 15% (0.46 ± 0.07, $p < 0.001$). We observed confident positive changes in rhythm of basic steps [7] ($p < 0.001$). In EG improvement of results was by 35.27% (14.00 ± 0.92points), in CG – by 19.25% (12.7 ± 1.08 points). Differences between groups also were of significance $p < 0.001$. Increment rates of jump rhythm in EG were 40.3% (4.70 ± 0.47points), and in CG – 20% (4.20 ± 0.52 points) ($p < 0.001$). The detected differences between EG and CG girl students in tapping test were statistically different at level $p < 0{,}01$ (right hand) and $p < 0.05$ (left hand). For example in EG increment rates were: right hand – 8.45% (214.25 ± 11.03 quantity of points), left hand – 5.88% (198.00 ± 10.73quantity of points). In CG they were accordingly 3.04% (203.157 ± 7.08 quantity of points) and 2.36% (191.00 ± 6.27 quantity of points).

Discussion

The conducted by us research expands the data about development of HEE girl students' motor skills. The research confirms the conclusions of specialists that aerobics permit to vary methodic depending on its purpose [15]. Application of various aerobic programs permits to obtain maximal use for minimal time [5].

In process of our work on the set problem we worked out and experimentally tested application of rope skipping in dance aerobic.

Analysis of scientific methodic literature witnesses that rope skipping permits to doze and regulate training load. As it is noted by scientists rope skipping is a men of training of general endurance [18]. Rope skipping under music accompaniment develops rhythm sense [14]. In certain modes of load they facilitate training of speed power and power endurance [11, 12].

Results of our research confirm it.

Conclusions

Thus, the received data witness about effectiveness of rope skipping implementation in dance aerobic trainings. Such approach increases training influence on practically all motor skills. For training quickness (in our opinion) it is necessary to use specialized exercises from light athletic or use rope skipping in mode, corresponding to development of this quality. We think to be purposeful to use more complex power exercises in ground part of the complex for development of maximal strength.

Acknowledgement

The research was conducted in compliance with scientific researches of department of physical education theory and methodic of Luhansk Taras Shevchenko National University – "Theory and methodic of senior pupils' profile training in sport directions in conditions of continuous education" (state registration number 108U002431).

Conflict of interests

The author declares that there is no conflict of interests.

Table 1. Dynamic of CG and EG girl students' motor skills progress by state tests

№	Tests	Period of testing	Statistic indicators					
			Control group		Experimental group		t	p
			n=20		n=20			
			X	σ	X	σ		
		beginning	17,53		17,54			
		end	17,30		17,09			
		t	7,452	0,77	14,673	0,63	-0,022	p1>0,05
1.	100 m run, *sec.*	p	**p3<0,001**	0,67	**p4<0,001**	0,59	1,049	p2>0,05
		increment of results	0.23		0.45			
		increment, %	1.31		2.57			
		beginning	12,00		12,02			
		end	11,77		11,03			
		t	6,920	0,51	66,359	0,65	-0,092	p1>0,05
2.	2000 m run, *min., sec*	p	**p3<0,001**	0,52	**p4<0,001**	0,62	4,105	**p2<0,001**
		increment of results	0.23		0.99			
		increment, %	1.92		8.24			
		beginning	13,9		14,1			
		end	15,6		18,5			
		t	-4,421	5,54	-11,000	4,15	-0,129	p1>0,05
3.	Flexibility, *cm*	p	**p3<0,001**	4,65	**p4<0,001**	3,79	-2,162	**p2<0,05**
		increment of results	-1.7		-4.4			
		increment, %	12.23		31.21			
		beginning	39,45		37,25			
		end	41,15		45,30			
		t	-5,840	2,21	-24,522	3,24	2,507	**p1<0,05**
4.	Torso rising in sitting position during 1 minute, *times*	p	**p3<0,001**	1,73	**p4<0,001**	3,26	-5,029	**p2<0,001**
		increment of results	-1.7		-8.05			
		increment, %	4.31		21.61			
		beginning	14,05		13,20			
		end	15,55		18,20			
		t	-4,943	8,14	-10,390	8,72	0,319	p1>0,05
5.	Pressing ups on the floor, *times*	p	**p3<0,001**	7,07	**p4<0,001**	7,06	-1,186	P2>0,05
		increment of results	-1.5		-5			
		increment, %	10.68		37.88			

6.	Shuttle run 4x9 m, *sec.*	beginning	11,43		11,5			
		end	11,40		10,81			
		t	1,045	0,50	20,673	0,37	0,538	p1>0,05
		p	p3>0,05	0,48	**p4<0,001**	0,35	-4,471	**p2<0,001**
		increment of results	0.03		0.69			
		increment, %	0.26		6			
		прирост, %						
7.	Long jump from the spot, m	beginning	1,68		1,66			
		end	1,69		1,77			p1>0,05
		t	-4,239	0,08	-27,341	0,13	0,651	**p1<0,05**
		p	**p3<0,001**	0,07	**p4<0,001**	0,11	-2,451	
		increment of results	-0.01		-0.11			
		increment, %	0.60		6.63			
8.	High jump from the spot, cm	beginning	34,25		33,75			
		end	35,10		38,05			
		t	-5,101	2,55	-15,253	2,15	0,670	p1>0,05
		p	**p3<0,001**	2,20	**p4<0,001**	2,11	-4,325	**p2<0,001**
		increment of results	-0.85		-4.3			
		increment, %	2.48		12.74			

Notes: p1 – confidence of differences of initial values
p2 - confidence of differences of final values
p3 – confidence of EG indicators' increment
p4 - confidence of CG indicators' increment

Table 2. Dynamic of CG and EG girl students' motor skills progress by additional tests

№	Tests	Period of testing	Statistic indicators					
			Control group		Experimental group		t	P
			n=20		n=20			
			X	σ	X	σ		
1.	Rope skipping, *times*	beginning end t p increment of results increment, %	55,25 59,45 -4,526 **P3<0,001** -4.2 7.6	8,22 6,92	54,45 73,35 -26,465 **P4<0,001** -18.9 34.71	5,34 3,56	0,365 -7,992	P1>0,05 **P2<0,001**
2.	Romberg's test, *sec.*	beginning end t p increment of results increment, %	5,30 6,45 -5,510 **P3<0,001** -1.15 21.7	2,60 2,54	5,55 13,35 -25,6 **P4<0,001** -7.8 140.54	1,99 3,07	-0,342 -7,746	P1>0,05 **P2<0,001**
3.	Integral coordination indicator, *m/sec.*	beginning end t p increment of results increment, %	0,40 0,46 -7,973 **P3<0,001** -0.06 15	0,06 0,07	0,39 0,72 -14,308 **P4<0,001** -0.33 84.62	0,09 0,09	0,219 -10,421	P1>0,05 **P2<0,001**
4.	Rhythm of basic steps, *points*	beginning end t p increment of results increment, %	10,65 12,7 -7,183 **P3<0,001** -2.05 19.25	1,18 1,08	10,35 14,00 -17,490 **P4<0,001** -3.65 35.27	1,35 0,92	0,748 -4,100	P1>0,05 **P2<0,001**
5.	Rhythm, of jumps, *points*	beginning end t p increment of results increment, %	3,50 4,20 -6,658 **P3<0,001** -0.7 20	0,51 0,52	3,35 4,70 -12,337 **P4<0,001** -1.35 40.3	0,49 0,47	0,946 -3,179	P1>0,05 **P2<0,01**

6.	Tapping test – right hand, *quantity of points*	beginning end t p increment of results increment, % прирост, %	197,15 203,15 -14,184 **P3<0,001** -6 3.04	8,27 7,08	197,55 214,25 -14,644 **P4<0,001** -16.7 8.45	13,25 11,03	-0,115 -3,788	P1>0,05 **P2<0,01**
7.	Tapping test –left hand, *quantity of points*	beginning end t p increment of results increment, %	186,60 191,00 -14,184 **P3<0,001** -4.4 2.36	6,89 6,27	187,00 198,00 -34,785 **P4<0,001** -11 5.88	10,96 10,73	-0,138 -2,519	P1>0,05 **P2<0,05**

Notes:
P1 – confidence of differences of initial values
P2 - confidence of differences of final values
P3 – confidence of EG indicators' increment
P4 - confidence of CG indicators' increment

References

1. Amosov NM, Muravov IV. *Serdce i fizicheskie uprazhneniia* [Heart and physical exercises], Kiev, Health; 1985. (in Ukrainian)
2. Bulkin VA, Popova EV, Saburova EV. Test dlia ocenki ballisticheskoj koordinacii dvigatel'noj deiatel'nosti [Test for assessment of ballistic coordination of motor functioning]. *Teoriia i praktika fizicheskoj kul'tury*, 1997;3:44–46. (in Russian)
3. Duliba OB. *Ocenka i optimizaciia umstvennoj i fizicheskoj rabotosposobnosti studentok sredstvami ritmicheskoj gimnastiki. Cand. Diss.* [Assessment and optimization of student's mental and physical workability by means of rhythmic gymnastic. Cand. Diss.], Lviv; 2000. (in Ukrainian)
4. Kostiunina LI. *Modelirovanie processa razvitiia ritmichnosti dvizhenij u studentok zanimaiushchikhsia ozdorovitel'noj aerobikoj. Cand. Diss.* [Simulation of rhythm training of students, who practice health related aerobics. Cand. Diss.], Ulyanovsk, 2006 (in Russian)
5. Kuper K. Aerobika dlia khoroshego samochuvstviia [Aerobics for good self-feeling],; 1989. (in Russian)
6. Martinova NP. Morfofunkcional'ni osoblivosti zhinochogo organizmu, shcho vplivaiut' na rozvitok rukhovikh iakostej [Morphological-functional characteristics of woman's organism, which influence on development of motor skills]. *Moloda sportivna nauka Ukraini*, 2014;18(3):128 – 132. (in Ukrainian)
7. Martinova NP. Novi vidi aerobiki, iak zasib rozvitku rukhovikh iakostej studentok VNZ [New kinds of aerobics as mean of HEE girl students' motor skills' training]. *Slobozhans'kij naukovo-sportivnij visnik*, 2014;1(39):62 – 65. (in Ukrainian)
8. Martinova NP. Viznachennia motiviv ta interesiv studentok VNZ do zaniat' z fizichnogo vikhovannia [Determination of HEE students' motives and interests to physical education classes]. *Naukovo-pedagogichni problemi fizichnoi kul'turi*, 2015;3(57, 15):218 – 222. (in Ukrainian)
9. Mil'ner E. Mozhno li zamenit' beg skakalkoj? [Can run be changed with skipping rope?], *Physical Culture and Sport;* 2008;12:2–5. (in Russian)
10. Nazarenko LD, Kostiunina LI, Krasnikova NV. Testirovanie urovnia razvitiia ritmichnosti pri zaniatiiakh ozdorovitel'noj aerobikoj [Testing of rhythm level at health related aerobic training]. *Teoriia i praktika fizicheskoj kul'tury*, 2005;4:57–63. (in Russian)
11. Pravdov MA. Vliianie zaniatij skippingom na fizicheskuiu podgotovlennost' studentov [Influence of rope skipping of students' physical fitness]. *Uchenye zapiski universiteta imeni P. F. Lesgafta*, 2010;7(65);64–67. (in Russian)
12. Pravdov MA, Korneva MA. Povyshenie effektivnosti zaniatij fizicheskoj kul'turoj so studentami na osnove skipinga [Increasing of physical culture students' training effectiveness on the base of rope skipping]. *Mezhdunarodnaia nauchnaia prakticheskaia konferenciia «Razvitie fizicheskoj kul'tury detej i uchashchejsia molodezhi», 2010, Shuya.* [International scientific-practical conference "Development of children's and students' physical culture" 2010, Shuya]. 2010. p. 174–176. (in Russian)
13. Red'ko TM. *Rozvitok rukhovikh iakostej studentok vishchogo navchal'nogo zakladu zasobami ritmichnoi gimnastiki. Cand. Diss.* [Training of HEE girl students' motor skills with means of rhythmic gymnastic. Cand. Diss.]. Chernigiv; 2012. (in Ukrainian)
14. Roters TT. *Muzykal'no – ritmicheskoe vospitanie i khudozhestvennaia gimnastika* [Musical-rhythmic education and calisthenics]. Moscow: Education; 1989. (in Russian)
15. Sinicia SV, Shesterova LIe. *Ozdorovcha aerobika* [Health related aerobics], Poltava: PNPU; 2011. (in Ukrainian)
16. Starkova EV. *Struktura i soderzhanie modul'noj tekhnologii razvitiia dvigatel'no-koordinacionnykh kachestv u studentok pedagogicheskikh vuzov* [Structure and content of module technology of motor skills' training in pedagogic HEEs girl students], *Teoriia i praktika fizicheskoj kul'tury*, 2009;5:31–36. (in Russian)
17. Krucevich TIu. *Teoriia i metodika fizicheskogo vospitaniia* [Theory and methodic of physical education], Kiev; 2003. (in Ukrainian)
18. Ter-Avanesian AA. *Pedagogicheskie osnovy fizicheskogo vospitaniia* [Pedagogic principles of physical education], Moscow: Physical Culture and Sport; 1978. (in Russian)
19. Fanygina OIu. *Korrekciia fizicheskoj podgotovlennosti studentok vuzov processe zaniatij ozdorovitel'nymi vidami plavaniia. Cand. Diss.* [Correction of HEEs girl students' physical fitness in trainings of health related swimming. Cand. Diss.], Kyiv; 2004. (in Ukrainian)
20. Chernenko OIe. *Pidvishchennia fizichnogo stanu studentok 18 – 19 rokiv zasobami fitbol – aerobiki. Cand. Diss.* [Improvement of 18–19 years old girl students' physical condition by fit-ball – aerobic means. Cand. Diss.], Dnipropetrovs'k; 2012. (in Ukrainian)
21. Beliak YuI, Zinchenko N. Dosing method of physical activity in aerobics classes for students. *Physical Education of Students,* 2014;5:8–13. http://dx.doi.org/10.15561/20755279.2014.0502
22. Bryukhanova NA, Bulgakova OV, Mokrova TI, Bogashchenko YA. Determination of possibilities of the use of high-intensive trainings facilities on lessons health aerobics. *Physical Education of Students*, 2013;2:25–29. http://dx.doi.org/10.6084/m9.figshare.156376

23. Furman YM, Salnikova SV. Improvement of aerobic energy supply processes in 37–49 yrs old women by means of complex aqua-fitness trainings' and methodic of endogenous – hypoxic breathing's application. *Pedagogics, psychology, medical-biological problems of physical training and sport.* 2015;7:59–63. http://dx.doi.org/10.15561/18189172.2015.0708
24. Kurmaeva EV. Fitness – programs as mean of forming of personality physical culture of students. *Physical Education of Students,* 2013;1:37–39. http://dx.doi.org/10.6084/m9.figshare.156355
25. Lambourne K, Hansen DM, Szabo AN, Lee J, Herrmann SD, Donnelly JE. Indirect and direct relations between aerobic fitness, physical activity, and academic achievement in elementary school students. *Mental Health and Physical Activity.* 2013;6(3):165–71.
26. Martyniuk OV. Justification for experimental methods for circuit training aerobics classes first mature age women. *Pedagogics, psychology, medical-biological problems of physical training and sports*, 2014;11:30–37. http://dx.doi.org/10.15561/18189172.2014.1106
27. Masliak IP. Physical health of young and middle age women under influence of step-aerobics exercises. *Pedagogics, psychology, medical-biological problems of physical training and sports.* 2015;10:45–50. http://dx.doi.org/10.15561/18189172.2015.1007
28. Pivneva MM, Rumba OG. Aerobics health as means of increasing somatic health of students of special medical group. *Pedagogics, psychology, medical-biological problems of physical training and sports*, 2013;8:74–87. http://dx.doi.org/10.6084/m9.figshare.747477
29. Pogrebniak IM, Kudelko VE, Nagovitsina OP. Effect of improving aerobics classes at the level of flexibility of female students. *Pedagogics, psychology, medical-biological problems of physical training and sports*, 2013;5:49–52. http://dx.doi.org/10.6084/m9.figshare.707099
30. Pop C, Ciomag V. The Influence of Aerobic Gymnastics on the Students' Body Image. *Procedia – Social and Behavioral Sciences.* 2014;117:129–35.
31. Rauner RR, Walters RW, Avery M, Wanser TJ. Evidence that Aerobic Fitness Is More Salient than Weight Status in Predicting Standardized Math and Reading Outcomes in Fourth – through Eighth-Grade Students. *The Journal of Pediatrics.* 2013;163(2):344–8.
32. Solanki R, Bhise A, Shukla Y, Prabhakar M. Effects of high intensity circuit training using body weight on aerobic fitness and muscular endurance in college students. *Physiotherapy*. 2015;101, Supplement 1:e1418–9.
33. Supilo IP. Biomechanical modeling of the physical training of girls during aerobic activities in non-school educational institutions. *Physical Education of Students,* 2014;6:73–76. http://dx.doi.org/10.15561/20755279.2014.0614
34. von Haaren B, Haertel S, Stumpp J, Hey S, Ebner-Priemer U. Reduced emotional stress reactivity to a real-life academic examination stressor in students participating in a 20-week aerobic exercise training: A randomised controlled trial using Ambulatory *Assessment. Psychology of Sport and Exercise*. 2015;20:67–75.

WORKING OUT OF HEALTH RELATED POWER LIFTING TRAINING PROGRAM FOR FIRST YEAR STUDENTS WITH MUSCULAR SKELETAL APPARATUS AFFECTIONS

Zhen Qiang San
Kharkov State Academy of Physical Culture

Abstract. *Purpose:* substantiation and working out of program for health improvement of first year students with muscular skeletal apparatus affections by power lifting means. *Material:* in experiment, which lasted one year, 24 first year students with muscular skeletal apparatus affections participated (two groups, 12 persons in each). The students' age was 18-20 years old. *Results:* optimal correlation of specific and non-specific loads – 60%:40% was found. The worked out complex of exercises for training of bench press barbell technique includes the following: special warming up exercises, exercises on special simulators and exercises with weights. As general physical training it is recommended to use complex of commonly accepted exercises. *Conclusions:* application of the worked out program ensures formation of steady interest to physical exercises' practicing, strengthening of health, replenishment of motor skills' base, training of motor qualities and functional fitness. Besides, it facilitates more effective students' social adaptation in collective.
Key words: experiment, health, power lifting, program, motor skills, students, testing.

Introduction

At modern stage of Ukraine development the problem of students' health improvement is still rather acute [7, 8, 20]. Diseases, connected with muscular skeletal apparatus (MSA) disorders, are the most often [19, 21, 29]. Such students additionally have problems with social adaptation in universities [11, 21]. Problem of social adaptation is the most acute for 1st year students with MSA affections. Sociological research, conducted by S.V. Korolinskaya (2011) [13] showed a number of social psychological factors, which determine effectiveness of students' adaptation to teaching educational process. The author recommends wide usage of physical culture for adaptation period's shortening and for increasing mental and physical workability.

The research by E.V. Makarova (2012) [16] permitted to mark out directions of students' adaptation to future profession. It was found that integrated and inclusive educational environment is an optimal form for provisioning of disabled youth with conditions for self expression, self-perfection and self-creation; for realization of rights and potentials, formation of personal significance and usefulness feeling.

Among many researches, devoted to problems of first year students' adaptation to HEE educational environment we can mark out the following works: Ye.L. Tomkiv (2008) [27], Ye.A. Belikova and O.L. Omelchenko (2010) [3], V.N. Kornilova and L.A. Prokopenko (2014) [12], T.Yu. Zharov et al. (2015) [10].

In the work by V.A. Druz et al. (2010) [9] directions of solution of re-socialization problems for disabled with MSA disorders are elucidated. The authors note demand in maximal consideration of kind of disease, degree of muscular skeletal apparatus disorders, individual features of physical loads' endurance. Besides, they supply recommendations on application of highly emotional exercises and games that facilitate more effective influence of used physical exercises.

As per specialists' recommendations one of ways of this problem's solution is practicing of different kinds of sports (power lifting, for example) [1, 8, 18]. In the work by Yu.V. Gordiyenko (2015) [6] it is shown, that power lifting trains girl students' ability to think independently; facilitates increase of self control and self analysis. It was found that correctly built training program facilitates strengthening of motivation for acquiring and mastering knowledge by girl students.

Internet information resources about power lifting are significant base for construction of training programs for students. For example, A.I. Stetsenko (2011) [25] thinks, that in Ukrainian speaking Internet environment power lifting is paid much more attention, comparing with other power kinds of sports. It promotes construction of students' power lifting program with better quality.

Speaking about students' power lifting, it is also necessary to pay attention to works by I.N. Manko (2009) [17], M.Yu. Minova (2010) [18], A.V. Gorbunova [5], Ye.V. Kurmayeva (2013) [14].

Alongside with it, power lifting trainings of students with MSA disorders have certain peculiarities. For example, in researches fulfilled by V.S. Lobko (2015) [15] we found distinctions between psycho-physiological characteristics, indicators of psychic state and features of students' personalities, depending on power lifting training experience. It was stated, that under influence of systemic power lifting trainings indicators of functional mobility and strength of nervous processes improve. The author also notes, that rising of students' sportsmanship is accompanied by noticeable improvement of practically all indicators.

By data of M.A. Al-Soub, R.V. Chudna and A.Kh. Khasan Faisal [2, 28, 29] it was found, that researches of the mentioned problem are of fragmentary character. Analysis of researches on problem of health related power lifting programs for first year students with MSA affections points at demand in additional researches.

Purpose, tasks of the work, material and methods

The purpose of the work is to work out program of power lifting health related trainings for first year students with affections of muscular skeletal apparatus.

Material and methods of the research: in experiment, which lasted one year, 24 first year students with muscular skeletal apparatus affections participated (two groups, 12 persons in each). The students' age was 18-20 years old

According to the tasks of the research we conducted experiment, which lasted one year. As a hypothesis we assumed possibility of working out of power lifting training program, which would consider correlation of specific and non specific training means in year cycle of first year students with MSA affections. In this connection we conducted pedagogic experiment with participation of two groups, consisting of first year students with MSA affections, who did not practice physical culture or sports before entering university. Both groups consisted of 12 students and had no confident differences by main indicators: functional, physical and psychological fitness. In the course of experiment groups 1 and 2 fulfilled different correlation of specific and non specific loads: in group 1– 60%:40%; in group 2 – 70%:30%.

Results of the research

More specific of training means in both groups is given in table 1.

Table 1. Year volumes of main training means of 1st year students – power lifters in group 1 and 2.

Min means of training	Group 1	Group 2
Quantity of trainings	120	120
Quantity of training hours	216.4	217.2
Quantity of competitions	4	4
Theoretical training, hours	4	4
Quantity of barbell lifting,	2411.5	2656.7
Including with intensity:		
up to 50% from maximal, %	40	32
up to 60% from maximal, %	20	22
up to 70% from maximal, %	20	22
up to 80% from maximal, %	10	12
up to 95% from maximal, %	10	12
Means of general physical training, including exercises by individual plan, hours	91.2	82.1
Exercises in game form and recreation, hours	3.5	3.5

In summer period of experiment as specific loads we used complex of exercises for training of barbell bench press technique, special warming up exercises, exercises on special simulators and exercises with weights. As general training means, in the course of all experiment, we used complex of commonly accepted exercises. Testing of 1st and 2nd groups' students, conducted at the end of experiment, permitted to register noticeable progress of functional, physical and psychological fitness indicators. For example, in 1st group volume of chest in inhale, exhale and in pause increased accordingly by 5.8; 5.7; 7.5% ($p < 0.05$). Vital capacity of lungs increased statistically significantly by 427.2 ml. Significant improvement of respiratory system's functional state was also registered in Stange's test –19.9% and in Genchi's test – by 37.9% ($p < 0.05$). Quantity of front and back claps (students' speed qualities) increased by 21.6% ($p < 0.05$). Final results in throw of medicine ball from behind the head – forward and from behind the head – backward increased accordingly by 16.8 and 13%. The highest progress (by 46.7%) was noticed in main competition exercise – bench press of barbell. Significant progress of motor and coordination potentials was accompanied by perfection of psycho-physiological indicators. For example, students of 1st group demonstrated reduction of simple visual response latent period by 22.2% ($p < 0.05$). Accordingly latent periods of choice of one from three irritators improved statistically significantly by 19.6 and 28.2%. Widening of students – power lifters' circle of conditional reflex links reflected in indicators of functional mobility (by 10.5%) and power of nervous processes (by 39%). At the end of experiment statistically significant positive changes were registered in 1st group by such, important for disabled, characteristics as psychic state and properties of personality.

Analysis of 2nd group students' psycho-physiological indicators also showed their improvement at the end of experiment. Though, we did not register statistically significant changes ($p > 0.05$). Experimental data permitted also to find that group 1 had noticeable superiority by indicators of respiratory system's functional state. For example, volume of chest at inhale, exhale and pause in 1st group was 82.7 cm, 72.4 cm, 77.3 cm in contrast to 79 cm, 70.1 cm, 72.4 cm in group 2. Also in group 1 there is higher level of vital capacity of lungs: 2718.9 ml in contrast to 2583.3 ml in 2nd group ($p < 0.05$). Comparison of students' physical fitness at the end of experiment showed the following (see table 2). Power lifters of 1st group demonstrated higher results in tests for quickness and speed power. With it differences between two groups were statistically significant. Statistically significant distinctions between groups were also registered in indicators of static endurance of strong and weak hands. In other tests we did not notice statistically significant difference ($p > 0.05$).

Table 2. Sport results and motor qualities indicators of students – power lifters with MSA disorders in group 1 and 2 at the end of experiment

The tested indicators		**Group 1 (n=12)**		**p**	**Group 2 (n=12)**	
		$\overline{X}$	**m**		$\overline{X}$	**m**
Front and back claps during 10 sec., quantity		23.15	0.21	<0.05	20.14	0.26
Forward throw of medicine ball from behind the head, m		4.52	0.03	<0.05	4.21	0.05
Backward throw of medicine ball from behind the head, m		4.38	0.03	<0.05	4,\.11	0.03
Bench press of barbell in lying position, kg		64.53	2.17	>0.05	66.91	2.11
Strong arm's mobility in shoulder joint, degrees		70.18	2.18	>0.05	70.92	2.46
Weak arm's mobility in shoulder joint, degrees		69.53	2.68	>0.05	69.87	2.84
Static endurance of strong hand, sec.		11.4	0.02	<0.05	8.1	0.03
Static endurance of weak hand, sec.		10.1	0.01	<0.05	6.9	0.02
Total indicator of strength of 5 muscular groups of strong arm, kg	absolute	169.8	3.96	>0.05	172.9	4.29
	relative	2.70	0.03	>0.05	2.79	0.04
Total indicator of strength of 5 muscular groups of weak arm, kg	absolute	157.5	3.75	>0.05	161.3	3.84
	relative	2.51	0.04	>0.05	2.61	0.03

At the end of experiment in both groups all psycho-physiological indicators improved. With it, more positive changes were in power lifters of group 1. Calculation of confidence of differences between indicators of group 1 and group 2 showed statistically significant superiority of group 1. Exclusion was indicator of latent period response when choosing one irritator from three (p> 0.05). Testing of psychic state and personalities' features in group 1 and group 2 at the end of experiment showed that in group1 there was higher level of nervous psychic stability in motivation for success and avoiding failure; besides there were statistically significant differences between groups.

Discussion

Final data of experiment confirmed actual materials of pedagogues, psychologists, medical workers, specialists in therapeutic physical culture, conches of sports for disabled about effective impact of regular physical exercises' practicing on physical health of disabled [1, 4, 7, 11, 21, 26, 31, 33]. In our experiment we realized, to some extent, principle, offered by L. Vygotskiy:

1) Observation of pedagogic actions' orientation on weakening of physical and psychic defects of children with health problems;
2) Active development of cognitive functioning, psychic processes, physical abilities and moral qualities of children [22-24, 30].

Results of our researches supplement the data of other authors (Trinkaus E., Rhoads M.L., 1999 [41]; Rossouw F., Krüger P.E., Rossouw J., 2000 [39]; Keogh J.W.L., Hume P.A., Pearson S.N., Mellow P., 2007 [36]; Jensen A.M., 2010 [35]; Hale B.D., Roth A.D., DeLong R.E., Briggs M.S., 2010 [34]; Kozub F.M., Brusseau T.A., 2012 [37]; Lewis C., 2015 [38]) about positive influence of power lifting specific loads on students' health.

Results of our researches also confirmed the data of V.S. Lobko (2015) [15] that systemic power lifting trainings facilitate improvement of functional mobility and nervous processes' power indicators.

The received by us results permit to speak about more effective influence of power lifting means on indicators of students with MSA disorders. Such influence is ensured by:

1) Correlation of specific and non specific loads – 60%:40%;
2) Application of worked out complex of exercises for training barbell bench press technique, which included special warming up exercises, exercises on special simulators and exercises with weights.

Conclusions:

1. It was found that recent years methodic of disabled health improvement through trainings in separate kinds of sports has been being prevailed. In our research we tried to substantiate program of health related power lifting trainings for first year students with disorders of muscular skeletal apparatus.
2. In the course of experiment we solved the task – determination of optimal parameters of physical loads in year cycle of power lifting training of students with MSA affections. The conducted during one year experiment permitted to substantiate optimal program of power lifting trainings for first year students with MSA disorders, which envisages application of specific and non specific loads in proportion 60% and 40%. Application of the worked out program ensures formation of steady interest to physical exercises' practicing, development of motor skills and functional fitness as well as facilitates more effective students' social adaptation in collective.

The prospects of further researches in this direction can be connected with studying of competition loads influence on students-power lifters' organism.

Acknowledgement

The topic of our research is an integral part of scientific research work's program of Kharkov State academy of physical culture. The work has been fulfilled in compliance with "Combined plan of scientific research work in sphere of physical culture and sports for 2011–2015" by topic 2.4 "Theoretical-methodic principles of individualization in education and sports" (state registration N 0112U002001) as well as in compliance with scientific-research project for 2013–2015 "Theoretical-methodic provisioning of formation of personality's healthy life style in conditions of educational establishment and in context of European integration" (state registration N 0114U001781) of Ministry of education and science of Ukraine.

Conflict of interests

The author declares that there is no conflict of interests.

References:

1. Vinnik DP. *Adaptivnoe fizicheskoe vospitanie i sport* [Adaptive physical education and sports], Kiev: Olympic Literature; 2010. (in Russian)
2. Al'-Soub MA. Kontrol' velichini fizichnikh navantazhen' futbolistiv z naslidkami ditiachogo cerebral'nogo paralichu [Control of physical loads values of football players with after-effects of cerebral palsy]. *Visnik Chernigivs'kogo nacional'nogo pedagogichnogo universitetu imeni Tarasa Shevchenka,* 2011;91:203–204. (in Ukrainian)
3. Belikova EA, Omel'chenko OL. K voprosu o sostoianii zdorov'ia studentov I kursa v period adaptacii k usloviiam VUZA [On the problem of s1st year students' health condition in adaptation period to HEE conditions]. *Zdorov'e i obrazovanie v XXI veke*, 2010;12(7):334. (in Russian)
4. Valeev N, Zakharova L, Ganzina N. Poisk novykh form fizkul'turno-rekreativnoj deiatel'nosti v processe reabilitacii invalidov s posledstviiami detskogo cerebral'nogo paralicha [Searching of new forms of physical culture – recreation activity in rehabilitation of disabled with after-effects of cerebral palsy]. *Mezhdunarodnyj Kongress "Chelovek v mire sporta"* [International congress "Man in the world of sports"]. Moscow; 1998. p. 524–525. (in Russian)
5. Gorbunov AV. Pauerlifting v sisteme fizicheskogo vospitaniia studentov [Power lifting in system of students' physical education]. *Izvestiia Volgogradskogo gosudarstvennogo tekhnicheskogo universiteta,* 2012;9(11,98):38–41. (in Russian)
6. Gordienko YV. Theoretical training in physical education of higher educational establishments' girl students. *Physical education of students*, 2015;4:3–9. http://dx.doi.org/10.15561/20755279.2015.0401
7. Guzij OV. *Zasobi fizichnogo vikhovannia u fizichnij reabilitacii ditej z cerebral'nim* paralichem [Physical education means in physical rehabilitation of children with cerebral palsy], Lviv: Ukrainian technologies; 2002. (in Ukrainian)
8. Denisenko N. Osoblivosti rivnia zdorov'ia, fizichnoi pidgotovlenosti, samopochuttia ta vedennia zdorovogo sposobu zhittia v uchniv zagal'noosvitnikh shkil i gimnazij [Specific features of health, physical fitness, self feeling and practicing of healthy life style of comprehensive schools' and gymnasiums' pupils]. *Slobozhans'kij naukovo-sportivnij visnik,* 2007;3:44–46. (in Ukrainian)
9. Druz' VA, Klimenko AI, Pomeshchikova IP. Social'naia adaptaciia lic s narusheniiami oporno-dvigatel'nogo apparata sredstvami fizicheskogo vospitaniia [Social adaptation of patients with muscular skeletal apparatus disorders by means of physical education]. *Physical education of students*, 2010;1:34–37.
10. Zharova TIu, Kulikov NM, Ekhlakova MA. Obshchestvennaia napravlennost' lichnosti studenta-pervokursnika v processe adaptacii k obucheniiu v VUZE [Social orientation of first year student's personality in process of adaptation to studying at HEE]. *Diskussiia*, 2015;1(53):127–131. (in Russian)
11. Ivanova IB. Do pitannia social'no-psikhologichnoi adaptacii molodikh invalidiv [On the problem of social-psychological adaptation of young disabled]. *Molodizhni problemi v Ukraini: stan ta shliakhi virishennia* [Problems of youth in Ukraine: situation and ways of solution]. Lviv; 1997. P. 81–84. (in Ukrainian)
12. Kornilova VN, Prokopenko LA. Adaptaciia studentov-pervokursnikov k obucheniiu v vuze cherez sredstva fizicheskoj kul'tury i sporta [Adaptation of first year students to studying at HEE through means of physical culture and sports]. *Mezhdunarodnyj zhurnal eksperimental'nogo obrazovaniia*, 2014;7(1):50–51. (in Russian)
13. Korolinskaia SV. Nekotorye problemy adaptacii inostrannykh studentov anglijskogo otdeleniia NFAU [Some adaptation problems of foreign students of English department of NPAU]. *Physical education of students,* 2011;4:48 – 51.
14. Kurmaeva E.V., Fitness – programs as mean of forming of personality physical culture of students. *Physical education of students*, 2013;1:37–39. http://dx.doi.org/10.6084/m9.figshare.156355.
15. Lobko VS. Psycho-physiological characteristics of students-powerlifters of different training experience, who have affections of muscular skeletal apparatus. *Pedagogics, psychology, medical-biological problems of physical training and sports,* 2015;5:22–26. http://dx.doi.org/10.15561/18189172.2015.0504
16. Makarova EV. Podkhody k povysheniiu effektivnosti processa obucheniia i budushchej professional'noj deiatel'nosti studentov s invalidnost'iu [Approaches to increase of effectiveness of training process and future professional functioning of disabled students]. *Physical education of students*, 2012;5:64–68.

17. Man'ko IN. Razvitie sily u studentov fizkul'turnykh vuzov na zaniatiiakh po silovoj podgotovke [Development of strength of physical culture HEEs' students at power training classes]. *Pedagogics, psychology, medical-biological problems of physical training and sports,* 2009;7:113 – 121.
18. Minov MIu. Pauerlifting kak effektivnoe sredstvo razvitiia fizicheskikh kachestv i ukrepleniia zdorov'ia studentov [Power lifting as effective mean of physical qualities' training and strengthening of students' health]. *Vestnik Krasnoiarskogo gosudarstvennogo pedagogicheskogo universiteta im. V.P. Astaf'eva*, 2010;2:47–51. (in Russian)
19. Perederij AV. Osoblivosti metodiki tekhnichnoi pidgotovki sportsmeniv-invalidiv z poshkodzhenniami oporno-rukhovogo aparatu [Specific features of technical training methodic for disabled sportsmen with disorders of muscular skeletal apparatus]. *Pedagogics, psychology, medical-biological problems of physical training and sports*, 1999;11:9–12. (in Ukrainian)
20. Platonov VN. *Obshchaia teoriia podgotovki sportsmenov olimpijskom sporte* [General theory of sportsmen's training in Olympic sports]. Kiev: Olympic Literature; 1997. (in Russian)
21. Prokopova LI. Deiaki problemi social'noi reabilitacii invalidiv zasobami fizichnoi kul'turi [Some problems of social rehabilitation of disabled by means of physical culture]. *II Vseukrains'ka naukova praktichna konferenciia "Koncepciia pidgotovki specialistiv fizichnoi kul'turi v Ukraini".* [2nd All Ukrainian scientific-practical conference "Conception of physical culture specialists' training in Ukraine"]. Kiev; 1996. p. 421–425. (in Ukrainian)
22. Romanova OL. Psikhologicheskoe izuchenie mekhanizmov formirovaniia lichnosti bol'nykh detskim cerebral'nym paralichom [Psychological study of personality's formation mechanisms of patients with cerebral palsy], *Narusheniia povedeniia u detej podrostkov* [Adolescents' behavior disorders], Moscow; 1982. p. 101–107. (in Russian)
23. Sermeev BV, Efimenko NN. Individual'no-differencirovannyj podkhod v processe korrekcii dvigatel'nykh narushenij u detej, stradaiushchikh cerebral'nym paralichom [Individual-differentiated approach in correction of motor disorders of children with cerebral palsy]. *Fizicheskoe vospitanie detej v special'nykh shkolakh* [Physical education of children in special schools], Bitter; 1980. p. 86–98. (in Russian)
24. Sin'ov VM, Kobernik GM. *Osnovi defektologii* [Principles of defectology], Kiev: High School; 1994. (in Ukrainian)
25. Stecenko AI. Teoretiko-metodicheskoe obespechenie uchebnogo processa studentov-pauerlifterov s pomoshch'iu internet-resursov [Theoretical methodic provisioning of students – power lifters' education with Internet resources]. *Pedagogics, psychology, medical-biological problems of physical training and sports,* 2011;11:118–123.
26. Tikhonova VA, Sidorko IV, Chesnokov GS. Vpliv rozvitku psikhomotornoi funkcii na formuvannia rukhovikh navichok na urokakh fizichnoi kul'turi [Influence of psycho-motor function's development on formation of motor skills at physical culture lessons]. *Teoriia ta praktika fizichnogo vikhovannia*, 2001;4:8–10. (in Ukrainian)
27. Tomkiv EL. Vzaimosviaz' social'nykh znachenij i cennostej [Interconnection of social meanings and values]. *Sovremennye gumanitarnye issledovaniia,* 2008;4:185–187. (in Russian)
28. Fajsal AKhKh. Kharakteristika izmenenij psikhofiziologicheskikh pokazatelej u studentov, perenesshikh zabolevanie cerebral'nym paralichom v processe mnogoletnikh zaniatij legkoatleticheskimi metaniiami [Characteristic of psycho-physiological indicators' changes of students with after effects of cerebral palsy in process of many years trainings of light athletic throws]. *Visnik Lugans'kogo nacional'nogo universitetu imeni Tarasa Shevchenka,* 2013;8:194–200. (in Russian)
29. Chudnaia RV. *Adaptivnoe fizicheskoe vospitanie* [Adaptive physical education]. Scientific opinion; 2000. (in Russian)
30. Shapkova LV. Opornye koncepcii metodologii adaptivnoj fizicheskoj kul'tury [Supporting concepts of adaptive physical culture methodology]. *Teoriia i praktika fizicheskoj kul'tury*, 1998;1:8–19. (in Russian)
31. Shtengerc S. Vpliv fizichnikh vprav na khvoru ditinu [Influence of physical exercises on sick child], *Koncepciia rozvitku galuzi fizichnogo vikhovannia i sportu v Ukraini*, 1999;1:57–59. (in Ukrainian)
32. Enoka RM. *Neuromechanical basis of kinesiology*. 2nd ed., Champaign, Leeds: Human Kinetics; 1994.
33. Gage JR. *Gate analysis in cerebral palsy*. London: Mac Keith Press; 1991.

34. Hale BD, Roth AD, DeLong RE, Briggs MS. Exercise dependence and the drive for muscularity in male bodybuilders, power lifters, and fitness lifters. *Body Image*. 2010;7(3):234–239.
35. Jensen AM. A mind-body approach for precompetitive anxiety in power-lifters: 2 case studies. *Journal of Chiropractic Medicine.* 2010;9(4):184–192.
36. Keogh JWL, Hume PA, Pearson SN, Mellow P. Anthropometric dimensions of male powerlifters of varying body mass. *Journal of Sports Sciences*. 2007;25(12):1365–1376.
37. Kozub FM, Brusseau TA. Powerlifting. *Journal of Physical Education, Recreation & Dance*. 2012;83(3):34–41.
38. Lewis C. Another sports drug-testing failure: Australian government policy and powerlifting. *International Journal of Sport Policy and Politics.* 2015;7(2):233–253.
39. Rossouw F, Krüger PE, Rossouw J. The effect of creatine monohydrate loading on maximal intermittent exercise and sport-specific strength in well trained power-lifters. *Nutrition Research*. 2000;20(4):505–514.
40. Tremblay L, Proteau L. Specificity of Practice: The Case of Powerlifting. *Research Quarterly for Exercise and Sport.* 1998;69(3):284–289.
41. Trinkaus E, Rhoads ML. Neandertal knees: power lifters in the Pleistocene? *Journal of Human Evolution.* 1999;37(6):833–859.

STUDY OF SPECIFICITIES OF ARM WRESTLERS' PSYCHOLOGICAL STATUS IN COMPETITION PERIOD

Podrigalo L. V., Galashko M. N., Galashko N. I.
Kharkov State Academy of Physical Culture

Abstract. *Purpose:* researching and analysis of psychological status dynamic of different qualification arm-wrestlers in competitions' condition. *Material:* in the research 21 students-sportsmen of 17-24 years' age participated. *Results:* before the beginning of competition experienced sportsmen are characterized by higher workability in comparison with beginners – (56.61±8.31) % against (23.23±11.93) %. After competitions among experienced sportsmen 57.14% had reduced anxiety; 71.43% - reduced activity and self-feeling; 50% - had worse mood. After competitions among sportsmen-beginners 73.73% demonstrated reduction of workability; 54.54% had weakened activity, mood and self-feeling. We established significant prevalence of statistically confident correlations among experienced sportsmen: 65.15% against 46.97%. Contribution of psychological components in system of sportsmen-beginners is significantly lower than of experienced sportsmen. *Conclusions:* we determined certain changes of psychological status of arm-wrestlers of different qualification under influence of competitions. For experienced sportsmen we confirmed more optimal status and favorable dynamic, illustrating high reliability of functioning.
Key words: arm-wrestling, psychology, inter-connections, students, competitions.

Introduction

Sport functioning is characterized by rather intensive impact on psychic, which is conditioned by its stress-genic influence. Factors of sport stress include: competitive character of sport struggle, oriented on record or victory; maximal tension of all physical and psychic forces of a sportsman; systemic sport training, which contributes serious corrections to mode of life; domestic conditions of sportsmen [2].

Success and rising of sportsmanship in every kind of sports are determined by complex, which includes (together with physical and functional components) psychic features [2, 15, 17, 20, 21, 25, 27, 28, 34]. With levels of physical fitness being nearly equal, exactly psychological fitness becomes a decisive factor for achievement of high results and ability to control it is a criterion of successfulness [4, 10]. We have determined certain distinctions in psychological status of sportsmen of different qualification; for example more experienced sportsmen are more aggressive than representatives of mass sport or people, who do not practice sports at all [12, 22, 32]. Development of sportsmen's skills of self-regulation is of great importance for maximal realization of their potentials [10, 13, 14, 23, 30, 31, 33]. Among factors, which condition formation of these mechanisms, central place is taken by self-assessment. It determines orientation and level of subject's activity, formation of his (her) personality [11, 24, 26, 29]. In martial arts competition result to large extent depends on sportsman's psychic status. Psychological training of a sportsman shall result in stability of combat fitness, i.e. in maximal mobilization for achievement of result [4].

For achievement of elite level in arm wrestling (AW) importance of sportsmen's morphological-functional state was confirmed [6, 7]. Considering specificities of this kind of sports (as martial art) psychological status acquires great significance; it's dynamic in process of training and competition loads. However, till present time there have been absent works, devoted to studying of this scientific task. It predetermined the urgency of our researches.

Purpose, tasks of the work, material and methods

The purpose of the work was research and analysis of psychological status dynamic of AW sportsmen of different qualification under influence of competition loads.

The participants of the research (21 AW sportsmen) were divided into two groups, depending on their sportsmanship: 1st group – 7 persons (mean age 23.71± 1.44 years), qualification – from 1st grade to master of sports; 2nd group – 11 participants (mean age 18.55± 0.68 years, 3 - sportsmen of mass grades.

The structure of the research implied studying and analysis of sportsmen's psychological status before and after competitions. As a test instrument we used complex test TPAHC, worked out by specialists of Kharkov national medical university. Choice of test was conditioned by researches, which proved its adequacy in studying of influence of intensive visual-information loads on schoolchildren's functional state and by available information about significant fluctuations of psychological status (as components of forming pre-nosological state) [3, 5].

The test permits to determine dynamic of such indicators as anxiety, workability, activity, mood and self-feeling. The tool for self assessment is a blank form, consisting of 40 lines. Information is presented as two adjectives, opposite by meaning as well as in the form of digits, which mean degree of expressiveness of every sign: 3 – strong expressiveness; 2 – middle; 1 – weak expressiveness of sign. Methodic of data processing is analogous to test SAM (Self-feeling, Activity, Mood) [9].

The research was conducted before and after competitions. Interval between tests was in group 1st - (3.47±0.55) hours, in group 2nd - (3.57±0.38) hours. It permits to speak about closeness of time intervals, to presuppose type-likeness of adaptation responses.

Statistical analysis of the received data was carried out with the help of license packages of electronic table Excel with determination of parametric and non-parametric criteria [1].

Results of the research

Results of the research (see table 1) permit to say about closeness of psychological statuses of the participants of the researches and witness about similar orientation of their changes in dynamic of competitions and depending on level of sportsmanship.

Table 1

Psychological status of arm wrestlers in dynamic of competitions

Indicators (%)	1st group	2nd group
Initial anxiety	47.09±11.62[3]	21.55±9.31
Final anxiety	52.37±4.88[1]	18.18±9.93
Initial workability	56.61±8.31[1]	23.23±11.93
Final workability	31.74±7.09[2]	21.55±9.64
Initial activity	38.08±13.38	21.97±10.16
Final activity	30.36±10.27	17.42±8.22
Initial state of mood	55.41±9.20	33.05±9.67
Final state of mood	46.75±15.99	24.52±12.33
Initial self feeling	62.71±11.89	41.53±11.43
Final self feeling	44.28±8.28	36.97±9.23

Notes: 1 – distinctions between groups are confident ($p<0.05$), 2 – distinctions in dynamic are confident ($p<0.05$), 3 – tendency to confidence of distinctions between groups ($p<0.1$).

Before competitions experienced sportsmen are characterized by higher workability, comparing with the beginners. It, in our opinion, shall be assessed as evidence of better readiness for competitions. At the same time anxiety in 1st group was confidently higher than in the 2nd. This fact, considering situational character of this quality shall be assessed as positive factor, illustrating response to results of performances.

Besides, in group of experienced sportsmen we found confident reduction of workability in dynamic of competitions with the help of parametric criterion (Student's criterion) and non-parametric indicators (the sign criterion). In our opinion it can be assessed as evidence of forming in the process of competitions fatigue and as indirect illustration of full dedication of sportsmen to this functioning. The determined tendency to increasing of anxiety level before competitions in the given context can be explained by experienced sportsmen's stress of expectation.

With regarding the question from position of reliability of systems' functioning studying of situational anxiety is more interesting. It is conditioned by the fact that sportsman can "adjust" to competition process, "to subdue" this anxiety at the account of experience and certain adaptation to stresses, appearing in connection with competition functioning. Thus, he can increase his psychological stability. It is known that the oftener sportsman "oversteps" his fear the more adequate his response in extreme situation is; the higher hid psychological stability (reliability) is [4].

Using conception "pre-nosological diagnostic" in context of sportsmen's functional fitness, it is necessary to regard initial state as reflection of functioning level. Final state shall be regarded as illustration of functional reserves [5]. In our case stability of output functional characteristics of system is the basis of its high reliability, ensuring effective achievement of goals of functioning.

Analysis of individual features also permitted to find out certain distinctions between groups. Before competitions experienced sportsmen did not demonstrate negative indicators of anxiety, workability, mood and self-feeling. Only one participant (14.29%) had negative value of activity. At the same time in 2nd group negative indicators of anxiety were intrinsic to 4 participants (36.36%), workability – to 3 (27.27%), activity, mood and self feeling – to 2 sportsmen (18.18%). After competitions in 1st group there were no negative indicators of anxiety, workability and self feeling. 1 participant (14.29%) was characterized by negative activity and 2 (28.58%) – by negative state of mood. At the same time, after competitions among sportsmen-beginners 3 persons (27.27%) had negative indicators of anxiety and mood, 2 (18.18%) – workability and self-feeling and 1 (9.09%) – activity. The received data permit to speak about worse psychological status of sportsmen-beginners and its more expressed aggravation under influence of competition loads, comparing with experienced colleagues.

Insufficient scope of samples conditioned increase of error of mean group values that does not permit to speak about confident shifts; however it gives basis for determination of tendencies of changes. For example we found out that after competitions in 1st group 57.14% of participants were characterized by reduction of anxiety, 71.43% had weakened activity and self-feeling and 50% - state of mood. These shifts confirm made earlier assumptions about formation of fatigue and tiredness against the background of optimizing of psycho-emotional status.

We received interesting data when analyzing results of two masters of sports, who participated in our researches. They were characterized by increasing of activity and state of mood with minima negative changes in self feeling and workability. One of them demonstrated reduction of anxiety, the second – its minimal growth. Thus, the presented data permit to assume that experienced sportsmen are characterized by optimizing of psychological status and high stress-resistance. Such level of stability ensures increase of reliability of organism's functioning in extreme conditions.

In 2nd group reduction of anxiety and workability was registered in 73.73% of participants, while 54.54% had reduction of activity, state of mood and self-feeling. I.e. sportsmen-beginners had more expressed negative changes of psychological status. They reflect not only already formed fatigue but also witness about lower level of psychological readiness for competition loads.

Our researches confirmed validity of correlation matrixes method for analysis of AW sportsmen's condition [6] that exactly conditioned its usage in the given case. Main indicators of correlation structures are given in table 2.

Table 2

Indicators of correlation matrixes of arm wrestlers' psychological status

Group	Specific weight of significant correlations (%)	Specific weight of confident correlations (%)	Indicator of labilization/synchronization (%)	Mean coefficient of correlation
1	65.15	18.18	22.22	0.56
2	46.97	30.30	16.56	0.56

Substantial prevalence of significant connections among correlations of 1st group sportsmen was established that shall be assessed as evidence of their more stable status, i.e. better fitness for competitions. In respect to specific weight of confident connections situation is opposite that conditioned by different quantity of groups' members. For example in 1st group minimal value of confident correlation ($p<0.05$) was 0.67. Then in 2nd group it was 0.55. It resulted in substantial differences between specific weights of the mentioned correlations. So it seems to be possible to compare correlation matrixes just by quantity of significant connections.

Increase of labilization/synchronization indicator in 1st group confirms mentioned earlier assumption about better functional state of experienced sportsmen. Their organisms are characterized by more balanced, more synchronized state. Lability of functions is less, comparing with sportsmen-beginners. It permits to predict high level of successfulness. The value of mean correlation coefficient in both cases was the same and related to interval of mean correlations. It permits to consider that in both cases systems were sufficiently stable, without rough violations, facilitating imbalance.

Thus, comparative analysis of correlation structures of psychological status's indicators of different qualification AW sportsmen permits to conclude that the studied psychological status's components are rather close. Absence of rough violations is confirmed by similar mean values of system's correlation, which is in interval of correlations of moderate strength in both groups. At the same time experienced sportsmen are characterized less label state. They have significantly less imbalance of regulation. Stability of system in this case is ensured by sufficient quantity of significant connections. They permit to minimize reduction of system's reliability, conditioned by influence of competition stress.

In order to study contribution of every of analyzed factors into system we determined indicators of system's formation (SI) (see fig. 1).

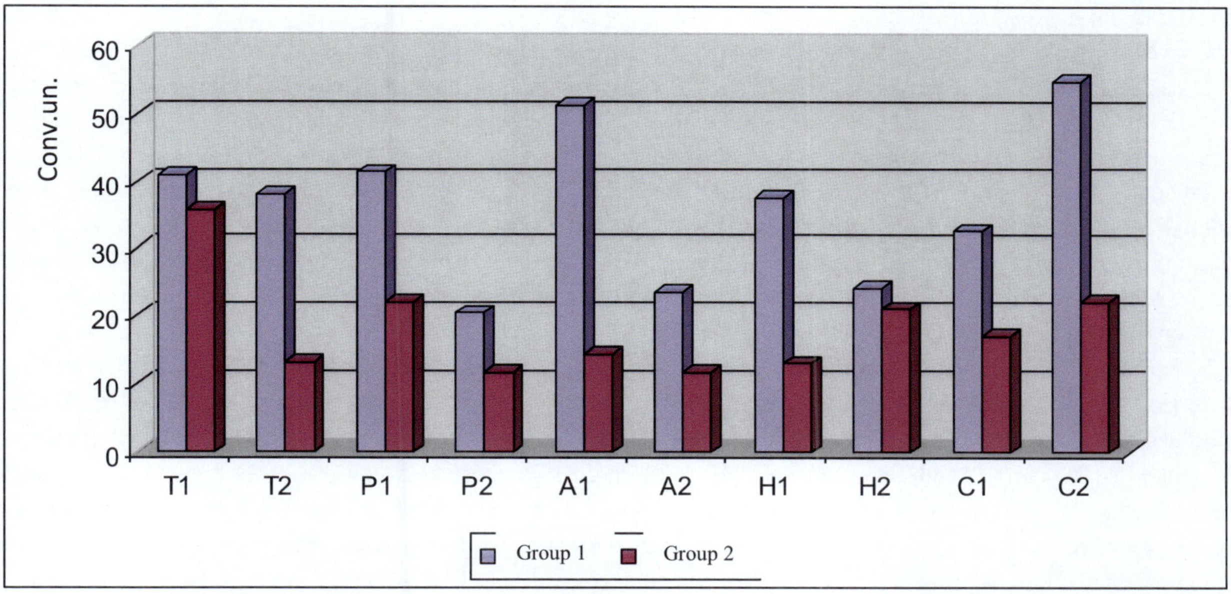

Fig.1. Dynamic of system's formation indicators of arm-wrestlers

Notes: T – anxiety, P – workability, A – activity H – state of mood, C – self-feeling, 1 – before competitions, 2 – after competitions.

First of all the following fact attracts attention: contribution of all components of sportsmen-beginners is significantly lower than of experienced sportsmen. It shall be assessed as one more proof of worse psychological fitness of 2nd group sportsmen.

It was found that the highest contribution to system of experienced sportsmen before competition is activity, i.e. psychological orientation on victory in future duels. Workability and anxiety are characterized by less, but rather significant values. It proves one more the made earlier assumptions about their importance for sportsmen's successfulness. Initial state of mood and self-feeling are lower and it can be interpreted as result of expectation stress. Dynamic of indicators confirms made earlier assumptions: reduction of workability, activity and state of mood reflect formation of fatigue. Practically stable anxiety illustrates post-stress state. Increase of self feeling is an indirect proof of successfulness of 1st group sportsmen.

In 2nd group we observed rather low contribution in initial state of all components except anxiety. Its increase undoubtedly proves formation of expectation stress. After competitions we registered reduction of contribution of anxiety and workability, insufficient reduction of activity and little increase of contribution of mood and self-feeling. These changes can be explained by peculiarities of sportsmen-beginners' state. Reduction of contribution of anxiety says about finishing of expectation stress. Workability and activity illustrate formation of fatigue. Mood and self-feeling shows optimizing of psycho-emotional status of sportsmen-beginners, which is connected with finishing of competition loads and certain "happiness", connected with it. Analysis of dynamic of psychological status indicators' contribution into sportsmen's condition proves made earlier assumption about changes in sportsmen's organisms under influence of competition loads. It permits to regard experienced sportsmen's condition as more resistant to competition stress.

Discussion

Changes in sportsman's psychological status appear in time and as a result of his professional functioning (trainings, competitions). It gives foundations for their studying and analysis. In our contest competitions shall be interpreted as extreme situations. Such situations put forward special requirements to sportsmen. They influence of psychological status, dynamic of which can be regarded as reflection of formation of adaptation. Analysis of available works, devoted to this problem, witnesses about similarity of literature data and results, received by us. Ermolaeva Y.S. thinks that levels of dancers' personal and situational anxiety is one of criteria of competition functioning's effectiveness [16]. High level of anxiety requires formation of self confidence and belief in success. Low level requires increase of activity, exiting of interest, responsibility in solution of training tasks.

On assessing of psychological status of chess players A.V. Khoroshavina, I.L. Udovenko, Ye.A. Strikalenko, O.G. Shalar conclude that chess players with high level of will self-regulation are characterized by calmness, self confidence, emotional stability, reliable self-control in different situations [10]. It is evident that these features of junior chess players influence positively on their competition results.

The data of Ivaskiene V.P., Skyriene V.V., Markevičius V.Z. witness that self-feeling, activity and state of mood of girl students in Judo and sambo in competition day permit them to achieve high results [20]. In its turn situational anxiety of most of these sportswomen is rather low. Researches of students, participating in Greco-Roman wrestling and boxing [18], Judo and sambo [19] resulted in the fact that self-feeling, activity and state of mood of sportsmen at eve of competitions was on high level. Situational anxiety was low.

V.A. Romanenko, N.V. Krayniaya, V.A. Mosenz, V.M. Prikhodko cinducted correlation analysis between parameters of anthropometric status and indicator of anxiety. They concluded that most of connections are characteristic for anxious girl students, comparing with not anxious ones [8]. In the first anthropometric and strength characteristics are interconnected ($0.31<r<0.83$) with anxiety positively. With indices of physical conditions by Erisman and chest they connected negatively ($0.62<r<0.64$). The second group girl students had body mass, strength of back and Ketle's index having negative correlation with anxiety. The rest indicators are positively connected ($0.36<r<0.53$) with this psychological characteristic.

At the same time results, received by M.F. Khoroshukha [11] are to certain extent opposite to the obtained by us. He thinks that higher level of anxiety and low level of aggressiveness are intrinsic to sportsmen-representatives of kinds of sports, oriented on higher endurance. For sportsmen of speed-power kinds of sports high aggressiveness is characteristic, to which lower indicators of anxiety correspond.

Thus, the received results deepen available information about peculiarities of psychological status of martial arts' sportsmen, its dynamic in process of competitions. The applied methodic of processing and analysis of data permit to more specifically differentiate condition of sportsmen of different qualification.

Conclusions:

The conducted researches permitted to determine certain changes in psychological status of different qualification AW sportsmen under influence of competition loads. Optimal condition of separate components of experienced sportsmen was confirmed as well as their favorable dynamic under competition loads. All these illustrate high level of functioning's reliability. The received results permit to regard specificities of psychological status as important factors, determining progress of sportsmanship. They give foundation for including of methodic, oriented on rising of stress resistance, into complex of AW sportsmen's training. The applied methods permit to promptly and adequately assess sportsmen's condition, prognosticate their successfulness and can be used in monitoring.

Acknowledgement

The research has been fulfilled in the frames of SRW "Theoretical and applied principles of construction of physical development, physical fitness and physical condition's monitoring in different strata of population"».

Conflict of interests

The authors declare that there is no conflict of interests.

References:

1 Antomonov MIu. *Matematicheskaia obrabotka i analiz mediko-biologicheskikh dannykh* [Mathematical processing and analysis of medical-biological data], Kiev; 2006. (in Russian)

2 Viatkin BA. *Upravlenie psikhicheskim stressom v sportivnykh sorevnovaniiakh* [Control of psychic stress in sport competitions], Moscow: Physical Culture and Sport; 1981. (in Russian)

3 Krivonosov MV, Podrigalo LV, Miteleva TIu. Profilaktika donozologicheskikh rasstrojstv zreniia u shkol'nikov [Prophylaxis of pre-nosological disorders of schoolchildren's eyesight]. *Gigiienichna nauka ta praktika na rubezhi stolit'* 2004;2:200-201. (in Russian)

4 Muntian VS. Optimizaciia rezul'tativnosti sorevnovatel'noj deiatel'nosti sportsmenov na osnove povysheniia urovnia ikh psikhologicheskoj ustojchivosti [Optimization of efficiency of sportsmen's competition functioning on the base of increase of their psychological stability]. *Physical education of students* 2010;3:55-58. (in Russian)

5 Podrigalo LV, Danilenko GN. *Donozologicheskie sostoianiia u detej, podrostkov i molodezhi: diagnostika, prognoz i gigienicheskaia korrekciia* [Pre-nosological states of children, adolescents and youth: diagnostic, prognosis and hygienic correction], Kiev: Genesis; 2014. (in Russian)

6 Podrigalo LV, Galashko MN, Galashko NI. Study and evaluation of indicators of relationships motor analyzer sportsmen of armsport. *Physical Education of Students* 2013;3:46-49. doi:10.6084/m9.figshare.669671

7 Podrigalo LV, Istomin AG, Galashko NI. *Monitoring funkcional'nogo sostoianiia sportsmenov v armsporte: mediko-gigienicheskie i sportivno-pedagogicheskie aspekty* [Monitoring of sportsmen's functional state in arm-wrestling: medical-hygienic and sport-pedagogic aspects], Kharkov: XNMU Publ.; 2010. (in Russian)

8 Romanenko VA, Krajniaia NV, Mosenz VA, Prikhod'ko VM. Lichnostnaia trevozhnost' – determinanta antropofunkcional'nogo statusa studentok [Personal anxiety as determinant of anthropological-functional status of girl students]. *Pedagogics, psychology, medical-biological problems of physical training and sports* 2011;11:95-98 (in Russian)

9 Sinajko VM, Gavenko VL, Sokolova IM. *Sposib ocinki trivogi, robotospromozhnosti, aktivnosti, nastroiu ta samopochuttia* [Mean of assessment of anxiety, workability, activity and self-feeling]. Patent 197(1). 2002. (in Russian)

10 Khoroshavina AV, Udovenko IL, Strikalenko EA, Shalar OG. Uverennost' v sebe, kak zalog uspeshnoj sorevnovatel'noj deiatel'nosti iunykh shakhmatistov [Self confidence as the pledge of junior chess players' successful competition functioning]. *Physical education of students* 2012;4:125-129. (in Russian)

11 Khoroshukha MF. Vivchennia vzaiemozv'iazku mizh agresivnistiu i trivozhnistiu u iunikh sportsmeniv 13-16 rokiv z riznoiu spriamovanistiu trenuval'nogo procesu [Study of interconnection between aggressiveness and anxiety of junior, 13-16 years' old, sportsm,en with different orientation of training process]. *Pedagogics, psychology, medical-biological problems of physical training and sports* 2011;4:154-156. (in Russian)

12 Shumakova NIu. Vzaimosviaz' fizicheskikh uprazhnenij s agressivnym povedeniem podrostkov [Interconnection of physical exercises with aggressive behavior of adolescents]. *Teoriia i praktika fizicheskoj kul'tury* 2002;9:53-56. (in Russian)

13 Asci FH. The effects of physical fitness training on trait anxiety and physical self-concept of female university students. *Psychology of Sport and Exercise* 2003;4:255–264. http://dx.doi.org/10.1016/S1469-0292(02)00009-2

14 Byrne AE, Byrne DG. The effect of exercise on depression, anxiety and other mood states. *Journal of Psychosomatic Research* 1993;37:565–574. http://dx.doi.org/10.1016/0022-3999(93)90050-P

15 Cocks M, Moulton C-A, Luu S, Cil T. What Surgeons can Learn From Athletes: Mental Practice in Sports and Surgery. *Journal of Surgical Education*. 2014;71(2):262–9.

16 Ermolaeva YS. Level of anxiety as one of the criteria of efficiency of emotional stability in sport dancing. *Pedagogics, psychology, medical-biological problems of physical training and sports* 2015;2:22-25. http://dx.doi.org/10.15561/18189172.2015.0204

17 Gorczynski P. Sport and Physical Activity for Mental Health. *Mental Health and Physical Activity*. 2010;3(2):102–3.

18 Ivaskiene V, Liaugminas A, Liaugminas S. Emotions in grecoroman wresters and boxers before the competition. *Education. Physical Training. Sport* 2010;3(78):29–33.

19 Ivaskiene V, Raskevicius K, Cepelioniene J, Markevicius V. *Emotions in sambo and judo athletes students before the competition. Physical Culture and Sport in Universities*. Kaunas: Technologija; 2012.

20 Ivaskiene VP, Skyriene VV, Markevičius VZ. Comparative analysis of prestart condition of students girls in Olympic and non-Olympic kinds of sport. *Physical education of students* 2013;4:27-30. http://dx.doi.org/10.6084/m9.figshare.669683

21 Jewett R, Sabiston CM, Brunet J, O'Loughlin EK, Scarapicchia T, O'Loughlin J. School Sport Participation During Adolescence and Mental Health in Early Adulthood. *Journal of Adolescent Health*. 2014;55(5):640–4.

22 Lueshen G. *Checting in sport. Social Problem in Atletics: Essays in the Sociology of sport*. Urbana Chicago-London: Univ. Illinois Press; 1976.

23 Massey WV, Meyer BB, Naylor AH. Toward a grounded theory of self-regulation in mixed martial arts. *Psychology of Sport and Exercise*. 2013;14(1):12–20.

24 McMahon JA, Penney D. (Self-) surveillance and (self-) regulation: living by fat numbers within and beyond a sporting culture. *Qualitative Research in Sport, Exercise and Health*. 2012;5(2):157–78.

25 Nezhad MAS, Besharat MA. Relations of resilience and hardiness with sport achievement and mental health in a sample of athletes. *Procedia - Social and Behavioral Sciences*. 2010;5(0):757–63.

26 Peckham AD, McHugh RK, Otto MW. A meta-analysis of the magnitude of biased attention in depression. *Depression and Anxiety* 2010;27(12):1135–1142. http://dx.doi.org/10.1002/da.20755

27 Perron A, Brendgen M, Vitaro F, Côté SM, Tremblay RE, Boivin M. Moderating effects of team sports participation on the link between peer victimization and mental health problems. *Mental Health and Physical Activity*. 2012;5(2):107–15.

28 Rogers RG. Mental Practice and Acquisition of Motor Skills: Examples from Sports Training and Surgical Education. *Obstetrics and Gynecology Clinics of North America*. 2006;33(2):297–304.

29 Rutter LA, Brown TA. Reliability and validity of the dimensional features of generalized anxiety disorder. *Journal of anxiety disorders* 2015;29:1–6. http://dx.doi.org/10.1016/j.janxdis.2014.10.003

30 Scoffier S, Gernigon C, d' Arripe-Longueville F. Effects of achievement goals on self-regulation of eating attitudes among elite female athletes: *An experimental study. Psychology of Sport and Exercise*. 2012;13(2):201–7.

31 Scoffier S, Paquet Y, d' Arripe-Longueville F. Effect of locus of control on disordered eating in athletes: The mediational role of self-regulation of eating attitudes. *Eating Behaviors*. 2010;11(3):164–9.

32 Snyder E, Spreitzer E. *Social Aspects of sport*. Englewood Cliffs (N.Y.): Prentice Hall; 1978.

33 Tamminen KA, Crocker PRE. "I control my own emotions for the sake of the team": Emotional self-regulation and interpersonal emotion regulation among female high-performance curlers. *Psychology of Sport and Exercise*. 2013;14(5):737–47.

34 Xiong J. The Functions and Methods of Mental Training on Competitive Sports. *Physics Procedia*. 2012;33(0):2011–4.

SUCCESSFULNESS OF GENERAL AND SPECIAL PHYSICAL QUALITIES' DEVELOPMENT ON DIFFERENT STAGE OF STUDENTS-BOXERS' TRAINING

Gaskov A.V.[1], Kuzmin V.A.[2, 3], Kudryavtsev M.D. [2, 3], Iermakov S. S. [4]
[1]Buryat state University, Russia
[2]Siberian Federal University, Russia
[3]Siberian State Aerospace University, Russia
[4]Kazimierz Wielki University in Bydgoszcz, Poland

Abstract. *Purpose:* to study indicators of general and special physical condition on different stages of macro-cycle training. *Material:* in testing qualified boxers - 28 sportsmen – participated. Characteristics of general and special fitness were registered. *Results:* it was found that structure of general and special physical qualities can be described by 9 factors, explaining about 80% of total sample variance. It was also determined that factorial structure of general and special physical fitness indicators does not change depending on stages of trainings. At every of the tested stages the marked out factors do not depend on each other. These factors are separate necessary sides of training. It was found that on general preparation stage of training these factors characterize sides of fitness: effectiveness of punches of strong and weak arms; special speed and power endurance; general endurance and strength of muscles (hands' flexors); specific sensor-motor reaction; condition of upper girdle muscles; general speed and power endurance; speed of punch movement. *Conclusions:* when distributing training means and loads it is necessary to uniformly doze correlation of means for all marked out factors. It ensures growth of boxers' spots results.
Key words: trainings, students, boxer, physical fitness, special, periods.

Introduction

Sphere of sports is characterized by exclusively intensive and continuous growth of sports achievements. It is a specific reflection of one of the most substantial and the least studied social phenomena – acceleration of social progress [1].

Increased level of competition's functioning at international sports forums forces coaches and sportsmen to seek more effective means and methods of training. Such approach will permit to solve specific tasks of boxing, directed on training of physical qualities and perfection of sportsmen's technical-tactic skillfulness.

At present development of boxing in the whole world and aggravation of competition gave powerful push to creative search of coaches and boxers. It gave birth to great number of new and original ideas in all links of sports training system. Recent time questions of building of training in boxing have been being paid more and more attention. It is not an occasional phenomenon, because boxers' skillfulness and their sports results to large extent depend on ability to conduct training. Application of elements of constant creative search in training makes it exciting and creative process.

At modern stage development of new methods of training searching of more effective means of workability's rising is the basis of boxers' sportsmanship increase. For example, there are some "reconstructions" in boxer's training: nowadays physical training is often oriented on application of special and general-training means of increased intensity.

The problem of optimal correlation of sportsman's general and special training has been being worked out and discussed for long ago. Recent time it again has attracted increased attention. It is explained by its extraordinary complexity. Sportsman's general and special condition change depending on level of his fitness, individual qualities, specificity of sports specialization, stages of many years' sports perfection process and training periods [5, 6, 15].

Modern theory of sports training does not specify any universal, quantitative standards of correlation of general and special training. The theory gives only principle landmarks. It admits rather wide range of definite correlations' variations, which are formed depending on different circumstances.

Modern level of sports achievements in boxing, intensity of boxers' functioning on ring set increased requirements to their general (GPF) and special (SPF) physical fitness. Rational building of training process in annual cycles on the base of optimal GPF and SPF correlations permits for sportsmen to achieve high results.

Analysis of scientific-methodic literature showed that in perfection of technical-tactic skillfulness in sportsmen's many years' training GPF and SPF level play the main role [2–4, 13, 23].

Purpose, tasks of the work, material and methods

The purpose of the work was to study indicators of GPF and SPF at different stages of qualified boxers' training.

The tasks of the research: 1. to detect interconnection of GPF and SPF means in qualified boxers; 2. to determine optimal correlation of GPF and SPF means in qualified boxers at different stages of macro-cycle.

Material of the research: qualified boxers (28 sportsmen) participated in testing. Preparatory period of training consisted of three stages: 1st stage- involving (18 days); 2nd- general-preparatory (20 days); 3rd – special-preparatory (21 days); 4th – recreational (18 days).

For determination of the most informative GPF and SPF indicators we registered the following characteristics:

General physical fitness: 100 m –100 meters' run; 3000 m – 3000 meters' run; LJ –long jump from the spot; PU – pressing ups in lying positions; CU – chin ups; SP 1– shot put (4 kg with stronger arm); SP2 - shot put (4 kg with weaker arm); HD1 – hand dynamometry of stronger arm; HD2 - hand dynamometry of weaker arm;

Special physical fitness: $V_{p.}$ – mean velocity of punch; SMR_1 – specific sensor-motor reaction in punch of stronger arm; SMR_2 – specific sensor-motor reaction in punch of weaker arm; t_1– time of achieving of maximal strength by stronger arm; t_2– time of achieving of maximal strength by weaker arm; t_3– t_1– time of achieving of strength by stronger arm; t_4– time of achieving of strength by weaker arm; F_1– strength of punch by stronger arm; F_2– strength of punch by weaker arm; S_1 – strength impulse of punch by stronger arm; S_2 – strength impulse of punch by weaker arm; N_5 – quantity of punches per 4 sec.; + F_5 – total of punches per 5 sec.; + S_5 – total of impulses of punches' strength per 5 sec.; F_{x5} – average strength of punches per 5 sec.; Sx_5 – mean impulse of punches per 5 sec.; N_{180} – quantity of punches per 180 seconds; + F_{180} – total strength of punches per 180 seconds; + S_{180} – total of impulses of punches' strength per 180 seconds; Fx_{180} – average strength of punches per 180 seconds; Sx_{180} – mean impulse of punches per 180 seconds; LS – level of sportsmanship.

The methods of the research: factorial analysis (principle component method with following rotation of reference axes by Varimax criterion) of the received experimental material was carried out. As a result, factors, determining boxers' GPF and SPF on different macro-cycle training stages were marked out.

On preliminary stage of data processing correlation analysis of indicators (34 GPF and SPF indicators per each boxer) was fulfilled. As a result we found the most informative GPF and SPF indicators for different stages of macro-cycle. We selected 31 the most significant indicators for factorial analysis.

Results of the research

Involving stage

Analysis of materials of 1st stage of training permitted to determine that structure of boxers' general and special qualities can be described by 9 factors, which explain 84.3% of total sample variance.

In 1st factor (36.8% of total sample variance) the most factorial significance belongs to indicators: N_{180}; F_{180}; S_{180}; Fx_{180}; SX_{180}; 3000 m (which characterize special power endurance and general endurance). In 2nd factor (9.8% from total sample variance) the most factorial significance belongs to equivalent indicators SMR_1, SMR_2 and SP. These indicators reflect specific sensor motor reaction when punching with stronger and weaker arms; condition of arms' muscles. In 3rd factor (8.6% of total sample variance) the highest factorial significance belongs to qualitative characteristics of single punches and general condition of muscle groups, participating in punch: t_1, F_2, S_2, LJ, SP. These indicators can be considered equivalent. In 4th factor (7.1% of total sample variance) high factorial loads were found by the following equivalent indicators: F_5, S_5, Fx_5, Sx_5, PU, CU. They characterize special velocity and general power endurance of muscles (arm's flexors and extensors).

5th factor (6% of total sample variance) highly correlates with t_2, N_5. These indicators characterize time parameters of punch by weaker arm and special speed motor skills. 6th factor (4.9% of total sample variance) – indictor of 100 meters run. It assesses general speed endurance. 7th factor (4.1% of total sample variance) correlates with F_1 and S_1, which characterize effectiveness of weaker arm's punches. 8th factor (3.9 % of total sample variance) correlates with indicator V. It characterizes mean velocity of punch movement. 9th factor (3.1% of total sample variance) correlates with equivalent indicators t_3 and t_4. These indicators characterize time of single punches by stronger and weaker arms and assess effectiveness of these punches.

General-preparation stage

Analysis of 2nd stage results showed that structure of general and special physical qualities can be described by 9 factors (explaining 85.1% of total sample variance).

In 1st factor (contribution 35.4% in total sample variance) high correlations of equivalent indicators F_1, S_1, F_2, S_2, F_5, S_5, Fx_5, Sx_5, F_{180}, S_{180}, 3000 m, HD_1, HD_2 were found. They characterize effectiveness of single punches by stronger and weaker arms, special speed and power endurance, general endurance and strength of hand's flexors. 2nd factor (12% of total sample variance) shows the highest correlation of indicators N_5, N_{180}, Fx_{180}, Sx_{180}. They characterize special speed endurance. In 3rd factor (9.6% of total sample variance) there is the highest correlation of equivalent characteristics t_1, t_3, t_2, t_4. They assess quantity of punches by stronger and weaker arms. In 4th factor (6.3% of total sample variance) the highest factorial significance belongs to equivalent indicators SMR_2 and SMR_3. They characterize specific sensor motor reaction when punching by stronger and weaker arms.

5th factor (5.6% of total sample variance) shows the highest factorial loads with LJ, SP_1 and SP_2. They characterize condition of muscular groups of upper girdle. In 6th factor (4.8% of total sample variance) the highest correlations were found with indicators of 100 meters' run and PU. They characterize speed and power endurance. In 7th factor (4.4% of total sample variance) indicators of arm's flexors' strength and CU were marked out.

8th factor (3.8% of total sample variance) shows one indicator - t. It characterizes quality of punch by stronger arm.

9th factor (3.2% total sample variance) shows the highest factorial significance of indicator V. It characterizes mean velocity of punch movement.

Special-preparation stage

Analysis of 3rd stage results showed that structure of general and special physical qualities can also be described by 9 factors (explaining 84.2% of total sample variance).

1st factor, with the highest contribution (35.7%) in total sample variance, correlates with equivalent indicators F_1, S_1, F_5, S_5, Fx_5, Sx_s, S_{180}, HD_1, HD_2. They characterize strength parameters of punch by stronger arm, special-speed and power endurance and general strength of muscles (arm's flexors). 2nd factor (10.4% of total sample variance) witnesses about high correlation with equivalent indicators SMR_1 and SMR_2. They characterize specific sensor motor reaction when punching by weakest and strongest arms.3rd factor (9.5% total sample variance) shows high correlation with equivalent indicators t_1, t_3, t_2, t_4, which characterize quality of punch by weaker and stronger arms.

6th factor (6.5% of total sample variance) shows the highest factorial coefficients with results V_p, 100 m. They characterize mean velocity of punch movement and general speed endurance.

5th factor (5.9% of total sample variance) highly correlates with indicators N_{180}, F_{180}, S_{180}. They characterize special power endurance. In 6th factor (5.2% of total sample variance) N_5, and CU have high significance. These indicators characterize speed motor skills and power endurance of arm's flexors. 7th factor (4.4% of total sample variance) correlates with LJ, SP_2 and SP_1. They characterize explosive poser of legs and condition of muscles, participating in punch. 8th factor (3.7% of total sample variance) correlates with PU, which characterizes power endurance of arms' flexors. 9th factor (2.9% of total sample variance) closely correlates with equivalent indicators F_2, S_2, Fx_{180}, Sx_{180}, and 3000 meters' run. They characterize qualitative characteristics of punch by weaker arm, special power and general endurance.

Recreational stage

Analysis of recreational stage results showed that structure of general and special physical qualities can also be described by 9 factors (explaining 86.2% of total sample variance).

1st factor (36.8% contribution in total sample variance) has high correlations with indicators N_{180}, 100m, SP_1 and SP_2. They characterize quantity of punches per one round, general speed endurance, condition of muscles, participating in punch. In 2nd factor (10.9% of total sample variance) we found high correlations with indicators SMR_1, SMR_2. They characterize specific sensor motor reaction when punching by weaker or stronger arms. In 3rd factor (8.9% of total sample variance) high significance was found in indicators t_1, t_3, t_2, t_4, which characterize quality of punches by stronger and by weaker arms. 4th factor (7.2% of total sample variance) correlates with 3000 meters' run indicator, which characterizes general endurance.

In 5th factor (6.2% of total sample variance) PU and CU have the highest significance. They characterize power endurance of arms' flexors and extensors. 6th factor (contribution in total sample variance 4.7%) shows high correlation with equivalent indicators F_2, S_2. They characterize quality of punch by weaker arm. 7th factor (4.3% of total sample variance) shows the highest correlation with indicator V, characterizing mean velocity of punch movement. In 8th factor (3.9% of total sample variance) equivalent indicators, S_1, N_5, F_5, S_5, Fx_5, Sx_5, F_{180}, S_{180}, Fx_{180}, LJ, HD_1, HD_2 are marked out. They characterize special speed-power endurance. 9th factor (3, 3% of total sample variance) factor of sportsmanship level was marked out.

Discussion

Indicators of general physical and special fitness of boxers are important elements, by which sportsman's fitness at different stages of macro-cycle is determined. It is witnessed by researches of different authors. For example Nykytenko A.O. et al. found interconnections between indicators of special preparation and general preparation exercises of sportsmen. It permitted to establish statistically confident correlations of: a) indicators of punches power with indicators of single movement; b) indicators of punches' velocity with indicators of distance of 300 grams' balls pushes; c) indicators of motion speed in combat stance with indicators of punches' velocity; d) indicators of punches' frequency with indicators of movements' on feet frequency (maneuvering) [21]. Martsiv V.P. determined correlations between indicators of special preparation and general preparation exercises. It was found that increase of boxers' sportsmanship is manifested in growth of punches' density in fight [19]. Kiprich S.B., Berinchik D.Y. registered absence of confidence distinctions in qualitative characteristics of apidemical shifts in organisms, which growth in process of fulfillment of test task. The authors determined that in different periods (rounds) of duel, in elite boxers there appear different manifestations and combinations of functional fitness's properties [16]. Aksutin V.V., Korobeynikov G.V. registered absolute and relative strength of serial and single punches. Their results witness that attacking style of fight is accompanied by high workability, reduction of fatigue, anxiety and dependence on status of vegetative functions [12]. Martsiv V.P. studied boxers' psycho-physiological state with usage of 9 kinds of anticipation responses at stage of specialized basic training. The author determined regularities of manifestation of every kind of response in given group of sportsmen; envisaged the ways of their application as criteria for assessment of boxers' psych-physiological state [20]. Kiprych S.V. et al. found that perfection of training process in boxing can be based on assessment of workability indicators and responsive characteristics of cardio-respiratory system of sportsmen [17].

Among many researches we can mark out the works, devoted to psychological training of Olympic teams; to boxing competence and practical experience; to processes of professional boxers' adaptation and other [22, 26–29].

In this aspect our researches supplement and expand information about successfulness of development of sportsmen's general and special physical qualities, which are determined by independent on each other factors. These qualities with high degree of confidence characterize the sides of sportsmen's fitness: strength of punch by stronger arm; special speed and power endurance, strength of hand's flexors; specific sensor motor reaction; time characteristics of punches by stronger and weaker arms. Results of our researches supplement our previous works [14, 18, 24, and 25] about purposefulness of optimization of fitness different sides, oriented on training of sportsmen's power abilities.

We assumed that problems in students' physical education can be corrected by means and methods of boxing. It was found that traditional system of physical education in state higher educational establishments does not realize to full extent the tasks of students' motivation for physical culture practicing. It is connected with absence of scientifically substantiated conception of formation of physical culture education [7–9].

Scientific and methodic worked, fulfilled in this direction, permitted to rather effectively organize learning regime in higher school, to weaken the problem of organism's overload in conditions of educational process; to maintain students' workability in relatively optimal frames in boxing circles [10–11, 18].

Conclusions

1. Basing on the above delivered we can conclude that in involving stage of training successfulness of development of general and special physical qualities is determined by independent on each other factors. These factors characterize sides of fitness: special and general endurance; total time of motor response and strength of arms' muscles, participating in punch; quality of single punches and general condition of muscular groups, participating in punch; special speed endurance and general power endurance of arms' flexors and extensors; time of punch by weaker arm and quickness of serial punches; general speed endurance; effectiveness of punches by weaker arm; velocity of punch movement; effectiveness of single punches by both arms.
2. From the said above we can conclude that in general-preparation stage successfulness of development of general and special physical qualities is determined by independent on each pother factors. These factors characterize the following sides of fitness: effectiveness of single punches by both arms; special speed and power endurance; general

endurance and strength of hand's flexors; specific sensor-motor reaction; condition of upper girdle muscles; general speed and power endurance; velocity of punch movement.

3. Analysis of special-preparation stage results permitted to find that successfulness of development of general and special physical qualities is determined by independent on each pother factors. These factors characterize the following sides of fitness: strength of punch by stronger arm; special speed and power endurance and strength of hand's flexors; specific sensor motor reaction; time characteristics of punches by stronger and by weaker arms; general speed endurance; special speed motor abilities; condition of muscles, participating in punch; power endurance of arm's flexors; strength of punch by weaker arm and general endurance.
4. Analysis of recreational stage results permitted to find that successfulness of development of general and special physical qualities is determined by independent on each pother factors. These factors characterize the following sides of fitness: condition of muscles, participating in punch; specific sensor motor reaction; time characteristics of single punches by both arms; general endurance; power endurance of arm's flexors and extensors; quality of punch by weaker arm; velocity of punch movement; special speed-power endurance; explosive power of legs and hand's flexors; level of sportsmanship.
5. Results of factorial analysis witness that factorial structure of GPC and SPC of qualified boxers does not change depending on stages of training. It should be noted that on every of the studied stages the marked out factors do not depend on each other and are separate, important sides of GPC and SPC. That is why, when distributing training means and loads it necessary to uniformly distribute and dose correlation of means for all marked out factors, characterizing different sides of fitness. It conditions increase of GPC and SPC level. As a result it ensures growth of sports results of students – qualified boxers.

Conflict of interests

The authors declare that there is no conflict of interests.

References:

1. Avdeev RF. *Filosofiia informacionnoj civilizacii* [Philosophy of informational civilization], Moscow: Vlados; 1994. (in Russian)
2. Gaskov AV. *Teoretiko-metodicheskie osnovy upravleniia sorevnovatel'noj i trenirovochnoj deiatel'nost'iu kvalificirovannykh bokserov. Doct. Diss.* [Theoretical methodic principles of control over competition and training functioning of qualified boxers. Doct. Diss.], Moscow: 1999. (in Russian)
3. Gaskov AV, Kuzmin VA. *Struktura i soderzhanie trenirovochno-sorevnovatel'noj deiatel'nosti v bokse* [Structure and content of training-competition functioning in boxing], 2004, Krasnoyarsk; KSU Publ.; 2004. (in Russian)
4. Gaskov AV, Kuzmin VA. *Metodologicheskie osnovy postroeniia effektivnykh modelej trenirovochnoj deiatel'nosti bokserov* [Methodological principles of construction of effective models of boxers' training functioning], Krasnoyarsk; SSAU Publ.; 2011. (in Russian)
5. Matveev LP. *Obshchaia teoriia sporta i ee aspekty* [General theory of sports and its aspects], Moscow: Doe; 2005. (in Russian)
6. Filimonov VI. *Boks: Sportivno-tekhnicheskaia podgotovka* [Boxing: sports-technical training], Moscow: Insan; 2000. (in Russian)
7. Kuzmin VA, Kudryavtsev MD, Kopylov Yu.A, Galimov I.G, Strelnikov VA. Konceptual'nye osnovy neobkhodimosti obnovleniia dopolnitel'nogo ozdorovitel'nogo fizicheskogo vospitaniia studentov [Conceptual principles of demand in students' health related physical education's renewal]. *Mezhdunarodnaia nauchno-prakticheskaia konferenciia "Molodaia sportivnaia nauka Belarusi", Minsk, 8–10 apr. 2014 g.* [International scientific-practical conference "Young sport science of Belarus", Minsk, April 8th- 10th, 2014], Minsk BGUFK; 2014;2. P. 162–165.]. (in Russian)
8. Kuzmin VA, Kudryavtsev MD, Galimov IG., Kopylov YA, Gaskov AV. Sovremennye podkhody k sozdaniiu koncepcii i obnovleniiu struktury i soderzhaniia ozdorovitel'nogo fizicheskogo vospitaniia studentov vuzov [Modern approaches to creation of conception and renewal the structure and content of health related physical education of HEE students]. *Vestnik Buriatskogo gosudarstvennogo universiteta*. 2014;13:34–41. (in Russian)
9. Kuzmin VA, Kudryavtsev MD, Kopylov YuA, Galimov IG, Strelnikov VA, Gaskov AV. Osobennosti formirovaniia social'no znachimykh lichnostnykh kachestv studentov-bokserov kak osnovy budushchej professional'noj

deiatel'nosti [Peculiarities of formation of students-boxers' socially significant qualities as the basis of their future professional functioning]. *Vestnik Buriatskogo gosudarstvennogo universiteta.* 2014;13:68–72. (in Russian)

10. Kopylov YuA, Jackowska LN, Kudryavtsev MD, Kuzmin VA, Tolstopyatov IA, Iermakov SS. The concept of structure and content of health related trainings for higher educational establishments' students. *Physical Education of Students*, 2015;5:23–30. http://dx.doi.org/10.15561/20755279.2015.0504;
11. Kuzmin VA, Kopylov YuA, Kudryavtsev MD, Galimov GY, Iermakov SS. Substantiation of effectiveness of trainings on health related methodic for students with weakened motor fitness. *Physical Education of Students*, 2015;6:43–49. http://dx.doi.org/10.15561/20755279.2015.0606
12. Aksutin VV, Korobeynikov GV. Psychophysiological states and special performance of boxers with different styles of fight. *Pedagogics, psychology, medical-biological problems of physical training and sports*, 2014;12:3–6. http://dx.doi.org/10.15561/18189172.2014.1201
13. de Garis L. Sometimes a bloody nose is just a bloody nose: play and contest in boxing, wrestling, and ethnography. *Sport in Society.* 2010;13(6):935–951.
14. Iermakov SS, Arziutov GN, Jagiełło W. Quick training of students to judo techniques. *Arch Budo,* 2016;12:15–24.
15. Ishioka T. Boxing, Poverty, Foreseeability – an ethnographic account of local boxers in Metro Manila, Philippines. *Asia Pacific Journal of Sport and Social Science.* 2012;1(2–3):143–55.
16. Kiprich SB, Berinchik DY. Specific descriptions of functional providing of the special endurance of boxers. *Pedagogics, psychology, medical-biological problems of physical training and sports,* 2015;3:20–27. http://dx.doi.org/10.15561/18189172.2015.0304
17. Kiprych SV, Donets AV, Makhdi Omar Ali. Improvement of management by training process of boxers at a stage of direct preparation for competitions. *Physical Education of Students*, 2013;6:20–24. http://dx.doi.org/10.6084/m9.figshare.840495
18. Kozina ZL, Iermakov SS, Kuzmin VA, Kudryavtsev MD, Galimov G.J. Change of cortisol and insulin content in blood under influence of special workability recreation system for students with high motor functioning level. *Research Journal of Pharmaceutical, Biological and Chemical Sciences,* 2016;7(2), 15–28.
19. Martsiv VP. Dynamics of psychophysiological state of the boxers influenced by the standard of specialized demands of specialized basic training. *Pedagogics, psychology, medical-biological problems of physical training and sports*, 2013;9:43–49. http://dx.doi.org/10.6084/m9.figshare.749697
20. Martsiv VP. Model characteristics of average skill boxers' competition functioning. *Physical Education of Students.* 2015; 4: 17–23. http://dx.doi.org/10.15561/20755279.2015.0403
21. Nykytenko AO, Nikitenko SA, Busol VV, Nykytenko AA, Velychkovych MR, Martciv VP. Intercommunications of indexes of speed and power qualities of sportsmen single combat on the stage of the specialized base preparation. *Pedagogics, psychology, medical-biological problems of physical training and sports*, 2013;1:49–55. http://dx.doi.org/10.6084/m9.figshare.106939
22. Okada M. Embodied interactional competence in boxing practice: Coparticipants' joint accomplishment of a teaching and learning activity. *Language & Communication*. 2013;33(4):390–403.
23. Ottoboni G, Russo G, Tessari A. What boxing-related stimuli reveal about response behaviour. *Journal of Sports Sciences.* 2015;33(10):1019–1027.
24. Podrigalo LV, Iermakov SS, Galashko NI, Galashko MN, Dzhym VY. Assessment of arm wrestlers' adaptation status on the base of saliva biochemical characteristics in dynamic of competition and training loads. *Journal of Physical Education and Sport*, 2015;15(4), 849–856. http://dx.doi.org/10.7752/jpes.2015.04131
25. Podrigalo LV, Iermakov SS, Nosko MO, Galashko MN, Galashko NI. Study and analysis of armwrestlers' forearm muscles' strength. *Journal of Physical Education and Sport*, 2015;15(3), 531–537. http://dx.doi.org/10.7752/jpes.2015.03080
26. Schinke RJ, Bonhomme J, McGannon KR, Cummings J. The internal adaptation processes of professional boxers during the Showtime Super Six Boxing Classic: A qualitative thematic analysis. *Psychology of Sport and Exercise.* 2012;13(6):830–839.
27. Schinke RJ, Stambulova NB, Trepanier D, Oghene O. Psychological support for the Canadian Olympic Boxing Team in meta-transitions through the National Team Program. *International Journal of Sport and Exercise Psychology.* 2015;13(1):74–89.

FEATURES OF CONSTRUCTION OF STRUCTURES IN LONG-TERM TRAINING ACROBATICS AT THE MODERN STAGE

Bachinskaya N.V.
Oles Honchar Dnipropetrovsk National University

Annotation. *Purpose:* the basic directions of the structure of long-term training in sports acrobatics are ground. The objectives of the study was to determine the leading requirements and criteria, the main stages of a multi-year training in acrobatics. *Material*: analysis of special scientific and methodical literature, revealing the specific features of the construction of long-term training in sports and gymnastics, acrobatic rock 'n' roll, a number of other sports. *Results*: general structure, goals, objectives and provisions of the basic stages of a multi-year training in sports acrobatics. Singled leading indicators and criteria for each of the main stages of long-term sports training in acrobatics. Recommended duration of training sessions and key requirements for the preparation of acrobats. *Conclusions*: outlines the main requirements and benchmarks that can guide the trainer in a training and competitive activity when working with acrobats all age groups and different sports qualification.
Keywords: stages, structure, long-term training, acrobatics.

Introduction

Nowadays competition program of sport acrobatics has rather complicated and reached certain limit. Dynamics and virtuosity of exercises increased, new original elements and combinations appear (S.K. Malinovskiy, 2003, O.V. Shebaldina, 2004) [8, 15].

All changes, which have happened, require significant correction of certain theoretical and methodic approaches to process of acrobats' many-years' training Все те изменения, которые произошли, требуют значительной коррекции определенных теоретических и методических подходов к процессу многолетней подготовки акробатов (S.K. Malinovskiy, 2003; M.I. Pyliuk, [8, 10].

The purpose of many years' training of acrobats, like in any other kind of sports, is maintaining of optimal dynamics of physical qualities and functional potentials as well as achievement of maximal for every sportsman sport result (I.G. Gibaddulin, 2005; A.A. Ruziyev, 1999; T.M. Absaliamov, 1996) [1, 4, 13].

Theoretical analysis and generalization of special literature showed that determination of perspective directions for perfection of many years training's structure in acrobatics have not nad proper scientific foundation and require additional work, considering the kind of sports.

Analyzing the above said we may state that on modern stage of sport acrobatics in Ukraine scientifically grounded conception of differentiated approach to training of acrobats, considering kinds of acrobatics, role in exercise, functional characteristics and gender distinctions of sportsmen.

Purpose, tasks of the work, material and methods

The purpose of the research is to give foundation for perspective directions of structure of many years' training in sport acrobatics.

The tasks of the research are to determine main indicators, criteria and main requirements of structure of many years' training in sport acrobatics.

The methods of the research: structural-functional analysis; synthesis; theoretical analysis of special scientific methodic literature and generalization; analogy and systemizing; pedagogic control over training and competition functioning of sportsmen; questioning, interviewing.

Results of the research

Analysis of a number of scientific publications, dissertations and programs for CJSS, SCJSS, devoted to acrobatics and other kinds of sports with complex coordination, permitted to form and mark out main directions of structure of many years' training in sport acrobatics (Ye.V. Bogatina, L.E. Pasmurova, "Crieria and orientations in sport acrobatics"/ Ye.V. Bogatina, L.E. Pasmurova, //Materials of V International students' electronic scientific conference "Students' scientific forum" URL: http://www.scienceforum.ru) [5-7, 9, 12, 16].

For realization of aims of many years' training it is necessary to fulfill the following conditions:

- Development of general plan of training and competition processes' construction on all stages of many years' training;
- Control of main parameters of training and competition loads, which are directed on achievement of the set aims, both intermediate and current;
- Planned and gradual increasing of scope of special physical training (SPT) in respect to general physical training (GPT);
- Compulsory consideration of age and gender characteristics;
- Development of acrobats' physical qualities in certain age periods.

In process of many years' training its integral part is pedagogic control. It is realized for determination of dynamics of multi-functional development, level of general and special physical fitness, correspondence of planned physical loads to potentials of trainees and to temp of their biological growth.

Stage-by-stage control in sport acrobatics, as a rule, is conducted at the beginning and at the end of academic year. Its main tasks are: dynamic of physical condition's progressing as well as sportsmen's general and special physical fitness; determination of results' increment during year in comparison with standard requirements.

Current control is carried out at every training lesson as well as at the end of week cycle of training for analysis of organism's functional changes. Main tasks of it: determination of degree of tiredness and sportsman's recreation after training loads; degree of sportsman's readiness to taking of planned loads.

For direct registering of results of one training exercise, combination, composition and training in general operative control if fulfilled [5, 12, 21].

Sport training in acrobatics is a many years' annual process, which includes comprehensive development, training, and education of trainees.

Main forms of trainings in sport acrobatics are:

- Trainings-lessons of practical and theoretical character;
- Intermittent (after competition and transitive period) and summarizing (after academic year) testing;
- Regular participation in different competitions;
- Studying of video-records of qualified acrobats' trainings and competitions;
- Trainings as home by individual program;
- Regular trainings at camps;
- Trainings at health related sport camps;
- Studying of refereeing [5, 6, 12].

On all stages of many ears' training in acrobatics main tasks are solved on the base of realization of curriculum, considering program schedule and standard requirements. Also mastering of training loads in compliance with curriculum is required.

Requirements and content of standards change depending of stage of training. Fulfillment of demanded criteria is compulsory for passing of trainees to next stage of many years' training.

Efficiency of many years' system of acrobats' training depends on a number of factors:

1. Age at beginning of sport acrobatic training. 2. Age at achievement of the highest results. 3. Consideration of regularities of formation of sportsmanship different sides in acrobats of different sex, formation of adaptation processes in main functions of organism. 4. Consideration of individual and gender distinctions of acrobats when planning training loads. 5. Means and methods of trainings, dynamic of training loads. 6. Peculiarities of building of training process's different structural formations.

In different kinds of sport acrobatics there are certain requirements to coach, videlicet:

- Presence of knowledge about methodic, practical and scientific achievements in acrobatics, about changes in classification and training programs;
- Knowledge about characteristics of motor, physical and functional development of trainees;
- Having techniques of sport exercises and means of teaching and sport training;
- умение анализировать и оценивать изменения в правилах соревнований.

With orienting of trainees on such exercises as jumps on acrobatic track coach shall be guided by the following principles:

- health condition and harmonious development of trainees;
- ability of trainees to effectively master acrobatic jumps;
- stability and reliability in fulfillment of exercises at trainings and competitions;
- high level of speed-power qualities, orientation in space and in time as well as integral sensor-motor coordination [2, 3].

In pair-group acrobatics trainees fulfill different functional roles, i.e. roles: upper, lower – in women, men and mixed pairs; upper, lower, central – in women groups; lower, first, central, second central, upper in men groups (four).

In every role acrobats need the following:

- prevailing development of strength, flexibility, quickness, endurance;
- balance in system of interacting bodies;
- space-time indicators of movements;
- reliable balance;
- sport techniques of supports, different stances (on one and two hands), throws, flights, catching, landing on hands and shoulders of partners;
- high level of choreographic fitness, musical abilities, artistry;
- presence of optimal weight-height indicators.

When completing of pair-group kinds of acrobatics coach shall compare biomechanically points of links (wrists-wrists), supporting points (shoulders-feet), working postures and consider sport techniques of such exercises with partners' combined actions [2, 3, 17].

Interconnections of kinds of training and main tasks are given in table 1 [5].

Table 1

Main tasks in kinds of sport acrobatics (generalized and processed data of L.V. Savonik, 2008)

Kinds of training	Tasks (requirements)
Physical	
General physical	Development of special physical qualities
Special physical	
Special motion	Development of abilities, required for mastering acrobatic exercises
Technical	
With objects	Mastering of basic exercises
Compositional	Training of competition programs
Choreographic	Perfection of elements of classic and other dances
Tactic	
In individual kinds	Training of competition program Working out of tactic for competition
In pair (group) exercises	Logic disposition of acrobats and training of their interaction in pairs (groups)
In team	Formation of team. Setting of team and personal tasks. The sequence of performances at competitions
Competition	
All kinds of acrobatics	Acquiring of experience of participation in competitions. Stability and reliability of fulfillment of competition program

Stage of initial training

As analysis of special scientific methodic literature shows certain difficulties of selection in sport acrobatics are connected with sharp rejuvenation of sports. At initial stage mainly boy and girls of 6-8 years age are enrolled in sport acrobatic groups. This age period is favorable for mastering of new movements and the more of them will be mastered, the better, in future, difficult elements will be trained. This stage lasts 1-2 years [10, 11, 14].

At this stage, in acrobatic, main role is played by anthropometrical and morphological characteristics of trainees [2, 8, 9, 11, 15].

When selecting children to acrobatic sport groups it is recommended by specialists to use a number of tests: balance, asymmetry of limbs' movements, latent period of motion response, quickness and frequency of movements, temp, posture. Sportsman's body height; size of foot, hand are important elements for choosing of sport acrobatic kind. Special accent is made on orientation of movements, which witnesses about physical condition and fitness, about condition of nervous system (strength, balance, mobility, dynamic) (Ye.V. Bogatina, L.E. Pasmurova, "Crieria and orientations in sport acrobatics"/ Ye.V. Bogatina, L.E. Pasmurova, //Materials of V International students' electronic scientific conference "Students' scientific forum" URL: http://www.scienceforum.ru); V.N. Boloban, 2008) [2, 3].

In connection with not stable in this age period attention it is recommended to use at trainings play form with methods of encouragement. Visual method of explanation is also widely used at trainings of such type.

On initial stage there is realized work, oriented on comprehensive physical progressing, teaching to principles of acrobatic techniques, fulfillment of tests for passing to next stage of training and cultivation of steady interest to sport acrobatic trainings.

Trainings are planned without usage of significant physical or psychological loads with accent on warming up exercises from different kinds of sports [7, 11, 14, 18-20, 22].

Main tasks of training at this stage are:

1. Selection of children for acrobatic training, considering morphological criteria and motor abilities. 2. Strengthening of health. 3. Harmonious physical development (removal of defects in physical condition). 4. Teaching to principles of acrobatic techniques' principles and to wide circle of motion skills. 5. Comprehensive development of physical qualities: flexibility, endurance, coordination, speed and power abilities. 6. Cultivation of moral-will qualities. 7. Formation of trainees' firm interest to systemic acrobatic trainings.

High level of trainings' effectiveness on this stage depends on a number of factors:

- Optimal age of starting of acrobatic trainings;

• Selection of children with characteristics of composition, which correspond to requirements of sport acrobatic requirements;

• Complex evaluation of motion abilities' correspondence;

• Individual level of mastering of simple and complex elements.

Elements for accuracy and coordination are gradually introduced in trainings. Acrobats master space, time and power characteristics of movements, fulfilled with high amplitude, quickness and temp.

The basis of program includes GPT and SPT exercises, special movements training (SMT) and special technical training (STT). GPT include general developing exercises, run, jumps, climbing. SMT tasks include development of coordination abilities both of static and dynamic character.

Main tasks of STT at initial stage are mastering of basic elements of acrobatic, choreographic elements as well as exercises on battue. Evaluation of individual achievements reduces to fulfillment of control tests by trainees, i.e. tests, close to program of physical and technical trainings [5, 6, 7, 15].

Stage of preliminary basic training. To this stage trainees, who were trained at initial stage not less than 1-2 years, pass.

Optimal age for the beginning of basic stage of initial specialization in acrobatics is 8-10 years. Duration of the stage is, in average, 3-5 years. Trainings take place in trainings groups [5, 6, 9, 12].

The necessary conditions are: fulfillment of special tests in general and special physical, technical trainings, which are determined by curriculum.

Main tasks of training are:

1. Strengthening of health.
2. Removal of defects in physical condition.
3. Perfection of level of general and specialized physical fitness.
4. Harmonious physical development.
5. Formation of steady interest to purposeful many-years' sport training.
6. Creation of firm motion potential for successful mastering of different motion skills.
7. Teaching to acrobatic techniques.
8. Preparation for tactical and psychological readiness.
9. Cultivation of moral-will qualities.

Stage of specialized training is especially important in formation of sportsmen. In this period main motion qualities are formed, great number of specific for acrobatic motion skills (elements and combinations) is mastered. Sportsmen acquire experience of participation in competitions. Basic elements are formed in basic combinations, which facilitate mastering of techniques in pair-group acrobatics. Some more difficult elements are mastered. For years of training at this stage the trainees are awarded with qualification sport grades.

Age of starting and finishing of this stage is influenced by individual temps of biological development.

Perfection of technique is based on material of the chosen kind of acrobatic. Comprehensive training with little scope of special exercises is characteristic for it. Such training results in formation of sportsmen's quick mastering of technique of the chosen kind of acrobatics.

Against the background of physical qualities' increment large loads shall not be planned at this stage.

Within this stage two periods are usually marked out: initial specialized training and profound specialized training. **In period of initial specialized training** acrobats master material of classification programs as well as perspective elements, links and combinations. In this period, as a rule, selection of acrobats in pairs or groups is conducted for more intensive deepened training.

In period of profound specialized training large scope of elements and combinations of technical training and SPT are criteria of acrobats' progress. Coaches conduct active pedagogic control for determination of promising sportsmen, who, in their age, go ahead of their peers. For starting of stage of profound specialization age of 10-12 year is considered to be optimal. This stage lasts 3-4 years.

Sportsmen are tested regularly by control tests for physical and technical fitness.

In this period sportsmen show increasing of physical fitness's level as well as sport results, considering individual features.

Main tasks of specialized profound training are: 1.Strengthening of health and comprehensive physical development. 2. Training and perfection of pair-group techniques. 3. Gradual leading of sportsmen to higher physical loads. 4. Dozed increase of training loads' intensity. 5. Mastering of complex elements and combinations, connected with combined rotations. 6. Moral will training, applied at competitions.

At this stage training means resemble competition exercises. We can observe increase of SPT and tactical training, means of power and special endurance.

There are certain factors, which restrict application of high physical loads at this stage: 1. Peculiarities of growing of junior sportsmen, i.e. functional specificities of organism. 2. Unevenness in morphological functional indicators and indicators of cardio-vascular system, body length and development of strength.

At stage of specialized training sportsmen, as a rule, master programs of candidate master of sports and even master of sports [5, 6, 9].

To **stage of sport perfection** usually sportsmen (as a rule 13-14 years old and older), who passed tests not less than for candidate master of sports, get. It is characterized by further deepening of specialized training, by mastering of standards for master of sports. Intensive increase of training loads coincides with active phase of acrobats' puberty. So individualized work is required; motor density of training increases. Coach work by individual plans in compliance with the set tasks.

Main tasks of this stage:

1. Planning of individual trainings (for every sportsman of acrobatic pair or group separately). 2. Perfection of technique of earlier mastered elements. 3. Mastering of elements of increased complexity.4.Successful performance of sportsmen by program of master of sports at competitions of different ranks (in particular at championships of Ukraine).5.Achievement of high and stable results and maintaining of results at high level for long time. 6. Fulfillment of tests for master of sports. 7. Making of competition program for participation in final of Ukrainian championships. 8. Selection and training of promising sportsmen for combined junior teams for participation in international competitions.

At this stage great physical loads are actively used; scope of fitness increases as well as integral and tactic fitness [5, 6, 9].

Stage of highest sport achievements is regarded for every separate sportsman or pair (group) individually. For some sportsmen the highest sport result can be performance by program of master of sports, for other – medals at international competitions of different ranks.

One of the most important indicator of training process's effectiveness is results of acrobats' fitness: level of their technique in acrobatic elements and combinations; complexity of exercises (as per tables of complexity); reliability of fulfillment of competition compositions.

At this stage it is necessary to plan scope and intensity of loads, considering reliability and stability of mastering of competition program.

Coaches work individually with every sportsman, pair or group, who are in national combined team. Level of acrobats' sportsmanship is on high level. At this stage main criterion of progress is mastering of new competition programs, introduction of new elements in compliance with rising requirements.

At stage of finishing of sport career it is important to gradually reduce great training loads for [preservation of sportsmen's health. Sharp reduction of loads can negatively influence on health of trainees. In acrobatics, after sport career, advanced sportsmen, after special casting, have opportunity to work in different show programs, in particular in famous Canadian circus "Dusseli".

However, usually acrobats, at the end of acrobatic career, shall pass to 3-5 trainings a week mode (maintaining mode). Also, sportsmen can pass to other kinds of sports.

Duration of trainings and most important requirements to training of acrobats are briefly given in table 2.

Table 2

Structure of many years' training in sport acrobatics

Training stages	Groups	Requirements	Q-ty of trainings
Initial training	Initial training	Fulfillment of tests for mass grades	2-3 times a week/ 1-2 hours
Preliminary basic	Training	III, II, I adult grade CMS	4-6 times a week/ 3-4 hours
Specialized basic	Sport perfection	CMS	6-8 times (1-2 times a week, double trainings)
Preparation for highest achievements	Of highest sportsmanship		
Maximal realization of individual potentials			
Maintenance of highest sportsmanship	National combined teams		6-8 times/ 3-4 hours a day
Gradual reduction of achievements		MS IMS	3-5 times a week / 2-3 hours

Conclusions:

Analyzing of main tasks of all stages of many years' training we may conclude about the following:

1. At initial stage leading indicators are: efficiency of selection of trainees in acrobatic groups; preservation as much of contingent of trainees as possible; control of indicators of expelling of not promising sportsmen.
2. At stage of specialized training the criteria are: quantity and quality of mastered and steadily fulfilled elements of basic technical and physical fitness, acquiring of sport grades by trainees.
3. At stage of sport perfection leading requirements are: presence of free and final program, corresponding to model characteristics of promising acrobats, pairs and groups.
4. At stage of highest achievements main bench marks are: high sport result, membership in national combined team; continuous growth of competition programs' complexity and achievement of personal peak.
5. At stage of sport career's finalizing one can observe stabilizing of sport results, when complexity (competition difficulty) of exercises shows no dynamic. Results gradually reduce.

Some differences in age indicators of sportsmen's results are explained by specificities of early specialization; by coming of sportsmen from adjoining kinds of sports, in particular from sport gymnastic to acrobatics; by specificity of role (upper, lower, central), by different periods of puberty.

Further researches are planned in direction of studying of morphological functional distinctions of acrobats of different age and roles.

References:

1. Absaliamov T.M. [Planning, control and management of training high-class athletes in cyclic sports]. *Nauchnye trudy VNIIFK* [Scientific papers VNIIFK], Moscow, VNIIFK, 1996, pp. 4-27. (In Russian)
2. Boloban V.N. *Metodika otbora detej dlia zaniatij akrobatikoj. Sportivnaia akrobatika* [Method of selecting children for training acrobatics. Sports acrobatics], Kiev, High School, 2008, pp. 18-32. (In Russian)
3. Boloban V. N. Obuchenie akrobaticheskim uprazhneniiam balansnogo tipa dvizhenij sistemy tel [Education acrobatic exercises balanced type motions of the system body]. *Nauka a olimpijskom sporte,* 2008, no.1, pp. 24 – 32. (In Russian)
4. Gibaddulin I.G. *Upravlenie trenirovochnym processom biatlonistov v sisteme mnogoletnej podgotovki. Dokt. Diss.* [Management training process biathletes in the system long-term preparation, Dokt. Diss.], Moscow, 2005, 309 p. (In Russian)
5. Savonik L.V. *Dopolnitel'naia obrazovatel'naia uchebnaia programma «Sportivnaia akrobatika»* [Additional educational training program "Sports acrobatics"], Murmansk, 2008, 39 p. (In Russian)
6. Berdinskikh S.Iu., Goncova E. Iu. *Dopolnitel'naia obrazovatel'naia programma fizkul'turno-sportivnoj napravlennosti «Sportivnaia akrobatika»* [Additional educational program of physical culture and sports orientation "sports acrobatics"], 2008, 96 p. (In Russian)
7. Kyzim P.N., Alabin V.G., Makurin Iu.K. *Akrobaticheskij rok-n-roll* [Acrobatic Rock and Roll]. Kharkov, Basis, 1999, 116 p. (In Russian)
8. Malinovskij S.K. *Metodika sovershenstvovaniia special'noj fizicheskoj podgotovki akrobatov na etape nachal'noj sportivnoj specializacii* [Technique of perfection of special physical preparation of acrobats on the stage of initial sports specialization]. Khabarovsk, 2003, 172 p. (In Russian)
9. Nesterova Tat'iana. Sovershenstvovanie sistemy mnogoletnej podgotovki sportsmenok v khudozhestvennoj gimnastike [Improving the system of long-term preparation of athletes in artistic gymnastics]. *Nauka v olimpijskom sporte*, 2007, no.1 pp. 66-73. (In Russian)
10. Piliuk N.N. *Postroenie i realizaciia sistemy sorevnovatel'noj deiatel'nosti akrobatov vysokoj kvalifikacii. Dokt. Diss.* [Construction and implementation of a system of competitive activity of acrobats of high qualification. Dokt. Diss.], Moscow, 2003, pp. 4-10. (In Russian)
11. Platonov V., Sakhnovskij K., Ozimek M. Sovremennaia strategiia mnogoletnej sportivnoj podgotovki [Modern strategy of long-term sports preparation]. *Nauka v olimpijskom sporte*, 2004; (1); 3-13. (In Russian)
12. Kan V.Ia., Belgrad S.V., Ivanov V.A., Iasharov S.G., Levkov K.G. *Programma sportivnoj podgotovki GBU «Sportivnaia shkola vol. 29 «Khamovniki» Moskomsporta po akrobaticheskomu rok-n-rollu* [The program of sports training "Sports School 29" Acrobatic Rock and Roll]. Moscow, 2013, 59 p. (In Russian)
13. Ruziev A.A. *Nauchno-metodicheskie osnovy mnogoletnej podgotovki kvalificirovannykh iunykh borcov. Dokt. Diss.* [Scientific and methodological foundations of long-term preparation of qualified young wrestlers. Dokt. Diss.]. Moscow, 1999, 30 p. (In Russian)
14. Sakhnovskij K.P. *Teoretiko-metodicheskie osnovy sistemy mnogoletnej sportivnoj podgotovki. Dokt. Diss.* [Theoretical and methodological bases the system long-term sports preparation, Dokt. Diss.]. Kiev, 1997, 318 p. (In Russian)
15. Shebaldina O.V. *Komplektovanie sostavov zhenskikh akrobaticheskikh grupp na etape specializirovannoj podgotovki s uchetom pokazatelej teloslozheniia, motoriki i lichnostnykh osobennostej sportsmenok. Cand. Diss.* [Recruitment compositions female acrobatic groups at the stage of specialized training based on indicators of body, motor skills and personality characteristics of female athletes. Cand. Diss.], Volgograd, 2004, 126 p. (In Russian)

16. Batieieva N.P. Optimization of the training process with skilled athletes acrobatic rock and roll in the annual preparation of macrocycles based on model characteristics. *Pedagogics, psychology, medical-biological problems of physical training and sports,* 2014, no.8, pp. 3-8. http://dx.doi.org/10.6084/m9.figshare.1022947
17. Bołoban W., Wiśniowski W., Płaza M., Niźnikowska E., Niźnikowski T. *The elements of sports orientation theory at the recrutrment for coordinationaly complex sports disciplines. Directions of development of scientific research in sports training*. Częstochowa: Faculty of management Technical University of Częstochowa, 2004, pp. 9 – 12. (in Polish)
18. Zaporozhanov V.A., Kochanowicz K., Kochanowicz A. Improvement of comprehensive assessment of specially trained childhood and adolescence gymnasts. *Pedagogics, psychology, medical-biological problems of physical training and sports,* 2014, no.10, pp. 3-7. http://dx.doi.org/10.5281/zenodo.10482
19. Kozhanova O.S. Compatibility of sports-women at a selection in commands on group exercises of calisthenics taking into account their technical and special preparedness. *Pedagogics, psychology, medical-biological problems of physical training and sports,* 2013, no.2, pp. 34-37. http://dx.doi.org/10.6084/m9.figshare.639188
20. Lyulina N.V., Zakharova L.V., Vetrova I.V. Effect of complex acrobatic elements in the development of physical skills of preschool children. *Physical education of students*, 2013, no.4, pp. 59-62. http://dx.doi.org/10.6084/m9.figshare.662618
21. Omelyanenko V.I. Complex integrated method of improvement of sports ballroom dance perfomance. *Physical education of students*, 2014, no.6, pp. 49-53. http://dx.doi.org/10.15561/20755279.2014.0610
22. Soronovich I.M., Chaikovsky E.V., Pilevskaya V. Features of functional support of competitive activity in sports dance given the differences prepared by partners. *Physical education of students*, 2013, no.6, pp. 78-87. http://dx.doi.org/10.6084/m9.figshare.840556.

RELATIONSHIP BETWEEN QUALITY OF LIFE AND RESILIENCE AMONG SPORT-ACTIVE SINGAPOREAN YOUTH

Michael Chia, Marcus Lee
Physical Education & Sports Science, National Institute of Education, Nanyang Technological University, Singapore

Abstract. *Purpose*: The study examines the relationship between paediatric quality of life (PEDSQL) and resilience, measured by the Singapore Youth Resilience Scale (SYRESS) among sport-active youth transiting from primary to secondary school education in Singapore. *Method*: The participants were 137 student-athletes aged 12.7 ± 0.3 years, height 156.0 ± 12.9 cm, and body mass 46.4 ± 10.2kg. PEDsQL and SYRESS questionnaires were administered at the start of the academic year and repeated again six months later. *Results:* Total health (PEDsQL) scores were significantly greater at baseline than when measured six months later (77.3±11.9 vs 72.1±11.8; $p<0.05$) but there was no significant change in the SYRESS score (198.2 ± 25.3 vs 194.0 ± 27.4; $p>0.05$). Total health in PEDsQL was significantly correlated to SYRESS scores at both time points (Baseline $r_s=0.61, p<0.01$; baseline plus 6 months $r_s=0.58$, $p<0.01$). *Conclusions*: The results reflect a linkage between student's resilience and PedsQL outcomes. Student-athletes perceived the transition from primary to secondary school to be a difficult period and sport-active youth are a unique population compared to normal school going youth.
Keywords: Quality of life, Resilience, sport-active youth, Singapore, secondary school transition.

Introduction

After six years of compulsory primary schooling (Primary1-6), beginning at age 6, Singaporean children transit to a secondary school education (Secondary 1-4 or 5), on the merit of nationalised examination results for another four to five years. In terms of academic coverage of subjects, there is a significant increase from 4 to 9 academic examinable subjects in the transition from Primary 6 to Secondary1. Additionally, in secondary school, youths are exposed to many different sports, where they are encouraged to enrol in 'after-school' co-curricular activities (CCA). CCAs complement the academic curriculum and contribute to students' holistic development. Participation in organized sports is a popular mechanism of achieving adolescent physical activity. It also brings about many health-related benefits which includes physical and psychosocial benefits (Côté, Strachan, & Fraser-Thomas, 2008). Recent statistics from the National Youth Council revealed that regular participation (1 to 2 times a week) of Singaporean youth aged 13 to 10 is at 64.8% which represents an increase from previous years (NYC, 2012).

The period of transition from primary to secondary school is believed to pose challenges or threats to adolescent well-being and quality of life (Seidman, Allen, Aber, Mitchell, & Feinman, 1994; Sirsch, 2003; Zeedyk et al., 2003). In a new environment, adjustments to social, academic and sporting factors would have to be made. Examples of such adjustments include an increase in disciplinary rules and regulations, an increase in opportunities to pursue different sport and activities, new teachers and coaches to interact with and also a new set of school peers (Seidman et al., 1994). In the Singaporean context, there is also an increase in academic workload from four to up to nine examinable subjects. Failure to successfully navigate and cope with it might have an impact on their well-being, mental health and also academic performance (Zeedyk et al., 2003). With changes and transition coming in quickly, there are always added challenges during this developmental adolescent phase both in the academic environment and also in sport competition. It is also in this period that quality of life (QoL) across several domains are affected (Seidman et al., 1994; Sirsch, 2003). QoL assesses an individual's perceptions of their position in life, in the context of the culture and value systems in which they live, in relation to their goals, expectations, standards and concerns. A Singaporean-based study on local primary schools pupils showed that increased school-based physical activity over a 40-week period improved the quality of life of students (Chia, Mukherjee, Nasrun., & Lim, 2013). On the other hand, adolescent athletes that are active in sport participation in inter-school or club sport reported better quality of life (QOL) compared to healthy individuals who do not participate in sport (Lam, Valier, Bay, & McLeod, 2013; Snyder et al., 2010).

Even though it may be logical to classify athletes as members of a healthy adolescent population, there is evidence, which show that athletes are a special and unique population where adolescent athletes scored better overall QoL than their non-athlete counterparts as well as enhanced mental, emotional and social health. Male adolescent athletes also have significantly higher scores compared to female adolescent athletes (Lam et al., 2013; Snyder et al., 2010). This suggests that sport and physical activities can be used as a means of improving the quality of life. Additionally youths who engage in sport on a regular basis should be treated as a different population group.

Sex differences in health outcomes on physical and psychological factors in early to mid-adolescence are documented (Sweeting & West, 2003). Regardless of the instrumentation used to measured health outcomes such as QoL, research shows that female participants usually score lower on the emotional scale rating (Jörngården, Wettergen, & von Essen, 2006; Reinfjell, Diseth, Veenstra, & Vikan, 2006; Upton et al., 2005). A Singaporean-based study on youths also supported the results seen in these Western populations (Yeo, Ang, Chong, & Huan, 2007). However, Yeo et al. (2009) reported that female adolescent reported higher positive adjustment towards school life and better interpersonal relationships compared to their male counterparts. The difference in emotional distress could be explained by gender role expectations in which femininity is associated with an expression of emotions, whereas masculinity is associated with active problem solving and a suppression of emotions (Ptacek, Smith, & Dodge, 1994). These male-female dispositions explain the difference in attitudes towards handling events and situations between genders. Furthermore, female participants tend to perceive stressful events more extremely than male participants, either positively or negatively and hence they respond differently to their emotional states (Newcomb, Huba, & Bentler, 1986).

Improving and developing the resilience of individuals are important for improving the well-being of youths. A key requirement of resilience is the presence of both risks, and factors that promote a positive outcome or reduce and avoid a negative outcome (Fergus & Zimmerman, 2005). In the context of the present study, the risk faced by participants is the transition from primary to secondary school while the positive outcomes are seemingly the holistic development of youths through the participation in school CCAs. A measurement of the outcome of resilience could indicate a positive adjustment (e.g. transition) as showed by a healthy development (e.g. quality of life). Having a high resilience would enable one to cope with change or stressors when the need arises (Davydov, Stewart, Ritchie, & Chaudieu, 2010). In the Singaporean context, the relationship between resilience and quality of life remains unknown.

Purpose, tasks of the work, material and methods

The aim of this study was to investigate and track the quality of life and resilience of sport-active youths within an academic year, following the transition from primary to secondary school. Secondly, it was to examine the relationship between quality of life and resilience in adolescence.

Method

Participants

The participants were Secondary 1 student-athlete intakes, via a convenience sampling approach recruited from two local secondary schools in the new academic year. Student-athletes are youths enrolled in the schools' sports team or sports core-curriculum (CCA). The students and parents were briefed about the research study and were allowed to opt out of the study if they did not wish to participate. Student and parents' assent and consent were obtained prior to participation in the study. Institutional ethics clearance for the study was sought and granted (IRB 12/04/17).

Conduct of the research

The study was conducted in a physical education setting where participants were monitored in two stages, six months apart within one academic year. The questionnaires were administered by the researcher in the presence of the physical education (PE) teacher before the start of their PE class or sport training. Students answered the questionnaire in a quiet classroom or in the multi-purpose hall of the school. For both occasions when the questionnaires were administered, the measurement conditions were the same- that is they were obtained at the same time of the day, and on same day of the week for both baseline and follow-up measurements.

The baseline data collection was conducted at the start of the academic semester at the beginning of the year where a total of 153 students were enrolled. Complete data from 151 students (compliance 98.7%) were used for the analysis of the baseline results. In the follow-up data collection, 10 students did not complete the follow-up and after adjusting for incomplete answers, a total of 137 (82 males, 55 females) matched pairs with complete data were used for the subsequent baseline-follow up analyses. Missing data were due to an absence from PE, or a failure to turn up on the test date or having incomplete questionnaire responses.

Measures

Health related quality of life (HRQOL) was measured by the PedsQL 4.0 (Pediatric Quality of Life Inventory Version 4.0). The PedsQL 4.0 is valid and reliable (Varni, Seid, & Kurtin, 2001) and were used in Singaporean school contexts (Østbye, Malhotra, Wong, Tan, & Saw, 2010). The PedsQL 4.0 is a 23-item questionnaire with Generic Scales that are designed to measure the core dimensions of health as delineated by World Health Organisation. The questionnaire takes less than 5 minutes to complete and covered four domains: physical (8 items), emotional (8 items), social functioning (5 items), and school functioning (8-items). The instructions enquire about how much of a problem each item has been during the last month. The items are reverse-scored and linearly transformed to a 0–100 scale (0=100, 1=75, 2=50, 3=25, 4=0), so that higher scores indicate better HRQOL. A total scale score is derived by the mean of all 23 items, which provides an overall measure of the HRQOL.

Resilience was measured by the Singapore Youth Resilience Scale (SYRESS) (Lim, Broekman, Wong, Wong, & Ng, 2007). The SYRESS is a self-rating scale of 50 questions that requires the respondent to indicate how much he/she agrees with each statement on a 5-point Likert scale ranging from "never" (1) to "always" (5). Scores range from 50 to 250 with higher scores denoting higher resilience. Anthropometric measurements are provided by the physical education teachers where measurements are taken yearly during PE class. BMI is derived from using the height and weight by the formula - Weight (kg) / [Height (m) x Height (m)]. Weight status is interpreted by the guidelines by the health promotion board (HPB, 2002).

Statistical Analyses

The mean score data are presented as mean ± SD. Data are separated into male and female. Gender differences are compared using independent-sample *t* test. Baseline and follow-up scores were compared using paired sampled *t* test with effect sizes (Cohen'd). The following criteria were adopted for interpreting the magnitude of change: 0.2 (small), 0.5 (moderate), and 0.8 (high). Associations between variables (PEDsQL and SYRESS) were assessed using Pearson's product-moment correlation coefficients and linear regression analysis. Statistical significance was accepted at $p < 0.05$.

Results

Participants

A total of 153 student athletes participated in the studies after parental consent. After adjusting for incomplete answers and matched pair samples of both baseline and follow-up measurements, a total of 137 (82 males, 55 females) paired-sample data were used for the analysis. To evaluate dropout bias, those data set dropped, were compared with the data set used for the analysis. There were no significant differences for mean PEDsQL scores (p=0.40-0.96) and no significant difference for mean SYRESS scores (p=0.12-0.16). The mean ages of the students were 12.7 ± 0.3 years; male 12.6 ± 0.3 years, and female 12.7 ± 0.3 years. Overall mean height was 156.0 ± 12.9 cm; male 155.5 ± 10.0cm and female 156.8 ± 16.5 cm. Overall mean weight were 46.4 ± 10.2 kg; male 44.7 ± 10.3kg, female 49.1 ± 9.5 kg. BMI-for-age for both genders was classified with the percentile chart by MOH. There are 7 (5.1%) severely underweight; 2 (1.5%) underweight; 121 (88.3%) acceptable weight; 6 (4.4%) overweight; and 1 (0.7%) severely overweight. Ranges of sports included were both individual based sports and team-based sports (track and field, netball, badminton, soccer and swimming).

Paediatric Quality of life & SYRESS

Descriptive statistics of PEDsQL are presented in Table 1. There is a gender difference in physical health. Male participants scored significantly higher than female participants in physical health both (p<0.05) at baseline and follow up time points. Male participants also scored significantly higher than female participants in SYRESS at follow up measurement (p<0.05).

Table 1:

Mean scores of PEDsQL of male and female participants at baseline and follow-up

	Overall (N=137)		Male (n=82)		Female (n=55)		*t*	*df*	*P* value
Variables	M	SD	M	SD	M	SD			
Physical health	79.9	11.4	81.8	10.7	77.0	11.9	2.43	135	0.02*
Emotional health	76.6	17.9	77.7	18.4	75.1	17.0	0.82	135	0.42
Social health	78.8	16.2	79.5	16.3	77.7	16.3	0.65	135	0.52
School Function	71.4	16.9	70.7	18.5	72.4	14.2	-0.57	135	0.57
Psychosocial health	75.8	14.4	76.0	14.6	75.1	14.1	0.35	135	0.73
Total health	77.3	11.9	78.1	11.9	76.0	11.9	0.98	135	0.33
SYRESS	198.2	25.3	200.6	25.6	199.5	25.4	1.37	135	0.17
Follow-up Scores									
Physical health	82.6	11.9	84.5	11.2	79.1	11.6	2.46	135	0.02*
Emotional health	70.9	18.1	71.8	19.8	69.7	15.3	0.68	132.16	0.50
Social health	77.3	16.8	77.3	18.2	77.3	14.5	-0.01	131.18	0.99
School Function	67.3	17.5	67.1	19.4	67.6	14.3	-0.20	133.62	0.85
Psychosocial health	66.5	13.9	66.8	15.8	66.2	10.6	0.27	135	0.79
Total health	72.1	11.8	72.9	13.2	70.8	9.1	1.11	134.90	0.27
SYRESS	194.0	27.4	194.6	24.6	185.6 ±	28.3	3.00	135	<0.05*

[a]Psychosocial health is the mean of the sum of emotional and social health and school functioning,
[b]Total Health is the mean of the sum of Physical And Psychosocial
*Sex difference is significant at p<0.05

Differences between baseline and follow-up PEDs & SYRESS scores

The magnitude of change from baseline to follow-up measurements for the PEDsQL and SYRESS is presented in Table 2. Figure 1 shows the differences in PEDsQL and SYRESS at baseline and follow-up measurements. Follow up physical health scores were significantly greater than at baseline measurement (M=-2.7, SD=12.1), t (136) =-2.6,

$p<0.05$. Follow up measurement of emotional health was significantly less than at baseline measurement (M=5.7, SD=16.1), t (136)=4.1, $p<0.05$. There was no difference ($p>0.05$) in baseline and follow up social health scores. Follow up school functioning was significantly lower than at baseline measurement (M=4.1, SD=17.9), t (136)=2.7, $p<0.05$. Follow up psychosocial health was significantly lower than at baseline measurement (M=9.1, SD=12.4), t (136)=8.6, $p<0.05$. Follow up total health was significantly lower than at baseline measurement (M=5.2, SD=10.0), t(136)=6.1 $p<0.05$.

Table 2

Magnitude of change in PEDs QL and SYRESS from baseline to follow-up measurement

	Baseline		Follow-Up		Change (%)	*t*	*df*	*p*	Cohen's d
Variables	M	SD	M	SD					
Physical health	79.9	11.4	82.6	11.9	+2.7	-2.62	136	0.01*	0.23
Emotional health	76.6	17.9	70.9	18.1	-5.7	4.13	136	<0.05**	-0.32
Social health	78.8	16.2	77.3	16.8	-1.5	1.01	136	0.32	-0.09
School Function	71.4	16.9	67.3	17.5	-4.1	2.67	136	<0.05**	-0.24
Psychosocial health	75.8	14.4	66.5	13.9	-9.3	8.59	136	<0.05**	-0.66
Total health	77.3	11.9	72.1	11.8	-5.2	6.07	136	<0.05**	-0.44
SYRESS	198.2	25.3	194.0	27.4	-4.2	1.87	136	0.06	-0.16

*Follow-up scores are significantly higher, **Baseline scores are significantly higher

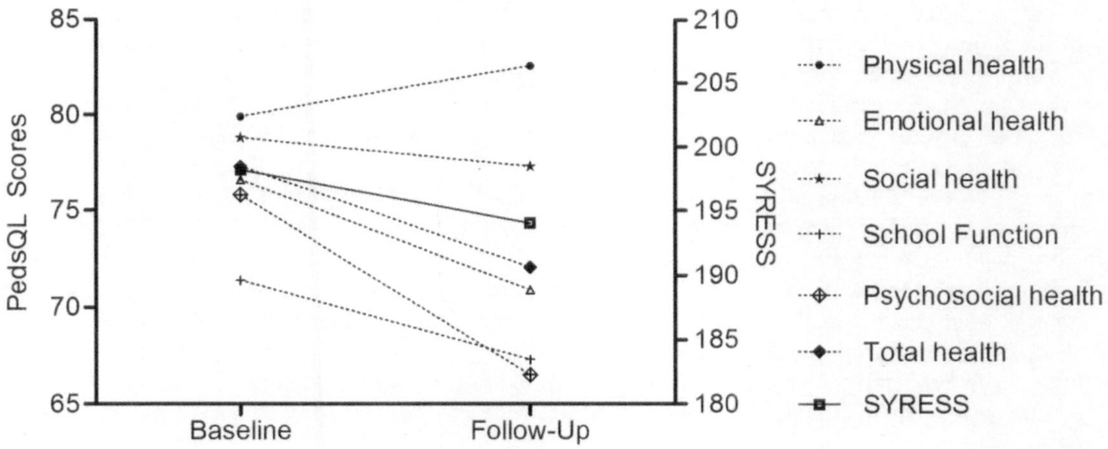

Figure 1. Changes in PEDs QL and SYRESS between baseline and follow-up. Follow-up PEDSQL scores for emotional, psychosocial and total health are significantly lower than at baseline ($p<0.05$). Follow-up scores of physical health are significantly higher than at baseline ($p<0.05$)

Relationship between PEDsQL and SYRESS

The association between PEDsQL and SYRESS is presented in Table 3. The PEDsQL sub-scale scores have moderate correlations with SYRESS (range 0.42-0.61) and are significant at $p<0.05$. Linear regression analysis showed SYRESS to be a significant predictor for PEDsQL at both baseline ($\beta=0.60$, $p<0.05$), follow up ($\beta=0.51$, $p<0.05$) measurements with an explained variance of 36.2% and 26.3% respectively (Figure 2).

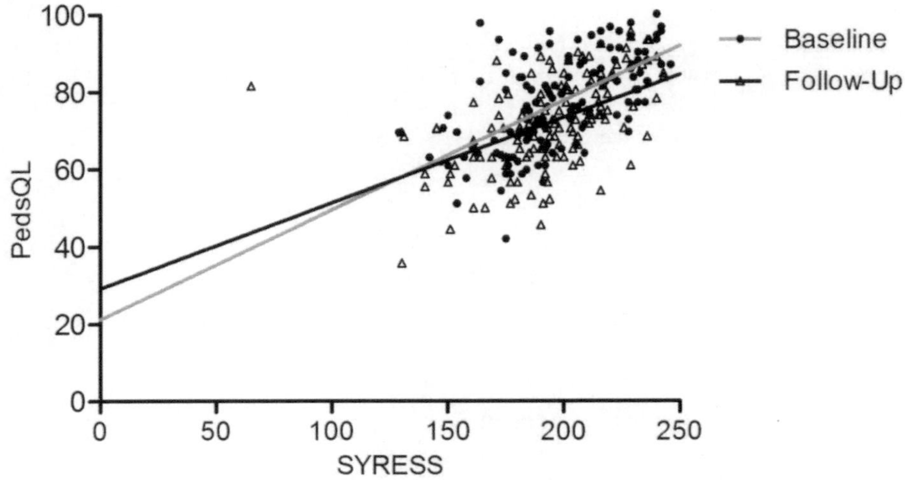

Figure 2. Spearman correlation between PedsQL and SYRESS at baseline and follow-up. The PEDsQL-SYRESS relationship at baseline is described by the linear equation (Y=21.27 + 0.28x; R2= 0.36, 95% CI (0.22-0.35) and the PEDsQL-SYRESS relationship at follow-up is described by the linear equation (Y=29.31 + 0.22x); R2=0.26, 95% CI (0.16 – 0.28).

Discussion

The objectives of the research were (i) to elucidate the quality of life of sport-active Singaporean youth in the transition from primary to secondary school and (ii) to examine the relationship between youth resilience and the quality of life of Singaporean youth.

Impact of school transition on quality of life

The transition from primary to secondary school is an important milestone for Singaporean children and their parents. An important finding of the present study was a lower PEDsQL score in all aspects, except for physical health of quality of life scores when compared to scores reported for healthy adolescents from Western countries of a similar age group (Varni, Limbers, & Burwinkle, 2007). PEDsQL (total health scores) at baseline and six months later were also lower when compared to scores for a wider age range group (age 11-18; N=1249) of Singaporean youths (Østbye et al., 2010). The differences between the two Singapore-based studies could be attributed to sample-specific differences (i.e. sample size and age-range) between the two studies.

Managing new peer relationships, increased workload of school and new school routines are among the common worries experienced by students who transit from primary to secondary school (Zeedyk et al., 2003), and a combination of these factors may help to explain the lower scores experienced by Singaporean youths at the beginning of the school year, only to be exacerbated six months later. Only physical health improved significantly over the same time period, more so in male, than in female youths. Sports-active youths in Singapore perceived their daily life to be difficult during this stage of transition from primary to secondary school, and it appears more so for female, than for male youths. The lower quality of life especially for emotional health reported by female adolescents in the present study is well supported by others (e.g. Upton et al., 2005; Yeo et al., 2007).

The present results are in agreement to those reported by others, albeit in an older age group of students. Varni and Limbers (2009) reported on the quality of life of new undergraduate students in the first year of university life where emotional and school functioning scores were distinctively lower compared to other sub-scale measures of quality of life. In the present study, the competing demands of school adjustment, coping with increased academic workload (primary-to-secondary school transition- an increase from four to eight examinable subjects) and coping with sport training and competition, continue to exacerbate the quality of life (social, emotional, psychosocial, school functioning), six months into the new school year. This is indicative that six months is still insufficient for sport-active youth to adjust to life as the quality of life (except for physical functioning) continues to drop.

In the present study, physical functioning scores improved over the six month period and this could be attributed to the participation and training in sport CCAs and also to the physical growth and maturation of the male adolescents in particular. Physical activity engagement and physical conditioning in sport, especially in a period of growth and muscle development (especially for male adolescents) contribute to one's physical ability and health such as improved fitness and strength. Furthermore, engagement in sport competition would bring about further gains due to a higher motivation in competing against or among peers in sport competition.

An unexpected finding in the present research was that the sport-active youth reported lower overall quality of life outcomes than one would expect. In the extant literature, sport-active youths are reported to have significantly greater quality of life, especially for emotional health compared to the general non-athletic population of youths, with female athletes reporting significantly higher social health compared to male athletes, and also higher social health than non-athletic female youths (Lam et al., 2013; Snyder et al., 2010). The reasons for this difference are not readily apparent, however, it is plausible that sport achievement is considered less important than academic achievement among Singaporean youth compared to the social contexts of other studies, especially when the results emanate from Western contexts. These assertions need to be further examined in future research. Nonetheless, it is apparent that sports-active Singaporean youth are a distinct population on its own, which is different from the general youth population and future research should take this into consideration.

Resilience of youth

The resilience score measured by SYRESS showed a comparable score compared to a healthy adolescent group (Lim et al., 2007). This confirms that there are no differences in terms of resilience between sports-active and healthy adolescent populations. The follow-up scores from baseline values decreased slightly but the decrease did not attain statistical significance. The result affirms that resilience in adolescent is fairly stable and that the mental attributes associated with an individual's resilience remain the same throughout the year despite a decrease in the perception of quality of life. This assertion is supported by research conducted by Masten et al (1999), who reported that resilience is relatively stable over an individual's lifetime. As not all individuals exposed to stressors experience negative psychological effects, the stable resilience scores in the present study indicate that Singaporean adolescents are able to cope with the new stressors brought about by the primary-to-secondary school transition period.

The use of the SYRESS is a useful gauge of the perceived resilience of students and this can help teachers or coaches to monitor the students' perceived resilience rather than using the traditional approach like observing students' behaviour, thereby avoiding observer bias and allow for objective monitoring and tracking over time.

Relationship between youth resilience and paediatric quality of life

The second objective of the study is to investigate the relationship between resilience and quality of life. Results showed a moderate association between SYRESS and the PEDsQL. The moderate positive relationship between Total Health score of PedsQL and SYRESS is seen where a higher resilience is associated with a higher PedsQL score. Linear regression analysis revealed that resilience is a significant predictor for PedsQL but accounts for only 36.2% and 26.3% of the shared variance. Although resilience is not substantially large enough to be used as a predictive outcome for gauging the quality of life of Singaporean youths, the association between SYRESS and PEDsQL showed that resilience plays a contributory role in the adolescents' total health. Previous researchers have discussed the linkage between quality of life and resilience (Lawford & Eiser, 2001). They highlighted the similarities and differences between the concepts of quality of life and resilience and that resilience can explain the variation in quality of life results across childhood and between individual children.

This is the first study that compared the PedsQL scores with a resilience measurement outcome for Singaporean sport-active youth. The positive relationship shown between the two constructs affirm the importance of identifying protective factors and promotion factors in the context of resilience that could predict and explain quality of life outcomes. Future research should examine and explain how a continued engagement in school sport affects these measurements.

Limitation of the research

A limitation of the current study is that it did not account for inter-individual differences in the evaluation of quality of life and resilience. As school transition is not always a negative event, several factors contribute to how well an individual deals with this transition and an identification of these factors would be crucial for a thorough evaluation of how well a student is adapted into his or her environment. Identification of the factors and reasons that contribute to the well-being of the students' school life may contribute to better understanding of the areas that are the causal factors for the quality of life. Another limitation is that the sample is specific to sports-active youth and may not represent the general non-athletic Singaporean youth population.

Conclusion

In conclusion, results of the study showed that sports-active adolescents perceived the transition from primary to secondary school to be difficult, and educators and school administrators may need to mitigate this by coming out with programmes or ways to help smoothen and ease the difficulties faces by youth in this transition. It is also suggestive that sports-active adolescent constitutes a unique population compared to non-sports active adolescent and might need to be evaluated differently compared to normal school-going youth who are not engaged in sport.

Declaration of Conflicting Interests

The authors declared no potential conflicts of interest with respect to the research, authorship, and/or publication of this article.

Funding

The research was supported by NIE Research Grant RS 2/12 MC.

We acknowledge and thank all teachers and students who participated in this research study. We also thank the students' parents for their support in the study.

References

Chia M., Mukherjee S., Nasrun. M., & Lim B. C. "Impact of daily physical education on the healthy related quality of life and academic performance of Singaporean primary school pupil", in Singal P. K. (Ed.), *Adaptation Biology and Medicine,* Narosa Publishing House, 2013, vol.7, Chapter, 26, pp.373-385.

Côté J., Strachan L., & Fraser-Thomas J. Participation, personal development and performance through youth sport. In N. L. Holt (Ed.), *Positive youth development through sport*, London, Routledge, 2008, pp. 34-45.

Davydov D. M., Stewart R., Ritchie K., & Chaudieu I. Resilience and mental health. *Clinical Psychology Review,* 2010, vol.30(5), pp. 479-495.

Fergus S., & Zimmerman M. A. Adolescent resilience: A framework for understanding healthy development in the face of risk. *Annu. Rev. Public Health,* 2005, vol.26, pp. 399-419.

HPB. Health Promotion Board Singapore. 2002, Retrieved 15th Feb, 2014, Available at: http://www.hpb.gov.sg/HOPPortal/health-article/HPB-039205 (accessed 10.03.2015)

Jörngården A., Wettergen L., & von Essen L. Measuring health-related quality of life in adolescents and young adults: Swedish normative data for the SF-36 and the HADS, and the influence of age, gender, and method of administration. *Health and quality of life outcomes,* 2006, vol.4(1), pp. 91-96. doi:10.1186/1477-7525-4-91

Lam K. C., Valier A. R. S., Bay R. C., & McLeod T. C. V. A unique patient population? Health-related quality of life in adolescent athletes versus general, healthy adolescent individuals. *Journal of athletic training,* 2013, vol.48(2), pp. 233-241.

Lawford J., & Eiser, C. Exploring links between the concepts of Quality of Life and resilience. *Developmental Neurorehabilitation,* 2001, vol.4(4), pp. 209-216.

Lim M. L., Broekman B. F., Wong J. C. M., Wong S. T., & Ng T. P. The development and validation of the Singapore Youth Resilience Scale (SYRESS). *Stress, vulnerability and resilience: a developmental approach,* 2007, vol.31, pp. 103-110.

Newcomb M. D., Huba G. J., & Bentler P. M. Desirability of various life change events among adolescents: Effects of exposure, sex, age, and ethnicity. *Journal of Research in Personality,* 1986, vol.20(2), pp. 207-227.

NYC. Youth Statistics In Brief, National Youth Council. 2012, Retrieved 1st March 2014, Available at: https://www.resourceportal.nyc.sg/nycp/ShowDoc/WLP%20Repository/nyc/resources_fs/Youth%20Stats%20in%20Brief%202012 (accessed 10.03.2015)

Østbye T., Malhotra R., Wong H.-B., Tan S.-B., & Saw S.-M. The effect of body mass on health-related quality of life among Singaporean adolescents: results from the SCORM study. *Quality of Life Research,* 2010, vol.19(2), pp. 167-176.

Ptacek J. T., Smith R. E., & Dodge K. L. Gender differences in coping with stress: When stressor and appraisals do not differ. *Personality and Social Psychology Bulletin,* 1994, vol.20(4), pp. 421-430.

Reinfjell T., Diseth T. H., Veenstra M., & Vikan A. Measuring health-related quality of life in young adolescents: Reliability and validity in the Norwegian version of the Pediatric Quality of Life Inventory™ 4.0 (PedsQL) generic core scales. *Health and quality of life outcomes,* 2006, vol.4(1), pp. 61-66.

Seidman E., Allen L., Aber J. L., Mitchell C., & Feinman J. The impact of school transitions in early adolescence on the self-system and perceived social context of poor urban youth. *Child development,* 1994, vol.65(2), pp. 507-522.

Sirsch U. The impending transition from primary to secondary school: Challenge or threat? *International Journal of Behavioral Development,* 2003, vol.27(5), pp. 385-395.

Snyder A. R., Martinez J. C., Bay R. C., Parsons J. T., Sauers E. L., & Valovich McLeod T. C. Health-related quality of life differs between adolescent athletes and adolescent nonathletes. *Journal of sport rehabilitation,* 2010, vol.19(3), pp. 237-248.

Sweeting H., & West P. Sex differences in health at ages 11, 13 and 15. *Social Science & Medicine,* 2003, vol.56(1), pp. 31-39.

Upton P., Eiser C., Cheung I., Hutchings H. A., Jenney M., Maddocks A., Williams J. G. Measurement properties of the UK-English version of the Pediatric Quality of Life Inventory™ 4.0 (PedsQL™) generic core scales. *Health and quality of life outcomes,* 2005, vol.3(1), pp. 22-26.

Varni J. W., Limbers C. A., & Burwinkle T. M. How young can children reliably and validly self-report their health-related quality of life?: An analysis of 8,591 children across age subgroups with the PedsQL™ 4.0 Generic Core Scales. *Health and quality of life outcomes,* 2007, vol.5(1), pp. 1-10.

Varni J. W., Seid M., & Kurtin P. S. PedsQL (TM) 4.0: Reliability and validity of the pediatric quality of life Inventory (TM) Version 4.0 generic core scales in healthy and patient populations. *Medical care,* 2001, vol.39(8), pp. 800-812.

Yeo L. S., Ang R. P., Chong W. H., & Huan V. S. Gender differences in adolescent concerns and emotional well-being: Perceptions of Singaporean adolescent students. *The Journal of genetic psychology,* 2007, vol.168(1), pp. 63-80.

Zeedyk M. S., Gallacher J., Henderson M., Hope G., Husband B., & Lindsay K. Negotiating the transition from primary to secondary school perceptions of pupils, parents and teachers. *School Psychology International,* 2003, vol.24(1), pp. 67-79.

OPERATIVE CORRECTION OF JUDOISTS' TRAINING LOADS ON THE BASE OF ON-LINE MONITORING OF HEART BEATS RATE

Liu Yong Qiang
Henan Polytechnic University, Republic of China

Abstract: *Purpose:* ensure increase of effectiveness of training process's control by means of operative correction of training loads of different qualification judo wrestlers' heart beats rate indicators. *Material:* the research was conducted on the base of Brest SCJSOR № 1. Judo wrestlers of different sport qualification (age 17-19 years old, n=15) participated in the research. Monitoring of judo wrestlers' heart beats rate was carried out with the help of system "Polar". *Results:* we have found factorial structure of functional fitness in every profile of sportsmen. Model characteristics of judo wrestlers were supplemented with the most important sides of functional fitness. Analysis of indicators of restoration effectiveness indicators (REI) in both groups of judo wrestlers showed high level of organism's responsiveness to training load of special and power orientation in comparison with speed power load. We have worked out algorithm of operative correction of training loads by indicators of heart beats rate in training process, depending on orientation and intensity of loads' physiological influence on judo wrestler. *Conclusions:* Telemetric on-line monitoring of sportsman's heart beats rate and calculation of REI permit to objectively assess effectiveness of training's construction and of micro-cycle in total and detect in due time the trend to development of over-loading and failure of adaptation.
Key words: operative control, judo wrestlers, restoration effectiveness indicator, heart beats rate, heart beats rate monitoring, over-load, factorial structure, algorithm, functional fitness.

Introduction

At present in judo there is observed intensification of training process, connected with implementation of new specialized means of training and control over their influence on sportsmen's organisms [1-4].

Modern system of management of judo wrestlers' sport training is based on interconnected functioning of three systems which are in mutual co- submission: purpose of functioning, system of functioning and system of training [4-6]. This combination of application of systemic-structural components is under control and, if necessary, is corrected in general or partially for rendering more substantial impact on prognostic assessment of sport training. In this connection control shall be understood as system of rational measures, based on effective means and methods. In this system means and methods are combined in progressive form of organization of training process in order to achieve prognosticated, planned and expected results.

Complexity of the regarded problem is still more evident, if substantiation of training programs' construction implies not fulfillment of oriented on maximum loads (that is characteristic for the present time) but rather receiving of programmed training effects [2, 7, 8].

At the same time, advanced experience of judo wrestlers' training witnesses, that excessive training and competition loads result in over-tension of organism's functional systems and increase of traumatism. It can be prevented from by rational construction of training process. It is conditioned by balanced correlation of work of different orientation, dynamic of training loads, alternation of tiredness and rest, means of workability's recreation, mobilization of functional reserves of judo wrestlers [1, 9, 10]. In system of control sportsmen's training important place is assigned to scientifically based control, which implies collection of stage-by-stage, current and operative information about object's condition and comparing of his actual condition with proper [2, 3, 11, 12]. With it, role of diagnostics in control system increases, because it permits to create required conditions for operative monitoring of training process and passing of rational adaptation changes in achievement of efficiency and reliability of competition functioning. That is why it is necessary to orient on such indicators, which adequately reflect organism's operative conditions: readiness for fulfillment of certain physical load, speed of recreational processes after trainings, effectiveness of functioning of different physiological systems [13-16].

Besides, in the course of operative control over training activity it is possible to realize the following assessment: sportsman's operative condition (i.e. urgent responses of his organism to loads); express-assessment of sportsman's condition at the moment or just after finishing of exercise. By results of such control it is possible to judge about correspondence of actual training effect with planned effect [7].

Basing on the a.m. we can say that the most informative, integrative and accessible for detection indicators of organism's functional state is heart beats rate (HBR). By its change it is possible to judge about urgent, relayed and cumulative effects of specific training loads [14, 17-19]. That is why control over training loads with monitoring of sportsmen's heart beats rate during fulfillment of different motor tasks by them will permit to achieve more perfect and informative forms of control over work fulfillment. In the future it will facilitate planning of training functioning in general with higher quality.

Thus, the choice of problem of our research was conditioned by ***actual scientific practical contradiction*** between existing system of control over different qualification judo wrestlers' training (on the one hand) and insufficient information about practiced training loads and their adequacy to judo wrestlers' individual potentials (on the other hand).

It is logical to assume that operative correction of judo wrestlers' training loads by indicators of their heart beats rate with the help of modern mobile telemetric means will be one of necessary components of training process's control during all period of training.

Purpose, tasks of the work, material and methods

The purpose of the work is to ensure increase of effectiveness of control over training process by means of operative correction of different qualification judo wrestlers' training loads by hear beats rate indicators.

The task of the work: working out of algorithm of operative correction sequence for training loads of different orientation on the basis of heart beats rate monitoring.

The methods and organization of the research:

In the research we used methods of theoretical study, experimental-empiric methods and methods of mathematical statistic. Mathematical processing of statistical parameters was conducted with the help of computer program STATISTIKA 6.0. For monitoring of judo wrestlers' heart beats rate we used multi-channel radio-telemetric system «Polar 400». With its help we corrected and optimized intensity of training on the base of record of HBR indicators in real time.

For determination of judo wrestlers' functional fitness and its dynamic under impact of training loads we used widely spread in practice of sport wrestling control tests [5].

For assessment of different qualification judo wrestlers' functional fitness we applied the following tests:

1. **Throw of dummy over hip during 1 minute** (special endurance). Description: the tested is in initial position – main stance and holds dummy by hands. By signal the tested shall as quick as possible and technically correctly fulfill throws over hip. Assessment of results: quantity of throws (n), HBR before and after the task and in 4 minutes of rest are registered.
2. **10 throws of dummy over hip** (speed-power endurance). Description: the tested is in initial position – main stance and holds dummy by hands. By signal the tested shall as quick as possible and technically correctly fulfill throws over hip. Assessment of results: quantity of throws (n), HBR before and after the task and in 4 minutes of rest are registered.
3. **Throw of dummy** (big weight) **over hip during 1 minute** (power endurance). Description: the tested is in initial position – main stance and holds dummy by hands. By signal the tested shall as quick as possible and technically correctly fulfill throws over hip. The weight of dummy is selected, considering the mass of the tested. Assessment of results: quantity of throws (n), HBR before and after the task and in 4 minutes of rest are registered.

For assessment of judo wrestlers' functional fitness in test tasks we used method of telemetric pulse metering. It was the simplest way to conduct urgent and current corrections of training session with the help of the so-called ***restoration effectiveness indicator (REI).*** This indicator permits to assess in the whole adequacy of load to sport form of sportsman as on the current moment of time.

Calculation of this indicator is conducted by formula (1), in which it is necessary to put values of pulse metering (HBR) just before fulfillment of training task (t_1), after the last main exercise (t_2) and after 4 minutes' rest (t_3). Processing of data was carried out with program Polar ProTrainer 5.0 (рис. 1).

$$REI = (t_2 - t_3)/ (t_3 - t_1)*100\% \quad (1)$$

Where:

Interpretation of REI depending on value REI = 50-60% – proper load; REI<50% – too high load (tiredness); REI>60% – training stimuli are too low.

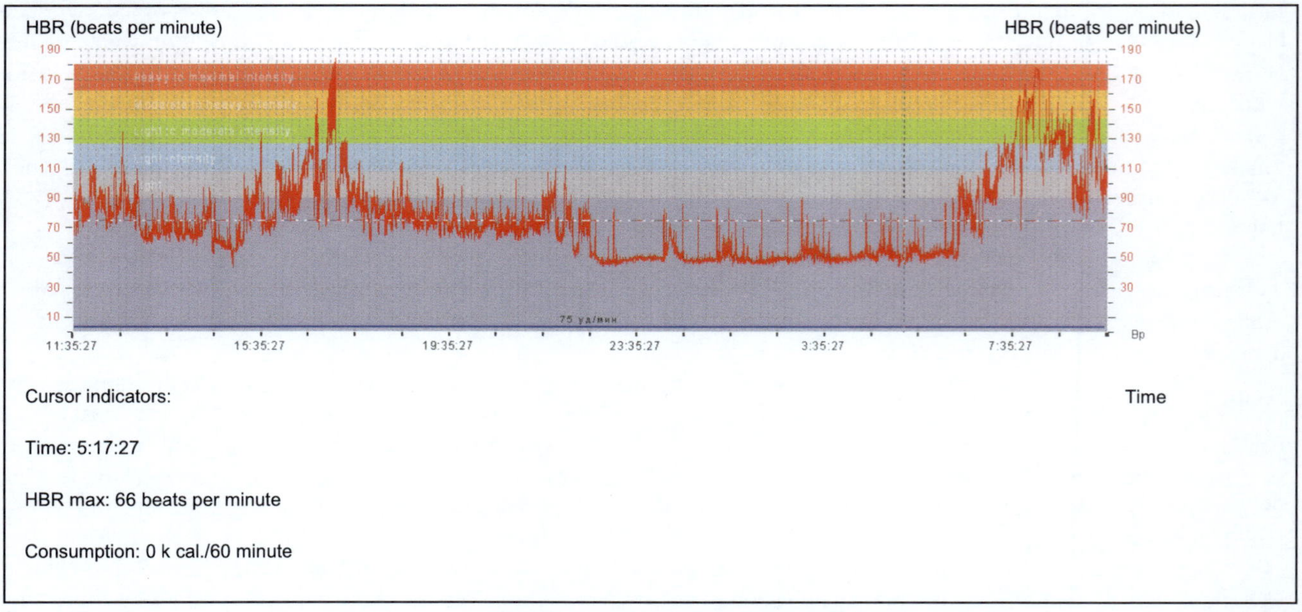

Fig.1. Application of software Polar ProTrainer 5.0.

Results of the research

Comparative analysis of functional fitness (see table 1) of judo different qualification wrestlers (1st group – 1st grade sportsmen, and 2nd group – candidates master of sports – CMS) permitted to reveal statistically unconfident differences (P>0.05) between results of tests "throw of dummy over hip during 1 minute" (special endurance: quantity of throws – t=0.77, HBR after the task – t=1.72, HBR after 4 minutes' rest – t=0.57); "10 throws of dummy over hip" (speed-power endurance: time of throws – t=1.02, HBR after the task – t=0.14, HBR after 4 minutes' rest – t=1.35); "power endurance, quantity of throws– t=0,82, HBR after the task – t=1.62, HBR after 4 minutes' rest – t=0.09);

Table 1

Comparative analysis of functional fitness of different qualification judo wrestlers

Test tasks	№	Indicators	Finalizing experiment						Difference t
			1-grade (7)			CMS (8)			
			M	σ	± m	M	σ	± m	
throw of dummy over hip during 1 minute	1	Quantity of times	14.14	3.39	1.28	15.50	2.29	0.87	0.77
	2	HBR after fulfillment of task	194.57	11.93	4.51	185.25	11.86	4.48	1.72
	3	HBR after 4 minutes	149.14	24.11	9.11	144.00	13.42	5.07	0.57
10 throws of dummy over hip for quickness	1	Time of throws*	28.71	3.77	1.43	27.38	4.19	1.58	1.02
	2	HBR after fulfillment of task	170.57	16.92	6.40	169.50	15.27	5.77	0.14
	3	HBR after 4 minutes	119.14	7.29	2.76	124.50	6.68	2.52	1.35
throw of big mass dummy over hip during 1 minute	1	Quantity of times	10.00	2.38	0.90	11.10	2.61	0.90	0.82
	2	HBR after fulfillment of task	200.57	11.41	4.31	195.75	11.41	4.31	1.62
	3	HBR after 4 minutes	150.00	16.97	6.41	150.00	12.69	4.80	0.09

In the process of factorial analysis of functional fitness structure of different qualification judo wrestlers we found the following characteristics (see table 2): total contribution in total dispersion of sample (TDS) was 85.33%; in 1st group (of 1st graders) we found 3 factors, total contribution of which was 87.15%; in second group (CMS) we found four factors with contribution in TDS – 83.04%; in 1st group (boys) we found 4 factors with total contribution of 94.18%; and in 2nd group (girls) – 3 factors with contribution of 79,87%

Table 2

Factorial structure of functional fitness of different qualification and sex judo wrestlers

Factors	Factorial structure of judo wrestlers	Indicators of factors	% of dispersion
Judo wrestlers (n=15)			
1	Morphological-physiological features	-weight/height indicators, HBR after 4 minutes' rest (accordingly 0.88, 0.77 and 0.82)	35.08
2	Quantitative characteristic	- quantity of throws of dummy (of appropriate mass), of higher mass	25.17

Factors	Factorial structure of judo wrestlers	Indicators of factors	% of dispersion
	of technical tactic actions (TTA)	and time of 10 throws of dummy (0.81, 0.85 and 0,93)	
3	Special power endurance	- HBR after throw of dummy (of proper weight) and (of higher weight) (0.90 and 0.97).	15.04
4	Restoration	- HBR after 4 minutes' rest after 10 throws of dummy with factorial mass 0.91	10.04
Judo wrestlers of different qualification			
1-group (1 graders) (n=7)			
1	Special power endurance	-quantity of throws of dummy and HBR after throw (of proper mass dummy) and (big mass dummy); factorial load (0.81, 0.80, 0.75 and 0.92)	40.28
2	Morphological-physiological characteristics	-weight/height indicators, HBR after 4 minutes' rest after throws (of proper mass dummy) and (big mass dummy); (0.98, 0.96, 0.81 and 0.82),	34.23
3	Speed-power endurance	-time of 10 throws of dummy, HBR after throw and after 4 minutes' rest, factorial load (0.70, 0.72 and 0.90)	12.64
2-group (CMS) (n=8)			
1	Morphological-physiological characteristics	- weight/height indicators, HBR after 4 minutes' rest (accordingly 0.77, 0.83 and 0.72)	36.69
2	Quantitative characteristic of TTA	-quantity of throws of dummy for quickness (of proper mass), (big mass) and time of 10 throws (accordingly 0.91, 0.85, and 0.83),	24.22
3	Special power endurance	-HBR after throw of proper mass dummy and (big mass) (0.96 and 0.97).	22.14
Judo wrestlers of different sex			
1-group (boys) (n=7)			
1	Morphological-physiological	- weight/height indicators, HBR after 4 minutes' rest after throws (of proper mass dummy) and (big mass dummy); time of 10 throws	43.07

Factors	Factorial structure of judo wrestlers	Indicators of factors	% of dispersion
	characteristics	(accordingly 0.80, 0.73, 0.94, 0.97 and 0.74)	
2	Quantitative characteristic of TTA	-quantity of throws for quickness (of proper mass dummy), (of big mass dummy) with load 0.92 and 0.99,	26.24
3	Special power endurance	-HBR after throw (of proper mass dummy) and (big mass dummy) with factorial weight 0.94 and 0.92,	15.88
4	Functional fitness	- HBR, start (0,94).	8.99
		2-group (girls) (n=8)	
1	Quantitative characteristic of TTA, considering weight category	- weight/height indicators, HBR after 4 minutes' rest after throws (of proper mass dummy) and (big mass dummy); (accordingly 0.92, 0.71 and 0.80)	51,29
2	Special power endurance	- HBR after throw (of proper mass dummy) and (big mass dummy) with factorial load (0.84 and 0.76)	18,13
3	Restoration	- HBR after 4 minutes' rest after 10 throws of dummy (0,92).	10.45

Factorial structure of functional fitness of different qualification and sex judo wrestlers has its own specificities in quantity of factors and their internal sense, which shall be considered with determination of judo wrestlers' functional fitness for training and competition functioning in certain conditions.

The received factorial structure of functional fitness in any qualification or sex profile permitted for us to supplement model characteristics of judo wrestlers with the most important sides of functional fitness.

In assessment of restoration efficiency indicator (REI) of different qualification and sex judo wrestlers (see fig.2) we registered a number of peculiarities:

– REI in process of "throw of dummy over hip during 1 minute" (of proper weight category and characterizing special endurance) witnesses that organism's response to training load was too high (that can result in tiredness of system) (38.71%).

- REI in process of "10 throws of dummy over hip for quickness" (of bigger mass and characterizing power endurance) witnesses that organism's response to training load was too high (that can result in tiredness of system) (52,71%).
- REI in process of "throws of dummy over hip" (of bigger mass and characterizing power endurance) witnesses that organism's response to training load was too high (that can result in tiredness of system) (40%).

Results of REI analysis witness, that for different qualification judo wrestlers training loads are too high in test tasks for special and power endurance. It can result in quick tiredness. In tests for speed-power endurance load was proper.

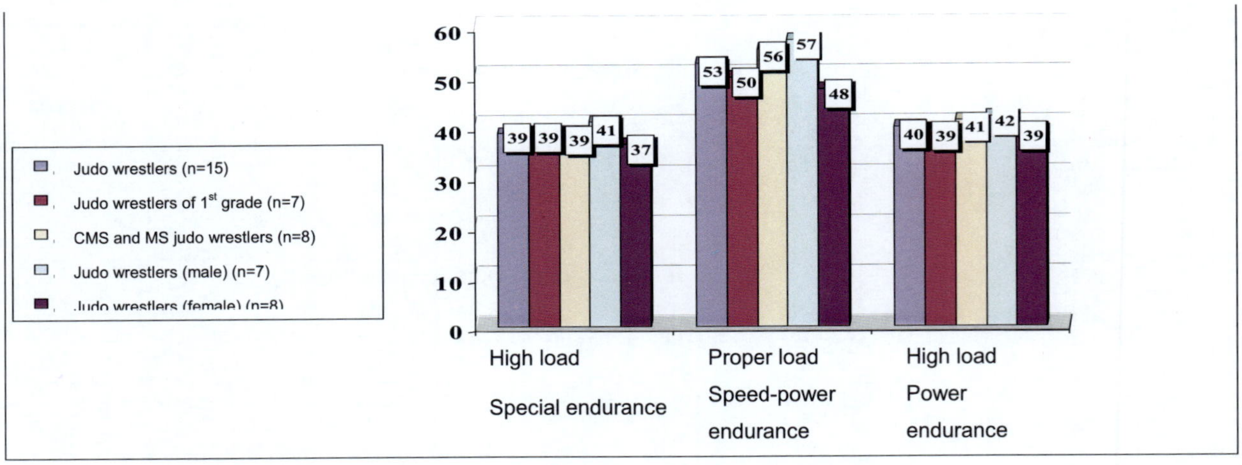

Fig.2. Restoration efficiency indicator of different qualification and sex judo wrestlers, %

Analysis of boys' REI results witnesses that training load was correct in tests for speed-power endurance. In control tests for special and power endurance load was excessive. It permits to say about tiredness and over-tension under such loads. For girls TEI in all tests was <50%. It also witnesses about too tensed organism's response to this loads. That is why it is necessary to recommend using in judo wrestlers' trainings REI, with the help of which it would be possible to reliably control parameters of scope and intensity of loads of different orientation.

For detection of signs of incomplete organism's restoration in separate training session we offer to apply the following algorithm of operative correction of differently oriented training loads:

1 STAGE – determination of purpose and task of training;

2 STAGE – determination of initial state of controlled system (by objective and subjective parameters of organism's fitness);

3 STAGE – working out of individual-differentiated program of influences (entering of load parameters by HBR and parameters of load orientation in «Polar»):

– ***Training exercises by HBR***

- 1 zone – load of low intensity, HBR up to 130-135 bpm;
- 2 zone – load of moderate intensity, HBR up to 155-160 bpm;
- 3 zone – load of high intensity, HBR up to 175-180 bpm;
- 4 zone – load of maximal intensity, HBR is not considered.
- ***Loads of purpose orientation***
- Aerobic, restorative (140–145 bpm)
- Aerobic developing (up to 160–175bpm)
- Mixed aerobic-anaerobic (up to 180–185bpm);
- Anaerobic hlycolitic (up to 180 – 200 bpm);
- Anaerobic-alactate (200 bpm and more)

4 STAGE – receiving of information as per definite system of parameters about condition of controlled system (feedback with «Polar») at every moment of control;

5 STAGE – processing of information, received by feedback channel and working out of correcting influences (transfer of information about realization of programmed purpose oriented information on display of "Polar" watch and sound signal);

6 STAGE – realization of correcting influences and plans on the basis of REI calculations (operative corrections are entered in "Polar" for further fulfillment of purpose orientation).

Discussion

As a result of conducted research we have the ground to state that ensuring of effectiveness of training loads' control for different qualification judo wrestlers is possible only with the help of operative registration of heart beats rate indicators. It is proved by researches of other authors [1, 4, 20-23].

In the works of specialists [23-25] functional fitness of judo wrestlers as holistic component are regarded. Just in our research we found factors, which determine structure of judo wrestlers' functional fitness. It permitted to define determinants of functional provision of different structural elements of special motor task, which simulates judo wrestlers' competition functioning.

Many authors [15, 21, 23] affirm that in connection with intensification of training process there appear still higher requirements to assessment of judo wrestlers' functional potentials with the help of telemetric registration of heart beats rate response to loads of different orientation. In this connection we used restoration efficiency indicator. This indicator permits to assess adequacy of physical load to organism's functional potentials as on current moment of time. On the basis of modern approaches to assessment of judo wrestlers' functional condition we worked out algorithm of operative correction of differently oriented training loads, which consists of six stages.

The received results are in agreement with researches of other authors [20, 23, 26]. These authors note high response of organism to training load of special and power orientation in contrast to load of speed-power orientation.

All these witness about demand in not only perfection of control system over judo wrestlers' functional state but also in realization of effective control system over training impacts at different stages of sportsmen's training.

Conclusions:

1. Control over training process on the basis of assessment of current training effects with the help of regulation of special exercises by their orientation and intensity of physiological impact on sportsman's organism permits to correct dozing of physical loads. Thus, functional fitness, effectiveness of training process and efficiency of competition functioning significantly improve.
2. Comparative analysis of different qualification and sex judo wrestlers' functional fitness permits to speak about statistically unconfident differences ($P>0.05$) of all researched parameters of functional fitness. This fact witnesses about relatively equal level of judo wrestlers' functional fitness, General laws and individual features of functional fitness's factorial model in context of judo wrestlers' motor fitness from the point of system-structural organization of motor functioning.
3. Permanent on-line monitoring of sportsmen's heart beats rate will permit for coach to correct training process during training session or after certain its parts (exercises): vary combinations and sequence of different training means' application; determine quantity of exercises' repetitions and intensity of their fulfillment; rationally determine rest intervals; set correspondence of exercise's intensity to solution of task. Constant recording of heart beats rate and REI calculation permit to objectively assess effectiveness of training micro-cycle's organization, to timely determine the trend to progressing of tiredness or adaptation's failure.

The prospects of further researches imply practical realization of the worked out algorithm of training process's operative correction in different kinds of martial arts.

Conflict of interests

The author declares absence of any conflict of interests.

References:

1 Bulatova M.M. *Teoretiko-metodicheskie osnovy realizacii funkcional'nykh rezervov sportsmenov v trenirovochnoj i sorevnovatel'noj deiatel'nosti. Dokt. Diss.* [Theoretical-methodic principles of realization of sportsmen's functional reserves in training and competitions' functioning. Dokt. Diss.], Kiev, 1996, 50 p.

2 Verkhoshanskij Iu.V. *Programmirovanie i organizaciia trenirovochnogo processa* [Programming and organization of training process], Moscow, Physical Culture and Sport, 1985, 176 p.

3 Godik M.A. *Kontrol' trenirovochnykh i sorevnovatel'nykh nagruzok* [Control of training and competition loads, Moscow, Physical Culture and Sport, 1980, 136 p.

4 Shiian V.V. *Planirovanie trenirovochnykh nagruzok u dziudoistov* [Planning of training loads for judo wrestlers]. Sportivnaia bor'ba [Sport wrestling], Moscow, Physical Culture and Sport, 1983, pp. 11-13.

5 Tumanian G.S., Kharacidis S.K. Sovershenstvovanie dziudoistov i sambistov [Perfection of judo and sambo wrestlers]. *Teoriia i praktika fizicheskoj kul'tury*, 1998, vol.4, pp. 59–61.

6 Little N.G. Physical performance attributes of Junior and Senior women, Juvenile, Junior and senior men judokas. *J Sports Med Phys Fitness,* 1991, vol.31(4), pp. 510–20.

7 Platonov V.N. *Teoriia i metodika sportivnoj trenirovki* [Theory and methodic of sport training], Kiev, High School, 1984, 352 p.

8 Shakhmuradov Iu.A., Sukhanov A.D. Programmirovanie sredstv i metodov trenirovochnykh vozdejstvij v sportivnoj bor'be [Programming of means and methods of training influences in sport wrestling]. *Aktual'nye problemy sportivnoj bor'by* [Urgent problems of sport wrestling], Moscow, FON, 1998, pp. 30-33.

9 Kulikov M., Rybakov V.V., Velikaia E.A. Sportivnaia trenirovka: upravlenie, sistemnost', adaptaciia i zdorov'e [Sportivnaia trenirovka: upravlenie, sistemnost', adaptaciia i zdorov'e], *Teoriia i praktika fizicheskoj kul'tury*, 1997, vol.7, pp. 26–30.

10 Sterkowicz S, Żuchowicz A, Kubica R: Levels of anaerobic and aerobic capacity indices and results for the special fitness test in judo competitors. *Journal of Human Kinetics*, 1999, vol.2, pp. 115–135.

11 Nabatnikova M.N. *Osnovy upravleniia podgotovkoj iunykh sportsmenov* [Principles of control over junior sportsmen's training], Moscow, Physical Culture and Sport, 1982. – 280 p.

12 Ahmaidi S., Portero P., Calmet M. Oxygen uptake and cardiorespiratory responses during selected fighting techniques in judo and kendo. *Sports Med. Training and Rehab*, 1999, vol.9(2), pp. 129–139.

13 Andreev V.M., Matveeva E.A., Sytnik V.I. Opredelenie intensivnosti trenirovochnoj nagruzki v bor'be dziudo [Determination of intensity of training loads in judo]. *Sportivnaia bor'ba* [Sport wrestling], Moscow, Physical Culture and Sport, 1974, pp. 13–16. Bulkin V.A. Teoreticheskie koncepcii upravleniia trenirovochnym processom v sporte vysshikh dostizhenij [Theoretical conceptions of control over training process in elite sports]. *Tendencii razvitiia sporta vysshikh dostizhenij* [Trends of elite sports progressing], Moscow, CNIIS, 1993, pp. 57–62.

14 Iordanskaia F.A. *Ocenka special'noj rabotosposobnosti sportsmenov raznykh vidov sporta: diagnostika, mekhanizmy adaptacii, sredstva korrekcii* [Assessment of special workability of different kinds of sports' sportsmen: diagnostic, adaptation mechanisms, means of correction], Moscow, Sport, 1993, 291 p.

15 Azevedo P.H.S.M., Drigo A.J., Carvalho M.C.G.A. Determination of judo endurance performance using the Uchi-Komi technique and an adapted lactate minimum test. *Journal of Sports Science and Medicine*, 2007, vol.6(2), pp. 10–14.

16 Muramatsu S., Horiyasu T., Sato S.I. The relationship between aerobic capacity and peak power during intermittent anaerobic exercise of judo athletes. *Bulletin of the Association for the Scientific Study on Judo Kodokan*, 1994, vol.8, pp. 151–160.

17 Tomlin D.L., Wenger H.A. The relationship between aerobic fitness and recovery from high intensity intermittent exercise. *Sports Med*, 2001, vol.31(1), pp. 1–11.

18 Volkov N.I. Pul'sovye kriterii energeticheskoj stoimosti uprazhneniia [Pulse energy cost criteria exercise]. *Fiziologiia cheloveka,* 2003, vol.29(2), pp. 91–97.

19 Kozyreva D.A., Varfolomeeva Z.S. Ocenka funkcional'nogo sostoianiia dziudoistov na etape nachal'noj sportivnoj specializacii [Assessment of judo wrestlers' functional condition at stage of initial specialization]. *Sovremennye problemy nauki i obrazovaniia*, 2013, vol.6, pp. 390.

20 Zebzeev V.V. Metodika ocenki funkcional'nogo sostoianiia dziudoistov na osnove sistemy kompleksnogo komp'iuternogo issledovaniia fizicheskogo sostoianiia sportsmenov «OMEGA-S2» [Methodic of assessment of judo wrestlers' functional condition on the base of system of sportsmen's complex computer study "OMEGA-C2"]. *Kul'tura: vospitanie, obrazovanie, trenirovka,* 2009, vol.5, pp. 41-43.

21 Zebzeev V.V. Metodika kontrolia i ocenka funkcional'nogo sostoianiia dziudoistov-iuniorov [Methodic of control and assessment of junior judo wrestlers' functional condition]. *Teoriia i praktika fizicheskoj kul'tury*, 2012, vol.8, pp. 75-77.

22 Zebzeev V.V. Metody ocenki funkcional'nogo sostoianiia i special'noj vynoslivosti borcov v sovremennom dziudo [Methods of assessment of functional condition and special endurance of wrestlers in modern judo]. *Materialy Vserossijskoj nauchno-prakticheskoj konferencii* [Materials of All-Russian scientific-practical conference], Kirov, 2014, pp. 223-228.

23 Potapova T.V., Namsrajn A. Funkcional'noe sostoianie iunykh dziudoistov na etape neposredstvennoj podgotovki k sorevnovaniiam [Functional condition of junior judo wrestlers at stage of direct preparation for competitions]. *Vestnik Iuzhno-Ural'skogo gosudarstvennogo universiteta*, 2008, vol.4(104), pp. 140-143.

24 Khor'iakov V.A., Mosenz V.A., Perekhrest A.N., Romanenko V.A. Problemy diagnostiki funkcional'nykh sostoianij v sporte [Problemy diagnostiki funkcional'nykh sostoianij v sporte], *Fiziceskoe vospitanie studentov tvorcheskikh special'nostej*, 2007, vol.4, pp. 89-94.

25 Vershinin M.A., Vershinin, Erofickij A.V., Novikov D.L. Fizicheskaia podgotovka vysokokvalificirovannykh dziudoistov na osnove differencirovannogo podkhoda [Physical training of elite judo wrestlers on the base of differentiated approach]. *Fizicheskoe vospitanie i sportivnaia trenirovka*, 2014, vol.3(9), pp. 5-10.

CAUSES OF DECLINING INTEREST OF STUDENTS TO EMPLOYMENT PHYSICAL EDUCATION AND SPORTS

Kondakov V.L., Kopeikina E.N., Balysheva N.V., Usatov A.N., Skrug D.A.
National Research University Belgorod State University, Russia

Annotation. *Purpose*: analysis of the main causes of the declining interest of students to the systematic physical training and sports. *Material*: The study involved 448 students (150 boys, 298 girls) conducted a questionnaire survey. Level of motor activity of students was determined using pedometers. *Results*: It was found that the transition of students in special medical groups inevitably entail a significant reduction in motor activity (it is almost 2 times lower than that of students of the main group of health). Notes the negative trend of increasing the number of students of both sexes who consume alcoholic beverages. Marked decrease of free time students because of the need to work. *Conclusions*: It is suggested to use a system of specific forms of organization of work and methods of influence that meet humanistic principles "to encourage, rather than compel." The function of such methods of influence should be to achieve the restructuring of the motivational sphere of students, the adequacy of their purpose activity.
Keywords: students, physical education, physical activity, personal orientation.

Introduction

Recent time great number of specialists in field of physical education raise question about need in increase of students' interest to physical culture and sports trainings [1, 3-7, 12-21]. As on to day program in discipline "Physical culture" for HEE envisages classes for 1st -3rd year students 2 times a week (2 academic hours every training). These classes shall be attended by all students, who have no medical counter indications, independent on the fact if they practice any kind of sports or physical culture in free time. However, analysis of physical culture academic records showed that about one third of students systematically miss planned trainings. With it, as it was cleared up as a result of questioning, 34.7% of respondents noted absence of interest to physical trainings as the main reason of their missing. It is undoubted that two training a week of 90 minutes duration can not replenish deficit of students' motion functioning (MF), more over actually duration of some trainings often shortens. This shortening is caused by many objective reasons (moving to places of trainings, changing of cloth, fulfillment of sanitary-hygienic requirements after trainings and so on) and by some subjective reasons (unfavorable weather conditions, students' delays caused by giving back of manuals, delays in cloak room, visiting of WC and other).

At the same time demand of young organism in motion is 14-19 thousand steps a day or 1, 3-1, 8 hours a day.

Purpose, tasks of the work, material and methods of the research

The purpose of the work is to clear up the reasons of students' interest to systematic practicing of physical culture and sports decay.

Achievement of our purpose was ensured by solution of the following *tasks:*

1. Theoretical analysis and generalization of problem of students' motion functioning.
2. Study specific features of students' motion functioning in condition of their studying and in everyday conditions.
3. Determine main reasons, facilitating weakening of students' interest to systematic practicing of physical culture and sports.

In order to understand the reasons, facilitating interest's weakening, in 2013-2014 teachers of physical education department of SRU "BelSU" conducted anonymous questioning of 1st-3rd year students of different specialties. In questioning 448 students participated: 150 boys and 208 girls.

Solution of tasks, determined by purpose of our research, conditioned selection of methods of the research: theoretical analysis and generalization of literature sources, questioning, talks, statistical methods.

Results of the research and discussion

Numerous researches [1, 2, 3, 5, 11], conducted in recent decade, witness that about 50% of students of Russian HEEs have health abnormalities. With every coming year increment of students, who, by their health condition, are allocated in special health groups (SHG), is registered, that is proved by our research (see fig.1). Quantity of students, for whom physical trainings are prohibited at all due to their health condition, significantly increased [1, 2, 8]. Actual scope of students' MF does not ensure full fledged physical development.

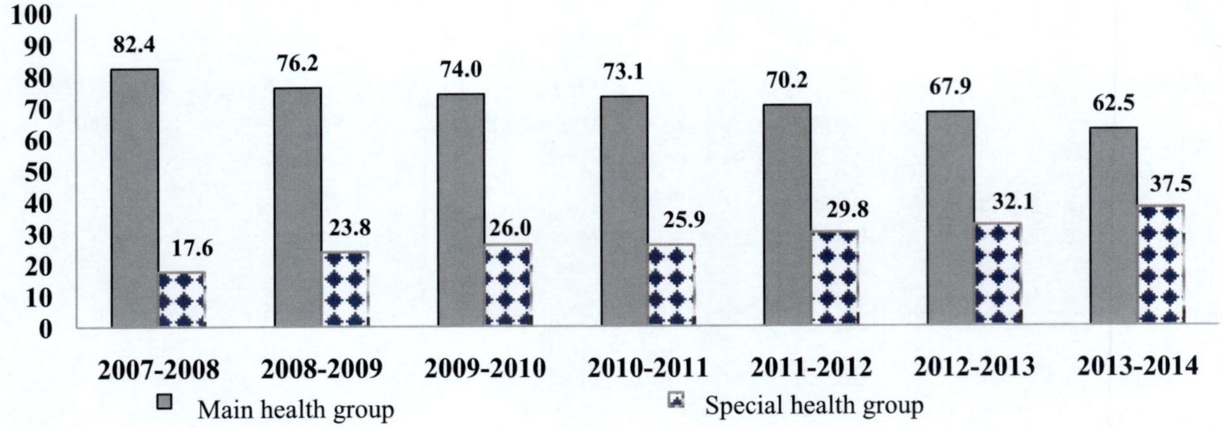

Fig.1. Correlation of students of main (MHG) special (SHG) groups in SRU "Bel SU" and

We analyzed level of students'from different health groups MF. We studied data of students' step-metering (main health group, special health group and students, released from trainings). These data are given in fig.2.

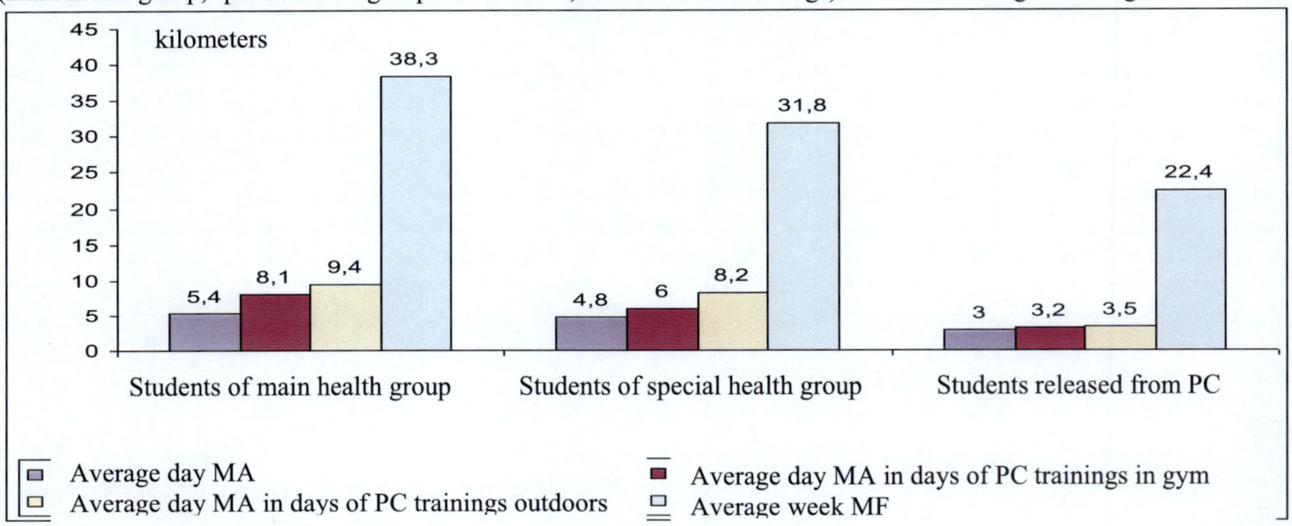

Fig.2. Motion functioning (MF) of students from different health groups (PC – physical culture)

Analysis of data witnesses that entering special health group and, more over, releasing from physical culture classes inevitably result in significant weakening of MF; with it in students, released from physical culture classes it is nearly 2 times lower than in main health group of students.

There appears certain contradiction: on the one hand MF is one of necessary components of healthy life style; it is a mean of health improvement; on the other hand young people, who have deviations in health, have indicators, reduced 2 times, while they especially need in improvement of health.

Contradiction is also in the fact that reduction of MF, being a result of health's weakening, simultaneously its reason. It is also proved by works of most of specialists [1, 10], as well as by our researches. For example quantity of students of Bielgorod HEEs, who additionally practice physical culture (in clubs or independently), reduces in proportion to increasing of students, who have health abnormalities of different heaviness (see fig.3).

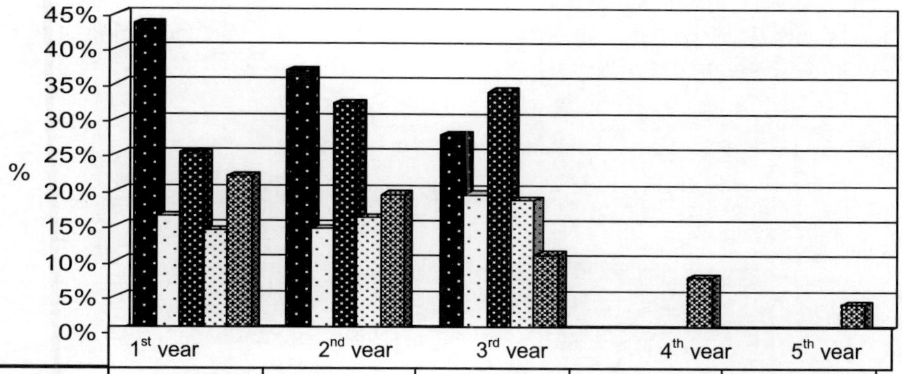

	1st year	2nd year	3rd year	4th year	5th year
Main group	43,7%	37,0%	27,8%		
Preparatory group	16,4%	14,6%	19,5%		
Special health group	25,4%	32,4%	34,0%		
Group of released from physical culture	14,5%	16,2%	18,7%		
Students, who practice physical culture	22,0%	19,5%	11,0%	7,8%	4,0%

Fig.3. Dynamic of distribution of students by health groups and quantity of students, who practice physical culture additionally (PE – physical exercises, PC – physical culture).

Analysis of students' answers to questions, which permit to asses their life style and determine factors, facilitating weakening of health, also cause trouble (see fig.4).

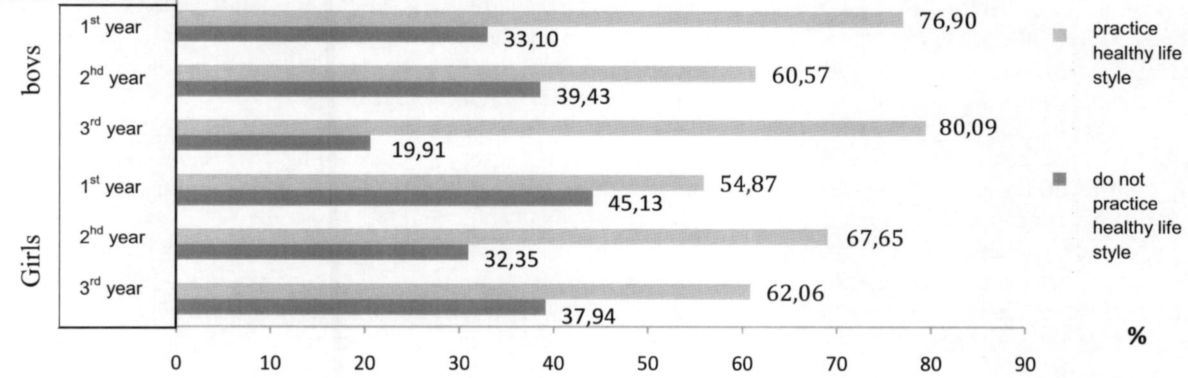

Fig.4. Self assessment of healthy life style by students of SRU "BelSU"

In spite of the fact that most of students declared their adherence to healthy life style we should note negative trend to increasing of quantity of students (boys and girls) who take alcohol (see fig.5).

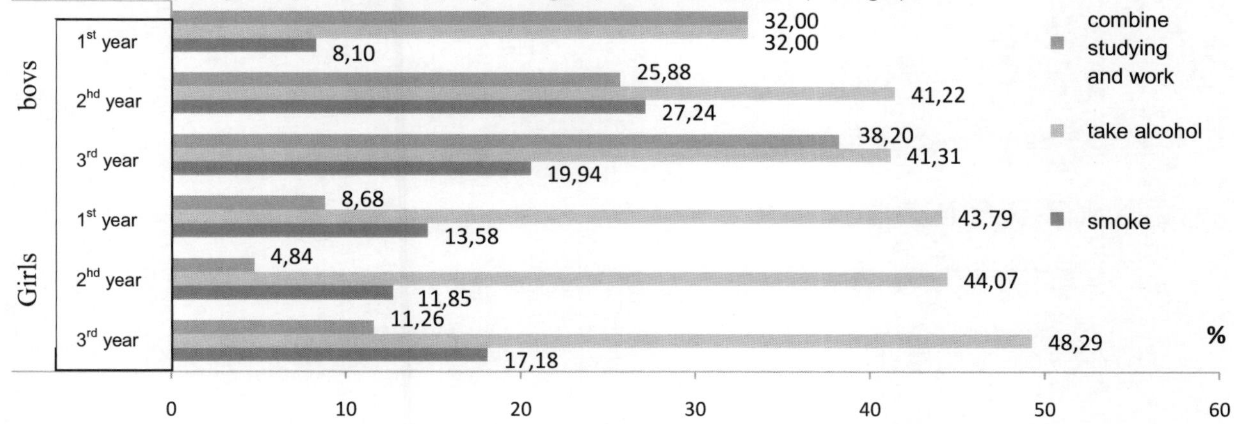

Fig.5. Negative factors in groups of SRU "BelSU" students

With it self-assessment of MF by students witnesses that their MF is not sufficient. For example most of boys characterize own MF as "above middle" and most of girls – as "middle" (see fig. 6).

The research, conducted by us in a number of Bielgorod HEEs showed that actual students' MF is obviously lower than their self assessment. Harmful habits, reducing of MF and shortening of free time, connected with necessity to work, do not facilitate increase of interest to practicing of physical culture and sports.

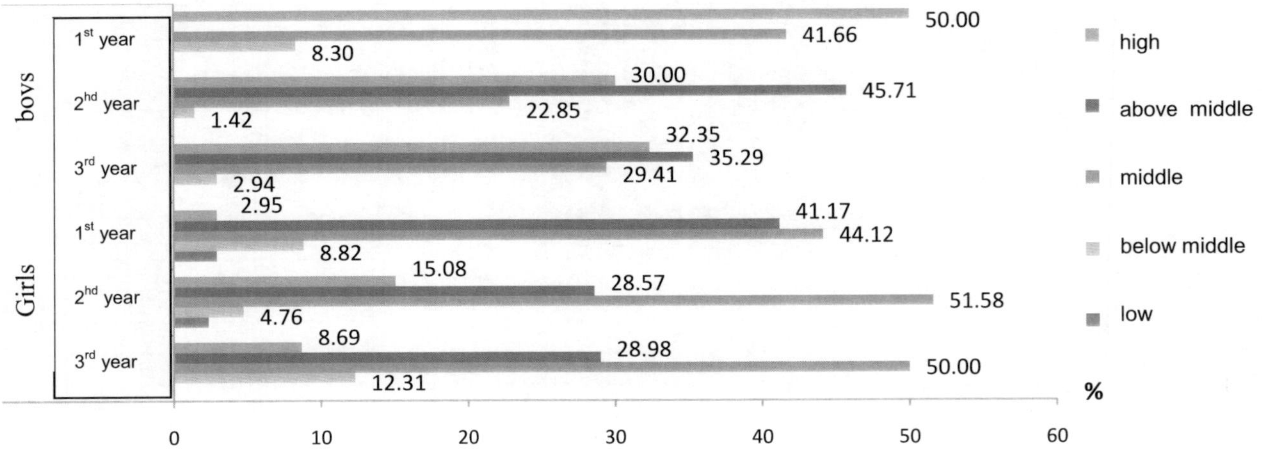

Fig.6. Self assessment of motion functioning of SRU "Bel SU" students

Analysis of formation of students' orientation on physical culture trainings permits to say that their orientation is, in the whole, poor. Among reasons of insufficient attention to own physical health, from 448 students 50% of boys and 54.5% of girls note absence of free time; indeed structure of free time to large extent influence on success of life targets', interests' and demands' formation. At present deficit of free time negatively influences on relation of youth to physical culture and sports' practicing, to taking them as desirable model of leisure.

It should be noted that 29% of girls and 4. 5% of girls have practiced sports at all. Most of students do not practice physical culture besides compulsory classes, though by the data of questioning 28. 5% of boys and 39% of girls point that just in their HEE there exist all conditions for physical culture and sports' practicing in convenient for them time. It was found that great majority of 1st year students, i.e. senior pupils of yesterday (75. 8%) – attend physical culture classes because it is required by curriculum and only 9. 4% attend these classes with wish.

In opinion of N.I. Ponomariov and V.M. Reisin [8] motives for physical culture practicing is the main condition of their effectiveness. Anonymous questioning of Bielgorod students showed that most of them have only one motive – to receive credit, less part of students want to improve health; however, percentage of wishing to improve health is increasing with every coming year. Thus, we can conclude that first, most of students do not understand significance of physical culture for their health and future professional and life progress and second, - for most of them (students who attend trainings and who miss them) content of these classes is not interesting (see fig. 7).

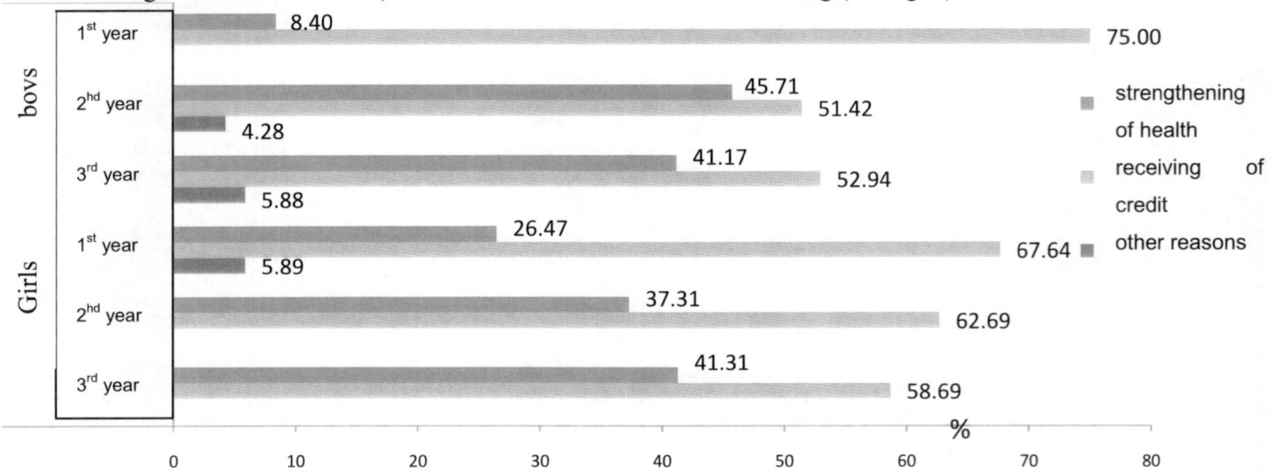

Fig. 7. Reasons of students' attendance of physical culture classes in SRW "BelSU"

The question what interest students manifested to physical culture at school, different years' students (boys and girls) was answered in somehow confusing way (see fig.8).

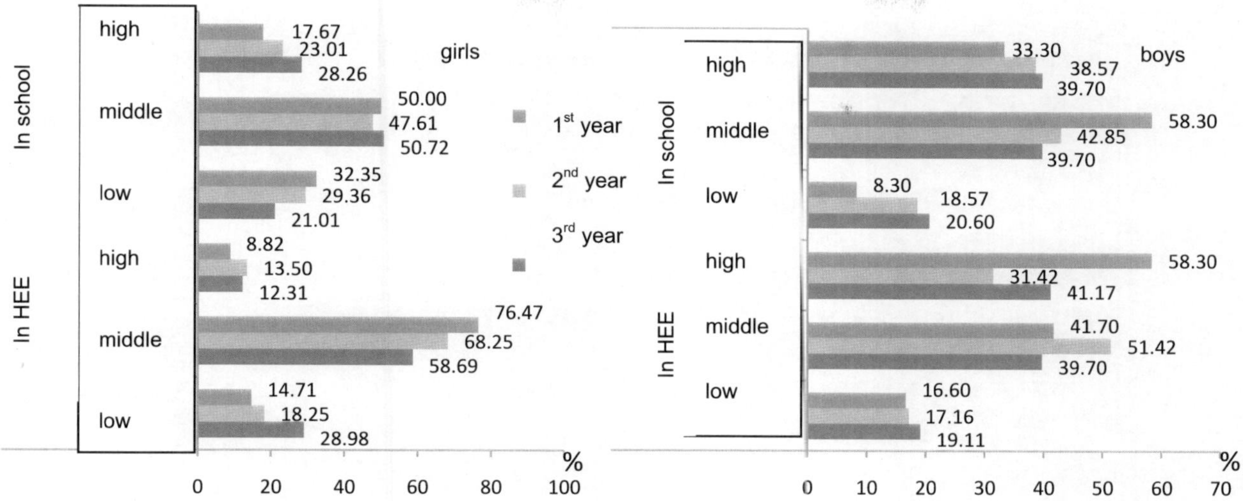

Fig.8. Interest of SRW "BelSU" students to physical culture at school and at HEE

At the first sight interest to physical culture should be equal and do not change with age. However, analysis of answers showed that with every year of studying at HEE students' interest to their physical classes at school increases. May be it is connected with some feeling of nostalgia, because it was interesting for them at school physical culture classes. Analysis of answers about interest to physical culture classes at HEE proves our assumption that with age both girls and boys loose interest to physical culture. For formation of positive emotions, increase of interest at physical culture trainings it is necessary: set clear, understood by students tasks; give, where it is necessary, scientific foundation of pedagogic and recommended methodic principles; avoid hackneyed patterns at classes, avoid monotony of used means; introduce novelty in exercises; use optimal loads and vary them; before new exercises give explanations to them; apply music (where it is possible) before exercises, in process of their fulfillment and in breaks between exercises as well as at the end of classes; consider commonality of trainees' purpose; regulate relations of trainees; form subgroups depending on their condition.

Reduction of students' MF is proved by comparison of results of answers to question about training in sport circles in school period and the, in period of study at HEE (see fig. 9). Girls stop practicing sports after school especially sharply. May be it is connected with deficit of free time, which they start to spend for preparation of home tasks, communication with new friends and so on.

Students' answers about kinds of sports, which were practiced by them in school period or are practicing at present time permitted to determine the most popular MF kinds. Most of boys marked out outdoor games. Girls also practiced often outdoor games in school period, but in student's life they start to pay attention to different aerobics.

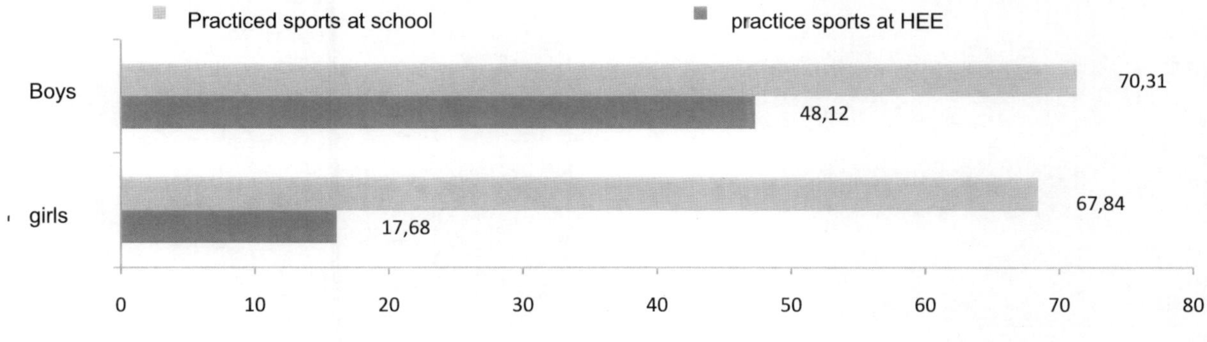

Fig.9. Attendance of sport circles by SRU "BelSU" students before entering HEE and at HEE

Students had different opinion in answers to question about changes in curriculum of "Physical culture" discipline. Most of students think it necessary to correct curriculum to some extent, the rest (minority) do not like any changes (see fig.10). In free time students can choose kinds of MF; different sport measures are organized for them at HEE sport sites. But, in spite of it, most of respondents answered that they do not participate in faculty's sport life. At senior years of studying quantity of students, participating in sport measures decreases.

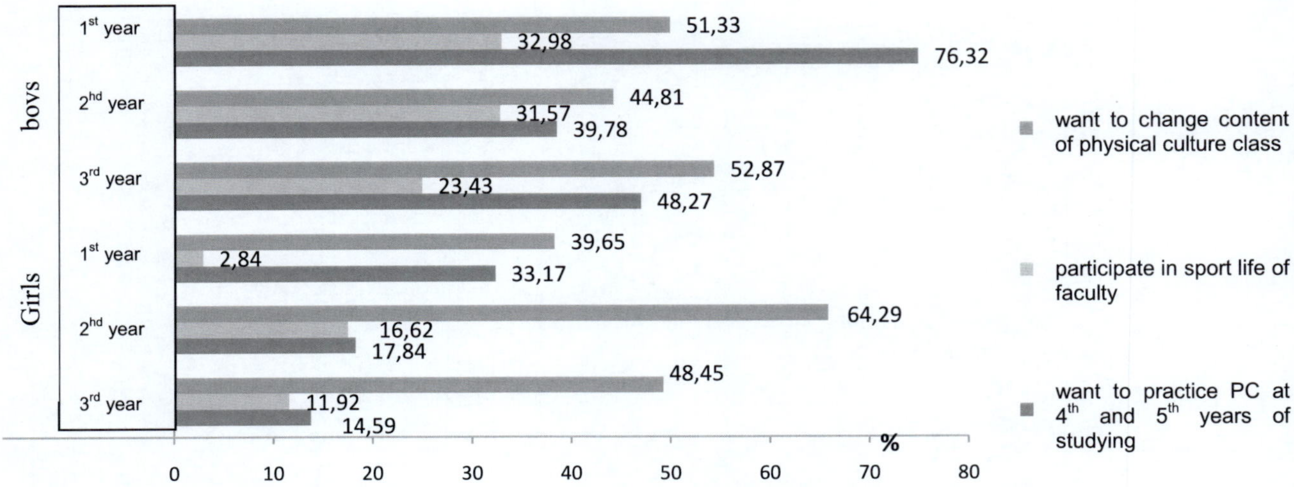

Fig.10. Opinions about changes in physical culture and participation in faculty's sport life

There is negative trend in students' attitude possibility of physical culture classes at 4th and 5th years of studying. And if 1st year students have obvious desire to continue physical culture trainings at 4th and 5th years, the, already 2nd and 3rd year students manifest weakening of such interest. Girls show even less interest to continuation of regular physical culture classes at 4th and 5th years of studying. Even among 1st year girl students there is quite a few of such persons and further this quantity even became less.

It is obvious that intensification of students' MF is impossible without formation of their sincere interest to physical culture practicing and without their conscious desire to practice physical exercises additionally. Analysis of answers to question what exactly kinds of physical exercises they would like to practice is given in figure 11.

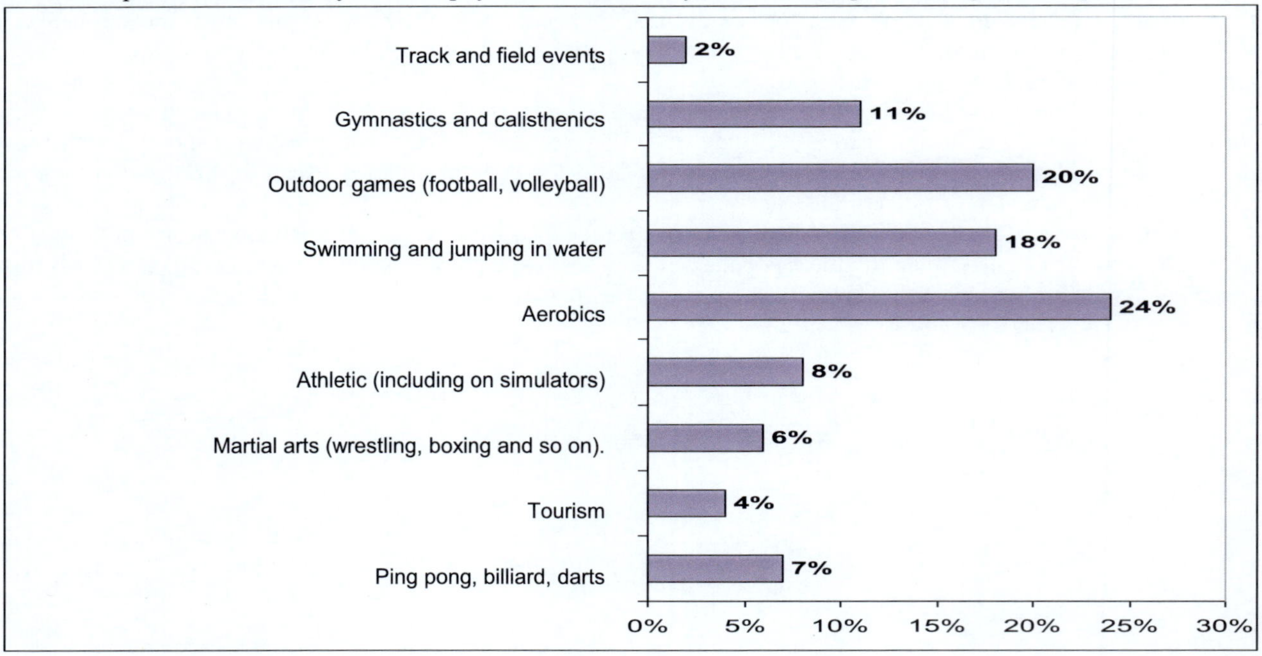

Fig.11. Kinds of physical exercises, preferred by students at physical culture classes

Significant part of the questioned (about 40%) noted that they would like to practice interesting for them physical exercises additionally, out of academic time. Results of questioning are rather optimistic in the sense that they witness about presence of interest to MF and readiness to practice physical trainings of most of students. At the same time these results call for seeking of possibilities and ways of re-organization of physical education departments' work so that students could practice interesting for them physical exercises and for which they would be ready to find spare time.

Conclusions:

Thus, demand in increasing of students' MF is undoubted. Generalizing results of researches, conducted in Bielgorod HEEs we can conclude that MF is a necessary condition of students' health and progress. With it with years of studying students' MF reduces that, in its turn, results in worsening of their health and academic progress. Quantity of MF depends, first of all, on presence (or absence) of additional physical culture trainings and secondly, on group of health, in which student practice physical culture. One of reason of students' low MF is that physical culture trainings are not interesting for them and as a result about one third of students regularly miss them. Most of students do not loose interest to MF, but they would like to practice interesting for them physical exercises. The most interesting are aerobics, outdoor games, swimming. About 40% of students are ready to practice interesting for them physical exercises additionally.

Analysis of MF of SRU "BelSU" students showed that, on the one hand, it is necessary component of healthy life style, mean of health strengthening and, on the other hand, MF of young people with health abnormalities is lower nearly 2 times. This contradiction is amplified also by the fact that weakening of MF, being a result of health's worsening, is simultaneously a reason of it. This conclusion is proved by conducted by us researches, which show that main health group's students, who practice physical culture additionally, have the least percentage of morbidity. The second place is engaged by main group students, who attend only academic classes of physical culture. However, in spite of good indicators of educational functioning they have rather high percentage of catarrhal diseases. It also witnesses about prevailing significance of health in successful mastering of HEE curriculum.

All above said witnesses about demand in serious measures on cultivation of students' interest to different kinds of MF, on formation of personality's orientation on physical culture practicing and, in the whole, formation of their motivation for healthy life style.

In modern situation it is important to re understand content, methods and techniques of personality's orientation on the base of personality-active approach with pedagogic researches, analysis of subjective factors in the center. Especially troubling is absence of students' positive motivation for practicing of physical culture and sports.

It should also be noted that physical culture classes will be more effective if students realize purposes of physical culture and personal value of such trainings. That is why it is necessary to seek such methods of physical culture classes' organization, means of influence, which could more effectively ensure formation of positive personality's orientation on physical culture trainings.

In this conditions application of only traditional methods and means of influence, which often are in discordance between each other and weakly consider individual-typological features of students, are insufficiently promising. It would be more purposeful to use such holistic system of specific forms of trainings' organization and means of influence, which would meet humanistic principle "awakening instead of forcing" and, thus, increase interest of trainees to functioning, to which pedagogue orients them. Function of such means of influence shall ensure reconstruction of students' motivation sphere, adequately accepted by them purpose of functioning, resulted in positive orientation on it.

References:

1. Balysheva N.V., Bogoeva M.D., Kovaleva M.V., Kopejkina E.N., Rumba O.G. Obshchaia kharakteristika problemy deficita dvigatel'noj aktivnosti studentov s ogranichennymi vozmozhnostiami kardiorespiratornoj sistemy [General characteristics of the shortage of motor activity of students with disabilities cardiorespiratory system]. *Kul'tura fizicheskaia i zdorov'e*, 2013, vol.4, no.46, pp. 85-90. (in Russian)
2. Gorelov A.A., Rumba O.G., Kondakov V.L. Analiz pokazatelej zdorov'ia studentov special'noj medicinskoj gruppy [Analysis of indicators of health of students of special medical group]. *Nauchnye problemy gumanitarnykh issledovanij.* 2008, no.6, pp. 28-33. (in Russian)
3. Gorelov A.A., Kondakov V.L., Usatov A.N., To the question about the use of independent physical training in educational space of modern higher institute. *Physical Education of Students*, 2013, no.1, pp. 17-26. http://dx.doi.org/10.6084/m9.figshare.156351.
4. Gorelov A.A., Rumba O.G. , Kondakov V.L. Opyt ispol'zovaniia sredstv fizicheskoj kul'tury dlia povysheniia umstvennoj i fizicheskoj rabotosposobnosti, snizheniia nervno-emocional'nogo napriazheniia studentov s narusheniiami v sostoianii zdorov'ia [Experience in the use of means of physical training to improve mental and physical performance, reduction of neuro-emotional stress of students with disabilities in the state of health]. *Nauchnye vedomosti Belgorodskogo Gosudarstvennogo Universiteta*, 2010, vol.6(77), no.5, pp. 185-192. (in Russian)
5. Gorelov A.A., Kondakov V.L., Rumba O.G. Fizkul'turno-ozdorovitel'nye tekhnologii kak sredstvo kinezioterapii v obrazovatel'nom prostranstve vuza [Sport and health technology as a means of physiotherapy in the educational space of the university]. *Physical Education of Students*, 2012, no.6, pp. 47-51. http://dx.doi.org/10.6084/m9.figshare.96568 (in Russian)
6. Kondakov V.L., Usatov A.N, Usatov V.N., Goverdovskaia E.V. O neobkhodimosti povysheniia dvigatel'noj aktivnosti studentov vuzov [On the need to increase motor activity of university students]. Kul'tura *fizicheskaia i zdorov'e*, 2008, vol.5, no.19, pp. 55-60. (in Russian)
7. Kondakov V.V., Kopejkina E.N., Usatov A.N., Balysheva N.V. Otnoshenie studentov k zaniatiiam fizicheskoj kul'turoj i sportom v obrazovatel'nom prostranstve sovremennogo vuza [The ratio of students to physical culture and sports in the educational space of the modern university]. *Ekonomicheskie i gumanitarnye issledovaniia regionov*, 2014, no.3, pp. 48-52. (in Russian)
8. Kondakov V.L. *Sistemnye mekhanizmy konstruirovaniia fizkul'turno-ozdorovitel'nykh tekhnologij v obrazovatel'nom prostranstve sovremennogo vuza. Dokt.diss.* [System design mechanisms of health and fitness

technology in the educational space of the modern university. Dokt. Diss.]. Sankt Petersburg,, 2013, 521 p. (in Russian)

9. Kondakov V.L. *Upravlenie formirovaniem napravlennosti lichnosti shkol'nika (na materiale fizicheskoj kul'tury). Kand.diss.* [Management of formation of orientation of the individual student (based on the physical culture). Kand.diss.]. Belgorod, 2000, 190 p. (in Russian)
10. Ponomarev N.I., Rejzin V.M. O formirovanii potrebnosti cheloveka v fizkul'turno-sportivnoj deiatel'nosti (teoreticheskij aspekt) [On the formation of the human need for physical culture and sports activities (theoretical aspect).] *Teoriia i praktika fizicheskoj kul'tury*, 1988, no.10, pp. 2-4. (in Russian)
11. Alekseev N., Kutergin N., Kulinichev A., Gorbatenko A. Integrated method development of general and special students stamina involved in the fight. *Physical Education of Students*. 2014, no.3, pp. 3-8. http://dx.doi.org/10.6084/m9.figshare.974476.
12. Edge K., Khamsi K. International school partnerships as a vehicle for global education: student perspectives. *Asia Pacific Journal of Education*. 2012, vol.32, no.4, pp. 455-472. http://dx.doi.org/10.1080/02188791.2012.739964.
13. Iermakova T.S. Peculiarities of forming health culture of pupils in Poland: historical aspect. *Pedagogics, psychology, medical-biological problems of physical training and sports*, 2014, vol.6, pp. 16-20. http://dx.doi.org/10.6084/m9.figshare.1004090
14. Harris J. Physical education teacher education students' knowledge, perceptions and experiences of promoting healthy, active lifestyles in secondary schools. *Physical Education and Sport Pedagogy*. 2014, vol.19, no.5, pp. 466-480. http://dx.doi.org/10.1080/17408989.2013.769506.
15. Hemphill S.A., Plenty S.M., Herrenkohl T.I., Toumbourou J.W., Catalano R.F. Student and school factors associated with school suspension: A multilevel analysis of students in Victoria, Australia and Washington State, United States. *Children and Youth Services Review*. 2014, no.3, pp. 187-194. http://dx.doi.org/10.1016/j.childyouth.2013.11.022.
16. Humphrey N., Lendrum A., Barlow A., Wigelsworth M., Squires G. Achievement for All: Improving psychosocial outcomes for students with special educational needs and disabilities. *Research in Developmental Disabilities*. 2013, vol.34, no.4, pp. 1210-1225. http://dx.doi.org/10.1016/j.ridd.2012.12.008.
17. Macleod G., Cebula K.R. Experiences of disabled students in initial teacher education. *Cambridge Journal of Education*. 2009, vol.39, no.4, pp. 457-472. http://dx.doi.org/10.1080/03057640903352465.
18. Maivorsdotter N., Lundvall S. Aesthetic experience as an aspect of embodied learning: stories from physical education student teachers. *Sport, Education and Society*. 2009, vol.14, no.3, pp. 265-279. http://dx.doi.org/10.1080/13573320903037622.
19. Mercier K., Doolittle S. Assessing Student Achievement in Physical Education for Teacher Evaluation. *Journal of Physical Education, Recreation & Dance*. 2013, vol.84, no.3, pp. 38-42. http://dx.doi.org/10.1080/07303084.2013.767721.
20. Oh H-K., Rizzo T.L., So H., Chung D-H., Park S-J., Lei Q. Preservice physical education teachers' attributes related to teaching a student labeled ADHD. *Teaching and Teacher Education*. 2010, vol.26, no.4, pp. 885-890. http://dx.doi.org/10.1016/j.tate.2009.10.027.
21. Prusik Krzysztof, Prusik Katarzyna, Kozina Zh.L., Iermakov S.S. Features of physical development, physical preparedness and functional state of boys and girls – students of Polish higher educational establishments. *Physical Education of Students*, 2013, vol.1, pp. 54-61. http://dx.doi.org/10.6084/m9.figshare.96415

STRUCTURAL ELEMENTS OF CONSTRUCTION OF INDIVIDUAL AND GROUP EXERCISES' COMPETITION COMPOSITIONS IN CALISTHENICS

Kovalenko Y.O., Boloban V.N.
National University of Physical Education and Sport of Ukraine

Abstract. *Purpose:* to analyze content of individual and group exercises' competition compositions in calisthenics. *Material:* in the research HEEs' girl students (n=20), junior sportswomen (n=10), experts (n=30), coaches with 10-40 years' working experience participated. *Results:* it was found that temporary indicators permit to assess level of female gymnasts' readiness for fulfillment of competition compositions' elements; facilitated rational correlation of body and object's elements of complexity. Quickness of preparation to elements and directly time of exercise's fulfillment acquire great importance. In individual and group exercises the most important are distribution of sportswoman's moving on all site with frequent change of directions. It was established that realization of structural elements facilitates full opening of female gymnast's artistic image. *Conclusions:* for building of competition compositions coaches shall fully use indicators of space and time structural elements.
Key words: female gymnast, composition, subject, building, coordination, space, time.

Introduction

Ukrainian female gymnasts have high sports achievements in the world. However, sports rivalry grows and new problems appear. Leading specialists connect these problems with building and demonstration of spectacular competition compositions [3, 5, 7, 12, and 14]. In modern calisthenics high requirements are set to competition compositions of sportswomen (Code FIG, 2013-2016). Female gymnasts shall fulfill complex elements at high technical level and their movements shall be graceful, plastic and artistic. The highest sports achievements in calisthenics imply artistic execution of composition under musical accompaniment with maximal demonstration of coordination abilities, flexibility, jumping, balance, and vestibular stability, consummate manipulation of object [3, 11, and 19].

During recent three Olympic cycles (2004-2016) a tendency of systematic increase of individual and group exercises' competition compositions complexity in calisthenics has being existed. Competition is constantly rising on world gymnastic platform. It is more and more difficult to win a victory. Only those female gymnasts, who will demonstrate artistry of competition programs' fulfillment against the background of perfect body control and object's manipulation, will be leaders. The problem of individual approach to training of sportswomen's motor abilities, basic technical fitness in formation of personality features. Solution of this problem is possible by building of competition compositions, by opening of female gymnasts' artistic and emotional skillfulness [6, 12]. In competition rules in many kinds of sports with complex motor coordination there are no clearly differentiated criteria of exercise spectacular level, sportswoman's artistry, technique's originality, complexity and sequence of exercise' fulfillment assessment. In many works it is noted that success of individual exercises' compositions in calisthenics (sports gymnastic, sports acrobatic) depends on skillful combining of all components in one as well as obeying of music's emotional content to this one [7,10,11].

There are rather few researches of methodic of competition compositions' building, considering FIG requirements. With the help of this document control over development of calisthenics in the world is realized (Code FIG, 2013-2016). In particular, new requirements have been set to space-time characteristics of exercises and combinations of exercises [19].

Purpose, tasks, material and methods of the research

The purpose of the research is to analyze content of individual and group exercises' competition compositions in calisthenics.

The tasks of he research:

1. To study theoretical-methodic status of the problem of competition compositions' building in individual and group exercises' of calisthenics.
2. To analyze space-time structural elements of individual exercises competition compositions' building for elite female gymnasts.

The methods of the research: for solution of the set tasks we used the following methods: analysis and generalization of scientific-methodic literature data; questioning; video-computer analysis of female gymnasts' exercises; analysis of competition records; methods of mathematical statistics.

Results of the research

For studying of competition compositions of girl students' individual exercises we fulfilled questioning. Analysis of data permitted to calculate time for composing and further correction of competition compositions [4]. Most of coaches (43%) answered in the following way: they spend 1 day for composing; 40% of coaches answered - 5-6 days and 17% – 2-3 days (see fig. 1). Coaches' opinions differed in question of competition compositions' correction: 13% of specialists' correct compositions during 1 day; 37% – during 5-6 days; 23% – during 3-4 weeks; 17% – during 2-3 months. Only 10% of coaches change competition programs during year. Coaches, who correct compositions during 1 day, base on their inspiration. In the future they correct programs and change them for perfection of exercises' elements.

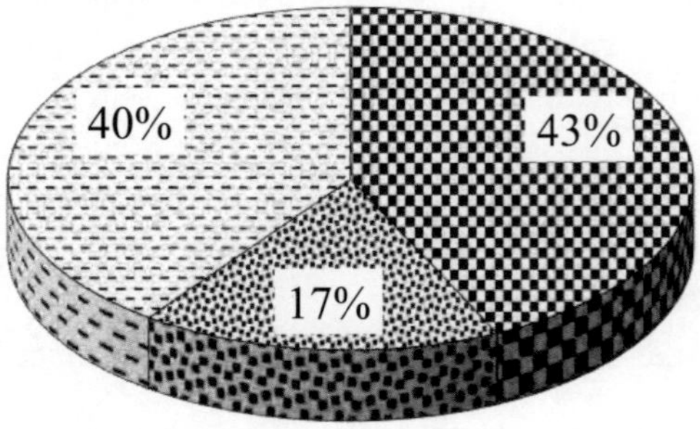

Fig.1. Percentage of correlation of time (days), spent by coaches for composing of competition compositions of individual exercises.

1day 2-3days 5-6 days

Questioning of coaches permitted to determine sequence of work on creation of artistic image of competition composition. At 1st place there is expressiveness of sportswoman, at 2nd – working out of new elements and their connections (in compliance with music); at 3rd place –watching video-records of competition compositions of the strongest in the world female gymnasts; 4th place – visiting of world competitions or international elite competitions; 5th – working out of leotard style; 6th – watching film (if musical accompaniment is soundtrack of film); 7th place – choosing of color gamma of object. In analysis of female gymnasts' answers to this question we found many similarities with coaches' answers. The only distinction is that female gymnasts put on the 1st place working out of new elements and their connections (in compliance with music) and on the 2nd place – expressiveness of female gymnasts.

Among the questioned respondents 93% said that they train female gymnasts' ability to compose compositions. It is a positive feature for development of female gymnasts' creative potential.

Competition rules dictate the following requirements: in competition composition it is necessary to demonstrate complexity of body movements (D); combination of dance steps, dynamic elements with rotation or throws of object, skillfulness in manipulation of object. Female gymnasts' motor actions shall be fulfilled in strict space-time frames, which are accessible for perception of spectators and assessment of referees.

For this purpose we analyzed competition compositions of female gymnasts.

In process of video-analysis we considered the following components:

1. Time, spent for fulfillment of body movements' complexity (D1).
2. Time, spent for fulfillment of object's complexity (D2).
3. Time, spent for fulfillment of risky elements (R).
4. Kinds of movements and covered distance in meters in competition composition.

In exercise with hoop we found the longest time, spent for fulfillment of body movements' complexity in Ukrainian and Byelorussian female gymnasts (35″). With it the shortest time was demonstrated by Russian female gymnast (23.01″). It was conditioned by the fact that Russian female gymnast fulfilled minimum of possible elements (7). It did not reflect in total sum of points for body movements' complexity. Female gymnast from Byelorussia shortened time for work with object by 6″ 2nd stage of research. Female gymnast from Azerbaijan increased time indicators of body movements' complexity by 18″. It permitted for sportswoman to show all skillfulness in handling object at the account of shortening of time spent for body work and dynamic elements with throws (see table 1).

Table 1. Comparative analysis of time indicators of time spent for fulfillment of body movements' complexity, object's complexity, dynamic elements in exercise with hoop (n=10)

Countries-participants	Body movements' complexity		Object's complexity		Dynamic elements	
	I	II	I	II	I	II
Azerbaijan	33	26.03	32.6	50.1	24.4	15.03
Bulgaria	20.99	28.03	52.01	43.01	15	17.12
Byelorussia	27.5	35.1	51.3	39.21	11.2	13.2
Russian federation	28.26	23.01	49	44.06	12.84	16.3
Ukraine	42.4	35.05	29.6	39.1	15	16.07

1st stage – performance of female gymnasts as per junior program at European championship 2012, Nizhny Novgorod
2nd stage – performance of female gymnasts by senior program (16 years and older) at World Championship, 2013, Kiev.

Analyzing space indicators of female gymnasts' movements in competition compositions on platform we researched types and kinds of sportswomen's movements on every composition.

For female gymnasts from Byelorussia and Ukraine semi-circumferential movements were characteristic. It widens possibilities of movements and opens all harmony of movements. Female gymnast from Russian Federation preferred multiple diagonal movements. It also witnesses about rational composition of jump and dynamic elements with throws. Female gymnast from Azerbaijan increased her distance indicator by 20 meters. She approached her result to leader's result in this parameter – female gymnast from Russian Federation (who covers 75 meters). The least distance was passed by Ukrainian female gymnast (45 meters). Most of composition she was in static positions and fixed elements of body movements' complexity. It is not a negative factor in technique of performance. When fulfilling several elements of body movements' complexity at the spot female gymnast loses opportunity to watch all range of movement (see fig.2).

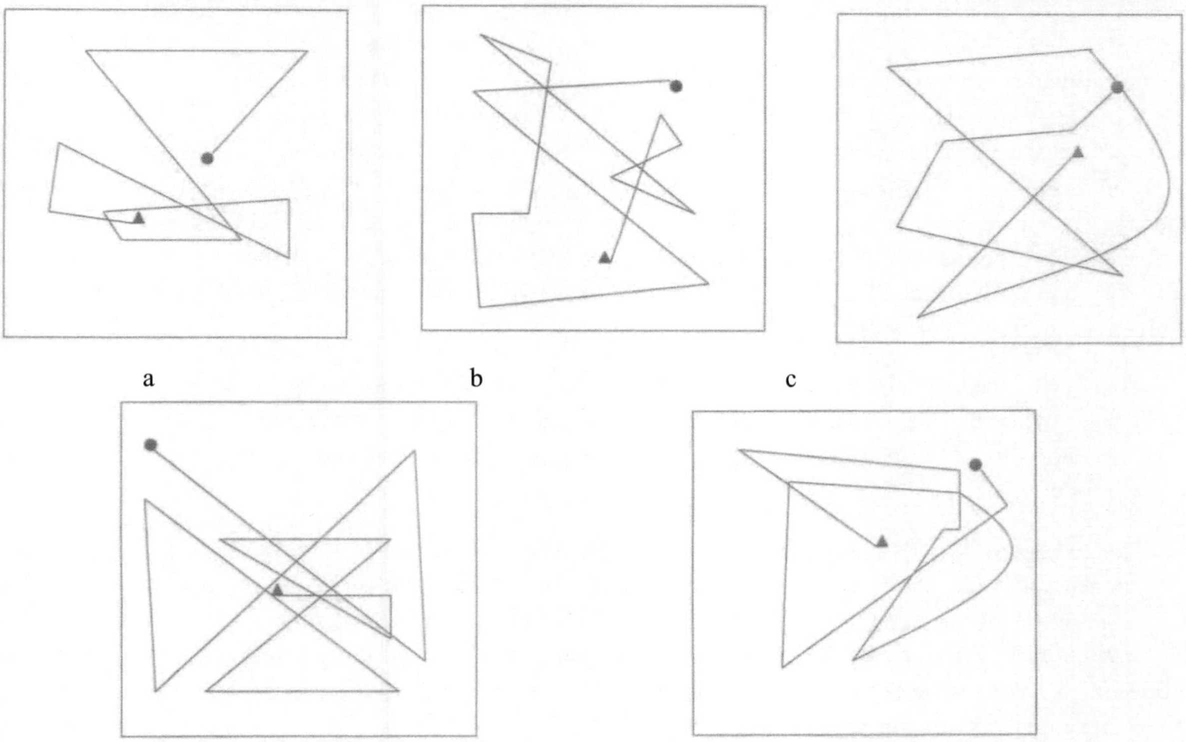

a b c

d e

Fig.2. Kinds of female gymnasts' movements on platform in competition compositions with hoop:
a – composition with hoop of female gymnast from Azerbaijan;
b – Composition with hoop of female gymnast from Bulgaria;
c – Composition with hoop of female gymnast from Byelorussia;
d – Composition with hoop of female gymnast from Russian Federation;
e – Composition with hoop of female gymnast from Ukraine;
▲- start of exercise
●- end of exercise

For studying of competition compositions we carried out video-analysis of performances of 10 strongest teams from 5 countries in group exercises: Spain, Italy, Byelorussia, Russian Federation and Ukraine.

The purpose of video-analysis was to study space-time indicators of group exercises' competition compositions building (n=10). In analysis we considered the following components:

1. Time, spent for fulfillment of body movements' complexity, throws, combinations of dance steps (D).
2. Time, spent for cooperation of female gymnasts (C).
3. Time, spent for fulfillment of risky elements (R).
4. Kinds of female gymnasts' positions at throws.

Analyzing video-records of group exercises' compositions of strongest teams (World Championship 2014) we studied duration of compositions. In average it was 2.30 ± 0.03″. With it there were registered no rough violations of rules. In group exercises with 10 clubs we found that all teams started their compositions with cooperation elements. It coordinated interaction of female gymnasts and increase spectacular character of performance. Elements of cooperation take in average 70-76″. Team from Byelorussia spent 79″. The team showed the highest quantity of interactions with the help of supports, multiple exchanges of objects, female gymnasts' passing under objects. Sportswomen used criteria of increasing of cooperation value: without visual control, without hands. In average fulfillment of risky elements by teams took 4-5″. Exclusion was team from Spain. This team spent 11″ for risky elements. It was conditioned by the fact that sportswomen fulfilled combination of elements turn by turn. It added dynamism to exercise and space movement of all female gymnasts during risky element's fulfillment. For elements of body movements' complexity gymnasts spend in average 50-70″. In exercise 10 complexities shall be presented: 5 with exchange of object and 5 without exchange [19]. The most wide-spread element of body movements' complexity ("fouette") was fulfilled by all teams. In average sportswomen fulfilled 6-8 rotations (it took 6-8″). Rotation "fouette", with its synchronous fulfillment, makes exercise effective and spectacular. Among jumping elements the most wide-spread is "jete anturnan". This jump permits to overcome big distance in movement and takes in average 2-3″. Team from Byelorussia fulfilled series of jumps, consisting of two "jete anturnan" (time - 3″). That is why in exercise of Byelorussian team more time was spent to interaction and cooperation. In Spain team 6″ were registered, which was not in any way marked in card of fulfillment of complexities and did not result in any points for fulfillment. Female gymnasts rhythmically moved with object but they did not interact. Probably it was purposeful to add 2″ for fulfillment of dance track, which, according to competition rules, shall take 8″. It would permit to receive 0. Points (see fig. 3).

We regarded female gymnasts' positions (orders) on platform during throws in group exercises with 10 clubs. In Ukrainian female gymnasts 2 throws one-by-one were registered. Pictures of throws were different. First throw was fulfilled with moving forward. It permitted for sportswomen to prepare for second throw, which was fulfilled in static position (see fig. 4).

Italian and Spanish sportswomen demonstrated similar types of positions for throws. They included: diagonal, vertical, horizontal, cross-like orders and circles. Byelorussian team did not demonstrate variety of throw orders. Three kinds of positions were noticed. With it, two throws were fulfilled consequently. Also position of throw start was changed in second throw. Female gymnasts started throw from initial position "on the floor". All throws of Byelorussian team were fulfilled at high speed, spontaneously with elements before and after throw of object. It visually increased effectiveness and complexity of competition composition.

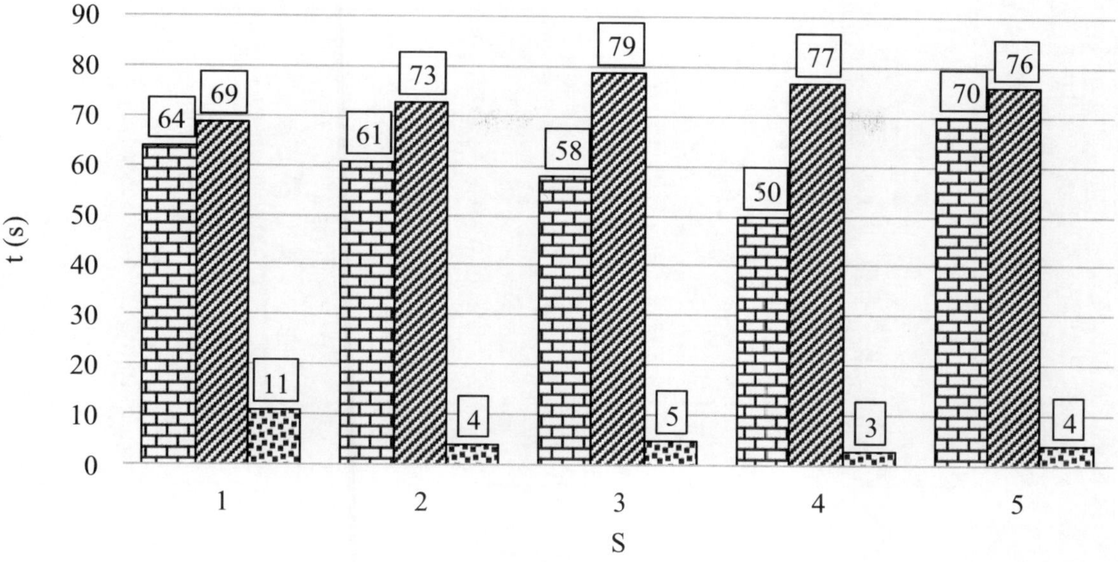

Fig.3. Indicators of time, spent for fulfillment of body movements' complexity elements (D), cooperation elements (C), risky elements (R), in group exercise with 10 clubs: t – time in seconds; S – team of country; 1 –Spain, 2 –Italy, 3 – Byelorussia, 4 – Russian Federation, 5 – Ukraine.

Elements of body movements' complexity (D)
Elements of cooperation (C)
Risky elements (R)

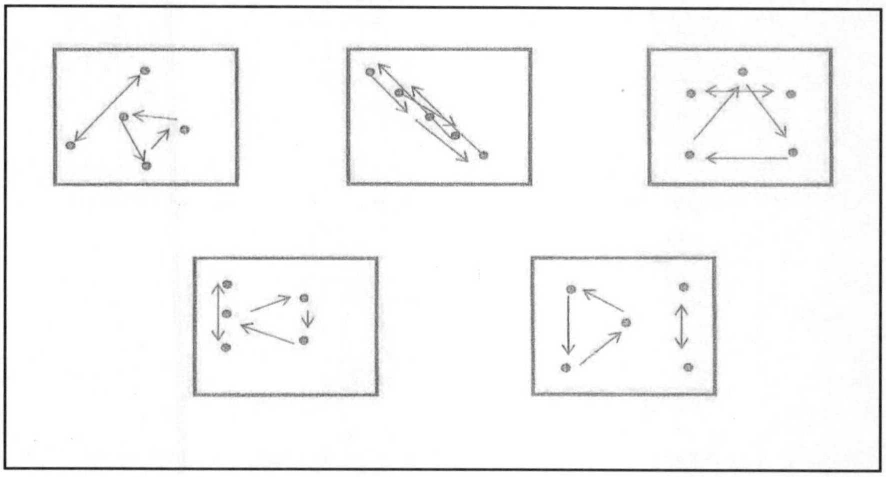

1

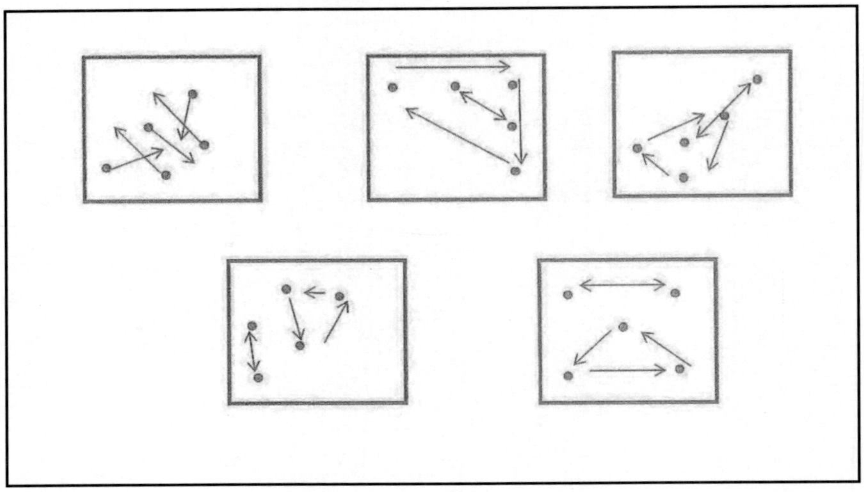

2

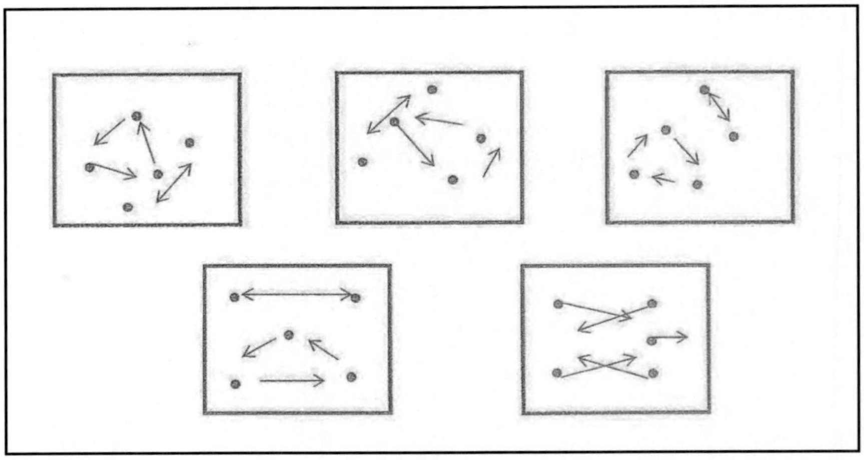

3

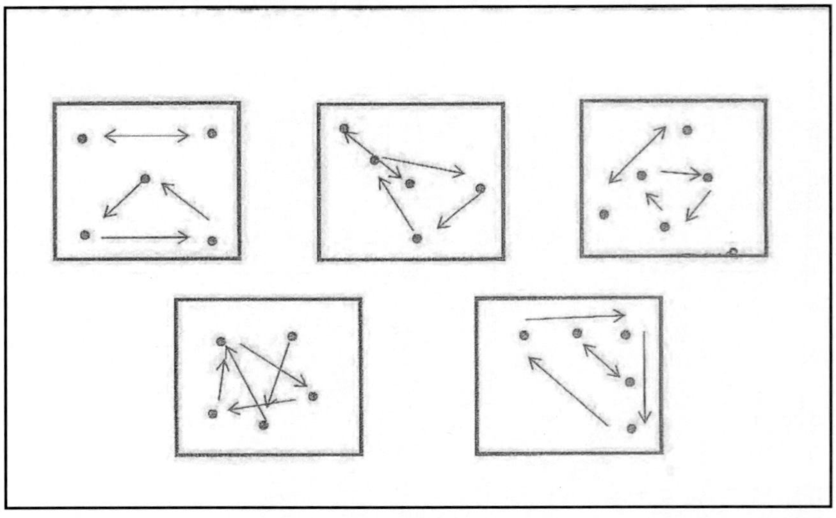

4

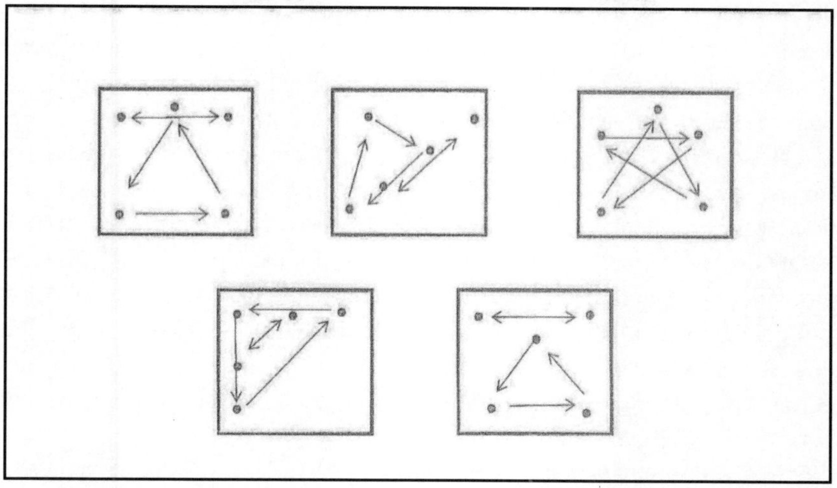

5

Fig. 4. Positions of female gymnasts (orders) on platform during throws in group exercises with 10 clubs in teams from: 1 – Spain; 2 – Italy; 3 – Byelorussia; 4 – Russian Federation; 5 – Ukraine.

Discussion

"Composition" implies composing of one from parts; building of artwork, conditioned by its content, character and purpose. In competition rules on calisthenics (principle document of International federation of gymnastics) high requirements to competition compositions of individual and group exercises are presented. New requirements to demonstration of space-time indicators in fulfillment of separate elements, their combinations, composition in the whole are set. These requirements concern: dynamic wholeness of exercises' phases; frequent change of movements' directions; rational distribution of elements in individual and group exercises (when moving by diagonal, by circle, by arch); distance, covered by female gymnast in composition; stability. Our researches showed that distance, covered by gymnast is the so-called indicators of female gymnasts' sportsmanship. For Ukrainian and Byelorussian female gymnasts, in compositions with hoop accentuated moving by circle were characteristic. It permits to move on platform and open technical potentials. In one composition gymnasts cover up to 45 meters. Female gymnast from Russian Federation covered twice bigger distance in exercise with hoop - 75 meters. In exercises with hoop sportswomen successfully add wide-amplitude movements by body and elements of complexity. It is an indicator of high sportsmanship, which was confirmed by high referees' marks. For example, gymnast Ya. K. Won title of absolute World Champion in calisthenics for 2013. Analysis of structural elements of group exercises' competition compositions shows complex constructions, functional cooperation and systemic motor interactions of gymnasts in exercise with 10 clubs. Video-analysis helped to study: time of fulfillment of complexity elements; combinations of dance steps; cooperation; fulfillment of risky elements; positioning and re-positioning of gymnasts for throws. It was found that in group exercises with 10 clubs all teams started their compositions with elements of cooperation. It should be noted that gymnasts of these teams are the best in the world. Actually we registered model indicators of structural elements. Analysis of researches' results showed that structural elements of space-time indicators of competition compositions are realized effectively in the following cases: high static-dynamic body balance; temp and rhythm of movements; flexibility; jumping; orientation in space, body balance in difficult rotations and rotations on one foot; motor interaction in system "gymnast-object". Materials of monograph [2] can serve as proof of these, as well as theoretical analysis and practical experience of specialists in sports gymnastics [1, 3, 7, 8, 12, and 15]. Gymnasts' active participation in composing of competition compositions brings elements of individuality in their content. In motor composition these elements become a "face" of all composition. They characterize performance skillfulness and are a mean of creation of artistic image [6, 7, and 11]. Analysis of scientific-methodic literature, devoted to effective building of individual and group exercises' competition compositions, witnesses about importance of this problem. The known specialists point at the fact, that composition is an artwork, free for creativity [14]. Restrictions are imposed only by competition rules. They concern time, sixes of platform and quantity of elements, determining value of all competition exercise.

Conclusions:

1. Analysis of scientific-methodic literature and practical experience of coaches permitted to mark out the most important components of the process as well as to accentuate ability of coaches and female gymnasts to consider space-time structural elements of exercises and fulfill them technically accurately.

2. Time indicators permit to asses the following: level of female gymnast's fitness; her ability to fulfill elements of competition compositions in individual exercises. Quickness of preparation to elements' fulfillment and directly time of their fulfillment are of great importance. In calisthenics sportswoman's ability to distribute movement on platform's area is also of great importance, as well as change of directions. For example, abrupt and jerky music is in harmony with change of directions under acute angles; soft music – corresponds to obtuse angles or to arch-like pictures of motion. To create impression of quickness and lightness direction from the left to the right is chosen. In this case spectator's look will as though "prod" the movement. When moving to other side it is more advantageous to use direction from the right to the left. Thus, correct and logical distribution of elements and combinations on platform; gymnast's movements create artistic completeness of composition.

3. Study of space-time characteristics of group exercises' compositions showed that the most permanent component of structure was cooperation and interaction. It is a basic normative foundation of compositions' building. Cooperation elements take 70-80″. It is 45-55% of total exercise's duration. Cooperation elements bring 40-45% of total basic mark for composition. That is why it is purposeful to fulfill different kinds of interactions, which can be supported by criteria of different complexity: for example, cooperation, when gymnast does not control object, or without help of hands. Kinds of supports and gymnasts' passing under or above object also are included in it. The research of content of modern group exercises' competition compositions permitted to find that important condition of their quality is logical character, variety and correspondence of positioning and re-positioning to gymnasts' fitness level.

Acknowledgements:

The researches have been fulfilled in compliance with combined plan of SRW in sphere of physical culture and sports for 2011-2015 by topic 2.15 "Control of body and system of bodies static-dynamic balance in kinds of sports with complex coordination of movements' structure" (state registration number 0111U001726). Scientific supervisor of the topic – doctor of pedagogic science, Professor V.N. Boloban.

Conflict of interests

The authors declare that there is no conflict of interests.

References:

1. Averkovich EP. *Kompoziciia uprazhnenij v khudozhestvennoj gimnastike* [Composition of exercises in calisthenics], Moscow: USRIPC; 1989. (in Russian)
2. Boloban VN *Reguliaciia pozy tela sportsmena* [Regulation of sportsman' body posture], Olympic Literature; 2013. (in Russian)
3. Viner IA. *Artistichnost' i puti ee formirovaniia* [Artistry and ways of its formation], Moscow: Human; 2014. (in Russian)
4. Denisova LV, Usichenko VV, Bishevec' NG. Analiz anketnikh danikh v sportivno–pedagogichnikh doslidzhenniakh [Analysis of questioning in sports-pedagogic researches], *Pedagogics, psychology, medical-biological problems of physical training and sports,* 2012; 1: 56–60 (in Ukrainian)
5. Karpenko LA. Komponenty sportivnogo i ispolnitel'nogo masterstva v gimnastike [Components of sports and performance skillfulness in gymnastics]. *Nauchno-prakticheskaia konferenciia, posviashchennaia 100–letiiu so dnia rozhdeniia L.P. Orlova* [Scientific-practical conference, devoted to 100 anniversary from birth of L.P. Orlov], Sankt Petersburg; 2001. P. 69–73 (in Russian)
6. Karpenko LA. *Khudozhestvennaia gimnastika* [Calisthenics], Moscow: Federation of Russia; 2003. (in Russian)
7. Miroshnichenko T. Metodika postanovki suchasnikh kompozicij grupovikh vprav u khudozhnij gimnastici [Methodic of composing of group exercises' compositions in calisthenics]. *Teoriia i metodika fizichnogo vikhovannia i sportu*, 2001; 4: 11-13 (in Ukrainian)
8. Morozevich-Shiliuk T. Artistizm akrobatov vysokogo klassa [Artistry of elite acrobats]. *Nauka v olimpijskom sporte*, 2012;1: 74-80 (in Russian)
9. Nachinskaia SV. *Matematicheskaia statistika v sporte* [Mathematical statistic in sports], Kiev: Health; 1987. (in Russian)

10. Nesterova TV, Bogorad OA. Sredstva vyrazitel'nosti sportivno-khudozhestvennykh kompozicij v khudozhestvennoj gimnastike [Means of expressiveness of sport-art compositions in calisthenics]. *Fizicheskoe vospitanie studentov tvorcheskikh special'nostej,* 2005; 5: 24-31. (in Russian)
11. Omel'ianchik O, Saliamin Iu, Dobrovol'skij E. Sravnitel'nyj analiz sorevnovatel'noj deiatel'nosti ukraiskikh gimnastov v olimpijskom cikle 2009 – 2012 godov [Comparative analysis of competition functioning of Ukrainian gymnasts in Olympic cycle 2009 – 2012]. *Nauka v olimpijskom sporte*, 2012; 1: 81–83. (in Russian)
12. Omel'ianchik-Ziurkalova OA. Model'noe postroenie kompozicij na vol'nykh uprazhneniiakh s uchetom khoreograficheskoj podgotovlennosti gimnastok [Simulation of compositions with free exercises, considering choreographic fitness of female gymnasts]. *Nauka v olimpijskom sporte,* 2015; 1: 63–67. (in Russian)
13. Sosina VIu. *Khoreografiia v gimnastike* [Choreography in gymnastics], Kiev: Olympic Literature; 2009. (in Russian)
14. Terekhina RN, Kriuchek ES, Medvedeva EN, Zenovka IB. Sovremennyj podkhod k processu postanovki sorevnovatel'nykh kompozicij v khudozhestvennoj gimnastike [Modern approach to composing of competition compositions in calisthenics]. *Uchenye zapiski*, 2014;8:180-185. (in Russian)
15. Tereshchenko IA, Otsupok AP, Krupenya SV, Liauchuk TM, Boloban VN. Coordination training of sportsmen, specializing in sport kinds of gymnastic. *Physical Education of Students*, 2015;3:52-65. http://dx.doi.org/10.15561/20755279.2015.0307
16. Boloban WN. Reaction time and motor time in an athlete's movements. *Pedagogics, psychology, medical-biological problems of physical training and sports,* 2009;10:295–301. (in Russian)
17. Zhulkevskaya GV. Gymnastics. Minsk: BGUFK; 2005.
18. Potop V, Grigore W, Marinesku S. Motor learning gymnastic exercises on the basic of transfer technologies. *Science in the Olympic sports*, 2012;1:47–57.
19. *Rules rhythmic gymnastics*. Federation international de gymnastique. Losana; 2012.

26

MODEL OF STUDENTS' SPORT-ORIENTED PHYSICAL EDUCATION WITH APPLICATION OF INFORMATION TECHNOLOGIES

Olkhovy O.M., Petrenko Y.M., Temchenko V.A., Timchenko A.N.
Kharkov National University

Abstract. *Purpose:* working out and practical application of approaches to perfection of physical education system's functioning. *Material:* in the research students (boys– n=92, girls– n=45) of 18-20 years old took part. *Results:* structural model of students' sport-oriented physical education with application of information technologies has been formed. The main purpose of such model's creation was cultivation of students' demand in physical functioning and formation of healthy life style in students' environment. The model of the process includes orienting, executive and control components. In this model groups of commonly accepted physical education and sport-oriented groups function. *Conclusions:* Main structural components of the created model have been determined: conceptual, motivation-active, resulting.
Key words: model, students, sport-oriented physical education, structure, information technologies.

Introduction

Recent years there has been observed substantial worsening of students' health and physical condition [22, 23, 26, 27, 32-34]. Most scientists connect this fact with unfavorable social economic life conditions and ecology as well as with significant reduction of students' interest to physical culture and sports, reduction of effectiveness of physical education (PE) system in higher educational establishments (HEE) [2, 12, 14, 20, 38-42]. Application of traditional approaches does not influence on students properly as well as influence on their strive for sport practicing, for constant self-perfection and physical functioning [1, 16]. Re-organization of PE in Ukrainian HEEs requires searching of new approaches to health related physical culture work with students [7, 8, 13, 19].

Analysis of researches and publications showed that nowadays in students' PE sport-oriented technologies are implemented more and more intensively. It facilitates increase of students' interest to physical culture in HEE's educational space [1, 10, 11]. Implementation of sport-oriented technologies in students' PE results in stage-by-stage increasing of physical culture classes' attendance, interest to chosen kind of sport, rising of motor functioning's level in class and out of class time [17, 18, 20].

In present conditions tendencies of education development imply transition of control over educational process to new technological level, envisaging application of information technologies [8, 21]. Such approach is a necessary condition of increasing of education's quality [7, 9, 13, 24, 25, 28-31]. However, at present there is no single approach to organization of students' sport-oriented physical education (SOPE) with application of information technologies (IT) influence of IT application both on organization and on effectiveness of SOPE functioning has been studied insufficiently [10, 21].

Purpose, tasks of the work, material and methods

The purpose of the research: is formation of SOPE with application of IT for perfection of PE system in HEE. Material: students of Kharkov national university (KNU), named after V.N. Karazine (boys– n=92, girls– n=45) of 18-20 years old took part. Methods of the research: theoretical analysis of scientific literature, simulation, forming pedagogic experiment.

Results of the research

Transition of discipline "Physical culture" to optional level (which is not included in curriculum and does not have final control) in Ukrainian HEEs requires change of approach to content of all learning process in present conditions of organization of higher education. Involvement of students in learning process becomes the main factor, determining functioning of PE departments in HEEs structure. For improving of physical fitness results and rising of students' psycho-physiological condition it is necessary to seek principally new approaches, methodic and technologies, which would comply with individual features, maximally facilitate effective realization of interests, demands and bents of students [7, 11, 12, 35-37, 43, 44].

Working out of SOPE model, based on students' motivation for PE trainings 12, 14, 15] provides opportunities to wider regard the tasks of such training process, to use specialists, assess quality of work of different links of education and to build model as a standard. Basing on such standard it would be possible to systemize and organize PE training process in HEE.

Let us formulate clearer the features of SOPE model, starting from conceptual principles of learning process. In this case PE training process will be provided with adaptive applied model, adequate in respect to object of the research, considering possible changes. The purpose of SOPE concept is presentation of theory in instructive and applied form. The most accessible is idea, based on achievement of useful final result – formation of healthy life style in students' environment. Criterion of such concept's substantiation is practicability of its application in HEEs. It will permit to determine disadvantages of existing in HEEs at present PE system [3-5, 12, 13, 16, 21, 23].

One of main ways of differentiated approach's and PE wholeness's realization in process of construction of SOPE model was approach, in compliance with which the following requirements to content of pedagogic model were put: didactic character (purposefulness, significance of training's content, dynamic character of its development, rationality of model's construction); methodic character (presence of logic and structure in reflecting of content; correspondence of scope of information to conditions of optimal functioning); connection of content with algorithm of the conducted measures; technical character (varying of information rendering temp, up-to date character of means of content's reflection, convenience of control over conducted measures) [13, 16, 19]. Content of training process shall be reflected in model systemically, with clearly outlined logic, special techniques and parts, Such approach attracts students' attention and causes positive emotions. With it, model of training process's content shall include orienting, executive and control components.

Orienting component contains main conceptual idea of training content and main positions of training. In this component program of actions' fulfillment is reflected, which ensures more efficient approach to students' mastering of training content and facilitates formation of their certain readiness to further professional functioning. Orienting component determines purpose, tasks, principles and sequence of appropriate actions of training.

Executive component is the main in the model. Its content is presented as organizational measures and conditions. They ensure effective course of realization of this content, methodic and technologies of organization of training process. It shows the ways of solution of the researched problem.

Control component is intended for determination of effectiveness of the created model, degree of correspondence of all changes in training variant of previous type. With its help required correction of orienting and executive components can be done.

It is purposeful to apply these conceptual approaches when using IT with introduction of all mentioned components and a number of changes in structure of commonly accepted in HEEs SOPE model. Main purpose of IT application in SOPE was cultivation of students' demand in physical functioning, rising of PE functioning in HEEs. As final result it is formation of student's healthy life style.

Conceptual tasks of SOPE with application of IT in HEE were the following:

– increasing of students' motivation for physical trainings with active usage of IT for this purpose (system of HEE's, physical education department's, sport clubs', organs of students self governing sites and etc.);

– increasing of effectiveness of general physical, technical and theoretical fitness of students in chosen kind of sports (motor functioning) with the help of IT for visualizing of training process.

Combination of correspondence of purpose and tasks, following the SOPE principles, simultaneity and complexity of their application, efficiency, create own orientation in compliance with conditions and specificities of sport orientation [22].

By the results of the conducted theoretical analysis of scientific sources [1, 9-11, 16-23, 46-49], considering basic principles of theory of physical education and sports (L.P. Matveyev, 1991; V.M. Platonov, 2004-2014; T.YU. Krutsevich, 2008-2014; Zaporozhanov V.A., 2009-2015) ad results of practical researches of PE departments of different HEEs, devoted to IT application in training process of students we optimized SOPE model. The model contains main structural components, shown in fig.1:

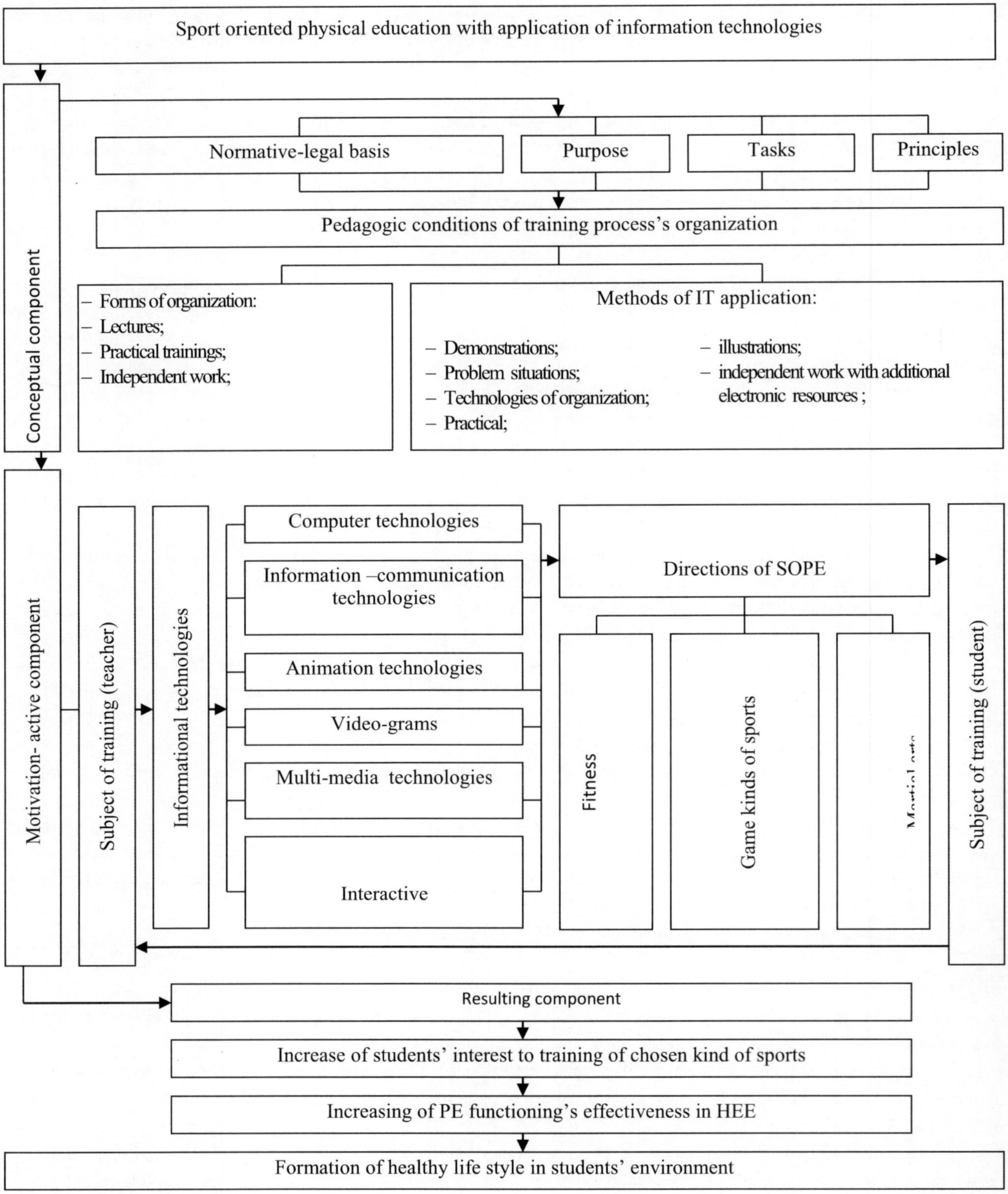

Fig.1. Structural model of SOPE with IT application

– conceptual, determining purpose, tasks, principles of targeted orientations, pedagogic conditions of control over training process in SPE, realized through organizational forms and methods of IT application;

– motivation-active – determines orientation and educational interaction of IT by directions of SOPE for students' mastering of training program, realization of purpose and tasks;

– resulting – determines effectiveness of PR process in HEEs by detecting of involvement level and interest of trainees in regular physical culture and sport trainings; formation of healthy life style in students' environment.

For determination of authors' SOPE model with application of IT on students' physical fitness, level of motor skills and skills in chosen kind of sports in period from September 2013 to May 2014 we conducted forming pedagogic experiment on the base of KNU. Control (CG – n=69) and experimental (EG – n=68) groups included students, training in sport-oriented groups: basketball CG-1 (n=14), EG-1 (n=14) – boys, CG-2 (n=10), EG-2 (n=11) – girls; football in doors CG-3 (n=21), EG-3 (n=19) – boys; ping-pong CG-4 (n=12), EG-4 (n=12) – boys, CG-5 (n=12), EG-5 (n=12) – girls.

In CG we used IT of open type (accessible for all sites and blogs) in EG we used both IT of open type and closed type (video- and multimedia-technologies for training of motor actions, which stipulated application of animation video-grams with accentuated demonstration of separate elements of technique; films on principles of theory and methodic of chosen kind of sports with real and animated heroes; published manuals with detail illustration of techniques' video-grams; video-materials, worked out by groups of authors and video-materials from Internet). Application of open and closed types' IT in our researches was used for activation of students' conscious attitude to training process.

Experimental researches proved that application of SOPE with IT in KNU there was positive influence on increasing of the following:

- Physical fitness of EG trainees (EG – $p<0.05$-0.001);
- Students' mastering of motor skills in chosen kinds of sports and motor functioning (EG – $p<0.05$-0.001);
- Final mark of trainees on discipline "Physical education" (EG-1 – by 7.7 points, $p<0.01$; EG-2 – by 6.8 points $p<0.01$; EG-3 – by 7.9 points, $p<0.01$; EG-4 – by 7.7 points, $p<0.01$; EG-5 –by 8.2 points, $p<0.01$).

In CG there were no confident changes by the mentioned above indicators.

Discussion

According to the presented conceptual apparatus, with the help of methodic of collection and processing of information on operative level the final purpose of our research was formation of structural model SOPE with application of IT (see fig.1). On the base of the regarded concepts of models' construction and requirements [1, 2, 9-14, 16, 22] we chose approach, in foundation of which direct and full studying of training process in HEE was embedded.

The conducted analysis of PE departments' work showed that at modern stage there are several variants of PE organization in HEEs, the main of which can be presented in the form of two models. The first – is traditional organization of PE, where teachers' staff organizes trainings of rooted general developing content. The second – is transition model: from traditional PE to SOPE. In this model, groups of traditional PE function side-by side with sport-oriented PE groups on different kinds of sports and motor functioning. These groups are practically not connected with each other.

Both models of PE organization are imperfect. In first case we have students' restricted choice of training's content that reduces their motivation and effectiveness. The second variant is a step ahead in comparison with traditional PE organization. Actually it is an attempt of SOPE realization. But such approach also has a number of disadvantages. In it there is no single form of assessment and construction of program material. IT is used insufficiently in training process or is not used at all. Solution of this problem implies perfection of organization of both: organization and training process itself (training of movements in every kind of sports or motor functioning). It is facilitated by application of IT, implying usage with visual printing and dynamic video and multi-media aids.

For creation of SOPE structural model with IT application we used techniques, oriented on achievement of maximal correspondence between theoretical construction of model, purposefulness and possibility of its practical realization. It should be noted that positive side of such approach was the fact that foundation of each of these ideas [1, 11, 13, 19, 20] in respect to perfection of training efficiency are certain changes. They consider urgent requirements of present time and motivation. Weak side of such approach is impossibility of 100% prognostication and objective preliminary assessment of the offered changes' after-effects.

Conclusions:

Basing on conception of achievement of useful final result (formation of healthy life style in students' environment) and systemic analysis of training process in higher educational establishments [1-20] we formed structural model of sport-oriented students' physical education with the help of information technologies. We determined general characteristics and main structural components of the created model: conceptual, motivation-active and resulting.

Experimental researches confidently proved purposefulness of SOPE model's application with usage of IT for achievement of useful final result of training in PE system in higher school – creation of necessary for formation of healthy life style in students' environment and cultivation of graduate's demand in physical (motor) functioning in further everyday life.

In the future we shall orient our researches on experimental determination of effectiveness of SOPE model's with IT application functioning.

Acknowledgement

The research has been conducted in compliance with combined plan of scientific-research works in sphere of physical culture and sports for 2013-2014 by topic "Theoretical-methodic principles of application of information, pedagogic and medical-biological technologies for formation of healthy life style" (State registration number 0113U002003).

Conflict of interests

The authors declare that there is no conflict of interests.

References:

1. Bal'sevich VK, Lubysheva LI. Sportivno orientirovannoe fizicheskoe vospitanie: obrazovatel'nyj i social'nyj aspekty [Sport-oriented physical education: educational and social aspects]. *Teoriia i praktika fizicheskoj kul'tury* 2003;5:19–22. (in Russian)
2. Iermakov SS, Ivashchenko SN, Guzov VV. Osobennosti motivacii studentov s primeneniem individual'nykh programm fizicheskoj samopodgotovki [Specificities of students' motivation with application of individual programs of physical self-training]. *Physical education of students* 2012;4:59–61. (in Russian)
3. Iermakov SS Issledovaniia v sporte: analiz informacii v seti Internet Ukrainy, Rossii i respubliki Belarus' [Researches in sports: analysis of information in Internet of Ukraine, Russia, Belarus]. *Pedagogics, psychology, medical-biological problems of physical training and sports* 2001;18:51-58. (in Russian)
4. Iermakov S. Osnovy sozdaniia informacionnoj sistemy obespecheniia nauchnykh issledovanij v kontekste edinogo obrazovatel'nogo prostranstva [Principles of creation of informational system for ensuring of scientific researches in context of single educational space]. *Nauka v olimpijskom sporte* 2005;2:117-127. (in Russian)
5. Iermakov SS, Krivencova IV. Perspektivi rozvitku navchal'noi disciplini «Fizichne vikhovannia» u vishchikh navchal'nikh zakladakh Ukraini [Prospects of development of discipline "Physical education" in higher educational establishments of Ukraine]. *Pedagogika ta psikhologiia* 2015;47:117-124. (in Ukrainian)
6. Zolochevs'kij VV. *Teoriia i praktika organizacii fizkul'turno-masovoi roboti iz students'koiu moloddiu u vitchiznianij pedagogici. Cand. Diss.* [Theory and practice of organization of mass physical culture work with students in domestic pedagogic. Cand. Diss.]. Kharkiv; 2009. (in Ukrainian)
7. Kamaev OI, Kamaeva EK. Osobennosti ispol'zovaniia kompetentnostnogo podkhoda v zdorov'eformiruiushchikh tekhnologiiakh v usloviiakh vuza [Specificities of usage of competence approach to health-formation technologies in HEE conditions]. *Physical education of students* 2010;6:37 - 39. (in Russian)
8. Kashuba VA, Valikov DP, Sergienko KN. Komp'iuternye tekhnologii v sisteme vysshego fizkul'turnogo obrazovaniia [Computer technologies in system of higher physical culture education]. *Fiziceskoe vospitanie studentov tvorceskih special'nostej* 2002;6:22–27. (in Russian)
9. Kashuba VA, Futornyj SM, Golovanova NL. K voprosu ispol'zovaniia informacionnykh tekhnologij v processe fizicheskogo vospitaniia studencheskoj molodezhi [On usage of informational technologies in process of students' physical education]. *Slobozhans'kij naukovo-sportivnij visnik* 2011;4:157–163. (in Russian)
10. Kolos NA. *Sovremennye informacionnye tekhnologii v fizicheskom vospitanii detej, podrostkov i studencheskoj molodezhi* [Modern information technologies in physical education of children, adolescents and students], Lutsk: Teren; 2011. (in Russian)

11. Krivcova MA. Interaktivnye metody obucheniia fizicheskoj kul'ture pri podgotovke specialista [Interactive methods of physical culture training in preparation of specialist]. *Trudy SPbGUKI* 2013;1:460–462. (in Russian)
12. Krucevich TIu, Nesterenko AN. Motivacionnye prioritety zdorovogo obraza zhizni studentok vuzov [Motivation priorities of healthy life style of HEEs' girl students]. In: *IX Mizhnarodnij naukovij kongress «Olimpijs'kij sport i sport dlia vsikh», 20–23 veresnia, 2005, Kiiv* [IX International scientific congress "Olympic sports and sports for all" 2005, September 20–23, Kyiv], Kiev; 2005. p. 581. (in Russian)
13. Kuz'min VA, Kudriavcev MD, Kopylov IuA, Galimov GIa, Strel'nikov VA. Konceptual'nye osnovy neobkhodimosti obnovleniia dopolnitel'nogo ozdorovitel'nogo fizicheskogo vospitaniia studentov [Conceptual principles of demand in additional health related physical education of students]. In: *Mezhdunarodnaia nauchno-prakticheskaia konferenciia. 8–10 aprelia, 2014, Minsk* [International scientific-practical conference. April 8-10, 2014. Minsk] Minsk: BGUFK; 2014. p. 162–165. (in Russian)
14. Liu Iun Cian'. *Motivaciia fizkul'turno-sportivnoj aktivnosti studencheskoj molodezhi v sisteme formirovaniia ustanovki na zdorovyj obraz zhizni. Cand. Diss.* [Motivation of physical culture – sport functioning of students in system of formation of orientation for healthy life style. Cand. Diss.], Minsk; 2011. (in Russian)
15. Moskalenko N. Pedagogichni innovacii u fizichnomu vikhovanni [Pedagogic innovations in physical education]. *Sportivnij visnik Pridniprov'ia* 2009;1:19–22. (in Ukrainian)
16. Ol'khovij OM. Stan funkcionuvannia sistemi fizichnogo vikhovannia zakladiv vishchoi osviti [Functioning of physical education system in higher educational establishments]. *Teoriia i metodika fizichnogo vikhovannia i sportu* 2014; 2:79 - 83 (in Ukrainian)
17. Poproshaev AV, Muntian VS. Preimushchestva sekcionnoj formy organizacii uchebnogo processa po discipline «fizicheskoe vospitanie» [Advantages of organization of circles' form of "physical education" discipline's training]. *Physical education of students* 2011;4:67–70. (in Russian)
18. Radaeva SV. *Fizicheskoe vospitanie studentov nefizkul'turnogo vuza na osnove sportivno-orientirovannykh tekhnologij. Cand. Diss.* [Physical education of students of not physical culture HEE on the base of sport-oriented technologies. Cand. Diss]; 2008. (in Russian)
19. Savin SV, Stepanova ON. Konceptual'nye i prikladnye aspekty tekhnologizacii proektirovochnoj deiatel'nosti v sfere ozdorovitel'noj fizicheskoj kul'tury [Conceptual and applied aspects of technologies' implementation in projecting functioning in sphere of health related physical culture]. *Podgotovka pedagoga po fizicheskoj kul'ture v usloviiakh modernizacii Rossijskogo obrazovaniia* [Training of pedagogue of physical culture in conditions of modernization of Russian education], Moscow, MGPU; 2007. p. 149–156. (in Russian)
20. Sadovnikova VV. Ispol'zovanie valeologicheskogo podkhoda v vuze dlia formirovaniia orientacij studencheskoj molodezhi [Application of valuelogic approach for formation of students' orientations in HEE]. *Aktual'nye problemy fizicheskoj reabilitacii i ergoterapii* [Urgent problems of physical rehabilitation and ergo-therapy], Minsk: BGUFK; 2008. p. 97–100. (in Russian)
21. Temchenko VO. *Sportivno-oriientovane fizichne vikhovannia u vishchikh navchal'nikh zakladakh iz zastosuvanniam informacijnikh tekhnologij. Cand. Diss.* [Sport-oriented physical education in higher educational establishments with application of information technologies. Cand. Diss.], Dnipropetrovsk; 2015. (in Ukrainian)
22. Futornyj S, Karavatskaia M. Informacionnye tekhnologii i Internet-resursy v formirovanii zdorovogo obraza zhizni studentov v processe fizicheskogo vospitaniia [Information technologies and Internet resources in formation of students' healthy life style in process of physical education]. *Molodizhnij naukovij visnik Skhidnoievropejs'kogo nacional'nogo universitetu* 2013;9:68–73. (in Russian)
23. Futornyi S. Actual issues of improving the process of student`s physical education through the application of modern health-saving technologies. *Molodizhnij naukovij visnik Skhidnoievropejs'kogo nacional'nogo universitetu* 2014;14:26–30.
24. Abar B. Promoting tobacco cessation utilizing pre-health professional students as research associates in the emergency department. *Addictive Behaviors* 2015;40;73–76.
25. Al-Hariri MT, Al-Hattami AA. Utilization of internet by health colleges students at the University of Dammam. *Journal of Taibah University Medical Sciences* 2015;10(1):66–73.

26. Belykh SI. Methodological foundations of individually oriented approaches to ground of physical education unprofessional university students. *Physical education of students* 2013;3:11-17. http://dx.doi.org/10.6084/m9.figshare.669662
27. Belykh SI. Structure of the concept of personality oriented physical education university students. *Physical education of students*, 2013;4:3-9. http://dx.doi.org/10.6084/m9.figshare.669663
28. Berger H, Franke GH, Hofmann F-H, Sperth M, Holm-Hadulla RM. Mental health of students and its development between 1994 and 2012. *Mental Health & Prevention*. 2015;3(1–2):48–56.
29. Dolan E, Hancock E, Wareing A. An evaluation of online learning to teach practical competencies in undergraduate health science students. *The Internet and Higher Education* 2015;24(0):21–5.
30. Hadden KB. Health literacy training for health professions students. *Patient Education and Counseling* 2015;98(7):918–20.
31. Holm-Hadulla RM, Koutsoukou-Argyraki A. Mental health of students in a globalized world: Prevalence of complaints and disorders, methods and effectivity of counseling, structure of mental health services for students. *Mental Health & Prevention*. 2015;3(1–2):1–4.
32. Iermakova TS. Peculiarities of forming health culture of pupils in Poland: historical aspect. *Pedagogics, psychology, medical-biological problems of physical training and sports* 2014;6:16-20. http://dx.doi.org/10.6084/m9.figshare.1004090
33. Kovaleva MV, Rumba OG. Active games in physical education students of special medical group with limited capacity of cardiovascular system. *Physical education of students* 2013;4:35-45. http://dx.doi.org/10.6084/m9.figshare.681644
34. Kramida IE. Exercises for students of different medical groups as factors of the weakening bad habits at students. *Physical education of students* 2013;4:46-50. http://dx.doi.org/10.6084/m9.figshare.669680
35. Lapkin S, Levett-Jones T, Gilligan C. Using the Theory of Planned Behaviour to examine health professional students' behavioural intentions in relation to medication safety and collaborative practice. *Nurse Education Today*. 2015;35(8):935–40.
36. Malenyuk TV, Kosivska AV. Training at sport circle as priority form of organization of students' physical education (on example of shaping). *Pedagogics, psychology, medical-biological problems of physical training and sports* 2015;4:38-42. http://dx.doi.org/10.15561/18189172.2015.0407
37. Michael Chia, Marcus Lee. Relationship between quality of life and resilience among sport-active Singaporean youth. *Physical education of students* 2015;2:29-36. http://dx.doi.org/10.15561/20755279.2015.0205
38. Mytskan BM, Fedynyak NV. Justification revitalizing body of persons third age by means of physical education. *Pedagogics, psychology, medical-biological problems of physical training and sports* 2014;10;18-23. http://dx.doi.org/10.5281/zenodo.10485
39. Pichurin VV. Psychological and psycho-physical training as a factor of personal anxiety at students. *Pedagogics, psychology, medical-biological problems of physical training and sports* 2015;3:46-51. http://dx.doi.org/10.15561/18189172.2015.0307
40. Pidpomoga AY. Dynamic of functional indicators' changes of students having harmful habits (on example of smoking) under influence of organized motion functioning. *Physical education of students* 2015;2:22-28. http://dx.doi.org/10.15561/20755279.2015.0204
41. Prusik Krzysztof, Prusik Katarzyna, Kozina ZhL, Iermakov SS. Features of physical development, physical preparedness and functional state of boys and girls – students of Polish higher educational establishments. *Physical education of students* 2013;1:54-61. http://dx.doi.org/10.6084/m9.figshare.96415
42. Roters TT. Physical improvement of students during interactive physical and aesthetic education. *Physical education of students* 2013;4:72-76. http://dx.doi.org/10.6084/m9.figshare.663624
43. Siri A, Rui M. Distance Education for Health Professions' Students. *Procedia - Social and Behavioral Sciences.* 2015;174(0):730–8.
44. Usher K, Woods C, Casella E, Glass N, Wilson R, Mayner L, et al. Australian health professions student use of social media. *Collegian*. 2014;21(2):95–101.

45. Yermakova TS. Individualization of forming health culture in schoolchildren of Polish schools. *Pedagogics, psychology, medical-biological problems of physical training and sports* 2015;1:29-33. http://dx.doi.org/10.15561/18189172.2015.0106
46. Zaporozhanov VA, Boraczynski Tomasz. Discussion on the concepts of "coordination" and "agility" in terms of physical education. *Pedagogics, psychology, medical-biological problems of physical training and sports* 2015;3:15-19. http://dx.doi.org/10.15561/18189172.2015.0303
47. Zaporozhanov VA. About reliable indicator of proprioception in agility control. *Pedagogics, psychology, medical-biological problems of physical training and sports* 2013;4:21-25. http://dx.doi.org/10.6084/m9.figshare.693023
48. Zaporozhanov VA, Borachinski T. On the transfer of skills skill in different conditions of motor activity. *Pedagogics, psychology, medical-biological problems of physical training and sports* 2013;9:25-28. http://dx.doi.org/10.6084/m9.figshare.749693
49. Zaporozhanov VA, Boraczynski T. Evaluation improvement of coordination abilities in physically active persons. *Pedagogics, psychology, medical-biological problems of physical training and sports* 2009;9:52 - 55.

PERSONALITY ORIENTED SYSTEM OF STRENGTHENING OF STUDENTS' PHYSICAL, PSYCHIC AND SOCIAL-MORAL HEALTH

Kudryavtsev M.D. [1,3], Kopylov Yu.A. [2], Kuzmin V.A. [1], Ionova O.M. [4], Yermakova T.S. [4]
[1] Siberian Federal University (SibFU), Krasnoyarsk, Russia
[2]The Federal State Scientific Institution of Russian Academy of education "The Institute of Age Physiology", Moscow, Russia
[3]Siberian State Aerospace University, Krasnoyarsk, Russia
[4]H.S. Skovoroda Kharkiv National Pedagogical University

Abstract. _Purpose:_ to work out content of individualized trainings, permitting to correct deviations in different aspects of physical, psychic and social-moral health of higher educational establishments' students. _Material:_ in experiment 105 boy students of 20-24 years' age participated. All students gave conscious consent to participate in experiment. The trainings were practiced 4 times a week, 45 minutes each. _Results:_ it is interesting that change of different personality's features is rather long process, which in some aspects resist to changes. We showed approaches to training vitally important skills and abilities, required for adaptation to modern social cultural medium; to the simplest techniques of organization of independent health related physical culture trainings; to means of health strengthening, formation of knowledge on health related physical culture. We developed personality-oriented system of formation of psychic and social-moral health. _Conclusions:_ the worked out approach permits to achieve real positive psychic and socially important qualities of student's personality during one academic year.
Key words: health, physical culture, physical training, psycho-regulation, breathing gymnastic.

Introduction

Recent years there have been observed worsening of higher educational students' physical, psychic and social-moral health [3, 17]. The found deviations in health are the results of many reasons: reduction of motor functioning against the background of increased academic loads; reduction of every day motor activity; violation of healthy life style rules [25].

Study of higher school students' psycho-physical indicators [16] showed that in most cases there is found weak condition of motor qualities with unsatisfactory state of different psychic indicators [14]. To avoid this situation it is necessary to implement different forms of health related physical culture, special, correcting and rehabilitating activity in system of higher educational establishment students' physical education. However, in this respect, pedagogues of higher educational establishments face great difficulties [6] because of absence of developed and scientifically grounded program of such trainings.

At present time problems of physical education of higher educational establishments' students are still more acute [37]. As it was found in [8], traditional system of physical education does not realize the tasks of health formation of educational establishments' students to the fullest extent. In such situation it is necessary to develop pedagogic technology [15] oriented on training of psycho-physical, social-moral health and important for learning students' qualities [5].

Formation of students' psycho-physical health can be realized in different directions. In opinion of V.V. Ismiyanov [13] such approach implies qualitative changes of students' physical fitness (improvement of motor qualities: general endurance, speed endurance, strength, flexibility, quickness), psycho-emotional state (personality's qualities, communicability, will power, feelings and emotions). It results in significant improvement of social status and life-building in system of higher education and further professional functioning of students. In such cases it is very important to determine students' ability to self-cognition of own psycho-physical and motor potentials [4]. Not less important is express-assessment of students' physical health level [27], substantiation of the used tests [28, 32].

The state of students' social-moral health is determined by several factors. A.A. Opletin and V.D. Panachev [21] found that students' will efforts facilitate stability of personality, psychic and physical health and increase of life tonus as well as workability and optimism. In process of pedagogic auto-training practicing at physical culture lessons psychological settings for formation of self development competence that facilitates formation of student's professional orientation. In the process of future functioning psychological settings are fixed and transform in social. In other works [19] it is shown that in the structure of students' temper low level of demand in mastering of objective world and strives for mental and physical labor prevails. With it is noted that there are good indicators of social activity and communicability.

Training of students' significant for studying qualities requires appropriate content of their psychological and psycho-physical fitness. The offered by V.V. Pichurin [24] content of students' such training is effective in respect to reduction of individual anxiety. The author points that application in physical culture lessons significant for boys kinds of sports – weight lifting and power lifting and for girls – aerobics and sakhadja yoga statistically significantly influenced on reduction of individual anxiety. For achievement of the set aims Yu.A. Osipov et al. [22] recommend using technologies of formation of social physical culture-sports medium, rating system of assessment of students' sports achievements; individualized and specialized programs of students' physical education.

In other works demand in the following is noted: rising of psychological comfort in students' groups in conditions of increase of their physical activity [38]; application of social constructive educational model for students' training [30]; demand in consideration of social demographic factors' influence on formation of students' healthy life style [33]; determination of health levels and physical condition, physical workability and physical fitness; students' psychic state [1, 26, 31]; constant monitoring of students' health condition [29, 32, 40]; appropriate substantiation of tests' usage [34].

In our previous researches we determined that content of additional (health related) physical culture training envisages prevailing orientation on health improving, general developing and sport-recreational tasks. With it, first attention is paid to formation of physical, psychic and social-moral health [15]. In such cases it is necessary to use adequate forms of control over students' health [32] with their appropriate substantiation [35]. Besides, it is necessary to consider the presence of possible deviations in students' health [36, 39]. Earlier we found that in training of future pedagogues it is important or realize salute-genetic approach [12]. This approach is based on anthroposophically oriented methodological principles and facilitates healthy, holistic development of students. With such approach main directions of students' training (academic learning, training by life experience, internal spiritual development) are oriented on activation of human internal intentions; awakening of students' will to study during all life; stimulation of independent work on own perfection in professional and personal spheres.

Testing of students elucidate a little individual peculiarities of such category. Such important aspects as physical, psychic and social-moral health of students are still out of scientists' interests. The absence of such data seriously hinders formation of students' comprehensive personalities and their social adaptation in modern society.

In connection with the above said it seems to be important to seek innovative approaches to new methodic and technologies' working out in the process of students' education and teaching. The purpose of such search is physical rehabilitation and pedagogic correction of students' health by means of health related physical culture and elements of sports activity [5].

Hypothesis: personality-oriented system of students' health formation shall consider their individual features. Such approach will permit to solve the following tasks:

- teaching to vitally important skills, required for adaptation in modern social-cultural medium;
- training the simplest techniques of organization of independent health related physical culture training;
- teaching to methods of health strengthening; formation of knowledge in health related physical culture.

The purpose of the research: is to work out personality oriented system of formation of students' physical, psychic and social-moral health.

The tasks of the research:

1. To work out complexes of physical exercises for correction of deviation in physical, psychic and social health of students.

2. To assess effectiveness of complexes of physical exercises for correction of deviation in physical, psychic and social health of students.

Material and methods

Participants: in experiment 105 boy students of 20-24 years' age participated. All students gave conscious consent to participate in experiment. The trainings were practiced 4 times a week, 45 minutes each.

Procedure:

Pedagogic experiment was conducted during one academic year on the base of pedagogic faculties of higher educational establishments. Experiment involved pedagogues, medical workers, specialists in physical education.

At each training, one from four training complexes was worked at:

1. Block "Attention", block "Gymnastic for eyesight" and block "Breathing gymnastic".
2. Block "Carriage" and block "Prophylaxis of flat-footedness".
3. Block "General physical training".
4. Block "Prophylaxis of cold" and block "Psycho-regulation".

Testing was fulfilled twice a week: at the beginning and at the end of pedagogic experiment.

Organization of health related exercises' training considered three main principles:

- Principle of consequent teaching from simple to complex;
- Principle of movement's temp and duration correspondence to targets and tasks of training process safety;
- Principle of safety of educational process.

Assessment of physical-metrical indicators: we studied right hand strength, kg; left hand strength, kg; vital capacity of lungs, l; body length (cm) and mass (kg); heart beat rate in rest (b.p.m.); chest circumference (cm) [18].

Assessment of significant for studying indicators: it was fulfilled by pedagogues by five points' scale. They assessed formation of interest to studying, mental workability, aggressiveness, emotional stability, degree of attention concentration, assiduity [10].

Assessment of formation of interest to physical culture and sports practicing: was fulfilled by students, who estimated each motive: health strengthening, communication, strive to be courage and resolute, preparation for future activity; self satisfaction with activity, self assertion and self realization by five points' scale [7]:

1. I practice physical culture for health strengthening.
2. I practice physical culture to communicate more with my fellow students.
3. Physical culture permits for me to manifest courage and resolution.
4. I practice physical culture to prepare for professional functioning.
5. I practice physical culture, because I like sports trainings.
6. I practice physical culture and sports to defeat my fellow students.

After it we calculated mean value of accounted points.

Assessment of formation of socially significant qualities [20]: in questionnaire students assessed statements about their qualities by five points' scale. In total 24 statements were used in questionnaire.

1. Respect most of people and my classmates;
2. I develop ability to see difficulties of other people and actively help them;
3. I am ready to sacrifice my interests in favor of collective;
4. I help my peers, not waiting for praise or award;
5. I want that my labor would be useful for people;
6. I have careful attitude to man made things;
7. I always strive to do my best in any work;
8. I strive to cope with all difficulties in work by myself;
9. I often invent my own approach to business, own means of achievement of the set target;
10. I like to offer and realize new deeds;
11. I am a purposeful person;
12. I am able to work in full strength for long time;
13. I am ashamed if I lazy to help my parents or friend;
14. Discontent with myself helps me to fight with my drawbacks;
15. I am responsible in respect to class interests, mutual success;
16. I feel sympathy toward peers, who are not able to do something;
17. I fulfill any unpleasant work, if it is useful for people;
18. I have careful attitude to animals, vegetation, nature;
19. I am scrupulous and diligent in any business;
20. I like independent, difficult work;
21. I like to do any work interesting and useful for myself and other people;
22. I like to master new activities, new knowledge and new skills;
23. I used to outline the main in any business without distracting to less important tasks;
24. I am able to control my temper and be tolerant in conflicts with people.

After calculation of collected by every student points we determined average level of social qualities' formation: activity, moral position (questions 1, 2, 13, 14), collectivism (questions 3, 4, 15, 16), civic consciousness – strive to be useful for people (questions 5, 6, 17, 18), diligence (questions 7, 8, 19, 20), creative activity (questions 9, 10, 21, 22) and will quality (questions 11, 12, 23, 24).

Assessment of motor qualities' formation: assessment of main motor qualities (strength, quickness, dexterity, flexibility, peed-power indicators, general endurance) we used tests for the following:

1) Quickness of movements – 30 meters' run from high start;
2) Dexterity – "shuttle run" 3x10 m;
3) Speed-power indicators – long jump from he spot;
4) Strength – chin ups;
5) Flexibility – forward bending from sitting position;
6) General (aerobic) endurance – run during 6 minutes.

Assessment of healthy life style indicators: components of healthy life style (in percents) were assessed with questioning method. Students informed about usage of the following components: morning exercises; independent practicing of physical exercises in any form; attendance of sport circle; hardening; normal night sleep. Every answer was assessed by five points' scale. The sum of collected points was calculated by eight test questions. Then mean value calculated.

Content of trainings: was oriented on strengthening of health different aspects [9].

Complex 1

1. Block "Attention" (25 minutes):

Walking on narrow support: gymnastic balance beam, gymnastic bench; walking by marks – with back forward, side forward.

Exercises for coordination and balance: juggling by big (volleyball) and small (tennis) balls (2-3 balls); moving on inclined, limited support with and without an object on head.

Exercise on gymnastic balance beam: walking with different amplitude of movements, with acceleration; walking with legs' waving and turns on toes; stance on toes; forward jump by pushing with two feet; balancing on one foot; squat with hands on floor; jumps down.

Multiple passes of basketball ball in pairs – up to 3-5 minutes.

Catching of volleyball (tennis) ball: from floor, rolling ball (standing on the spot and in motion), flying high, making step.

Throw of basketball ball in basket by two hands from below.

Throw of small balls to target from the spot and in motion.

2. Bock "Gymnastic for eyesight" (10 minutes)

The exercises are fulfilled in convenient sitting position with head resting on chair's back and maximally relaxed muscles.

"Eyeball movements to the right and to the left" – shall be fulfilled without excessive tension, as slow as possible.

"Eyeball movements upwards and downwards" – shall be fulfilled with maximal amplitude with head upright. Repeat 4-6 times to each side. Close eyes and relax muscles for 30-40 seconds.

"Fixing of eyes on tip of nose" – shall be fulfilled with maximally relaxed muscles and calm, even breathing, during 10-20 seconds. After exercise, close eyes and relax body muscles for 30-40 seconds. If student feel fatigue, rest time can be prolonged.

"Eyes' rotation" – rotate eyes by circumference: first clockwise, then – counterclockwise. Make 3 rotations to each side. Rotations shall be smooth, without jerks. Head shall be unmovable. Relax muscles for 30-40 seconds.

"Blinking": quickly press and part eyelids (blink) during 15-20 seconds. After it, close eyes and relax muscles for 30-40 seconds. This exercise is useful after durable reading; in breaks between exercises for eyesight.

3. Block "Breathing gymnastic" [2] ***(10 minutes)***

Lungs' ventilation: deeply inhale and exhale as quickly as possible. Make 5-7 cycles. After exercise, relax muscles in lying position with closed eyes.

Cleaning breathing: take main stance and deeply inhale through nose, make 2-3 seconds' pause. Exhale by "portions" (3-4 portions in one cycle).

Expansion of chest: in main stance stretch arms forward. Fulfill deep inhales/exhales: during inhale move arms backward aside; at exhale – return arms in forward position. Repeat 10-12 times. This exercise expands chest that is very important for good breathing. Children with narrow chest have weak breathing muscles. This exercise helps to form elementary skills of rational breathing movements.

Complex 2

Block "Carriage" (35 minutes)

Hatha Yoga exercises [11].

Bow posture: lie on abdomen, feet together. Bend legs and seize ankles. Arms shall be stretched. Try7 keep legs and feet together. Slowly raise shins. Backbend so that only abdomen is in contact with floor. Look upward. Keep the posture for 10 sec. and slowly take initial position. Relax all body. The posture is useful for all body, especially for backbone and abdomen; it perfectly eliminates defects of carriage.

Stand on one foot: - initial position – stand on one foot with left ankle on the base of right thigh. Or you can place left sole on inner surface of right thigh. Keep palms together in front of chest. Keep balance. Slowly raise palms above head, keeping them together. Part hands aside like tree branches. Arms shall be stretched. Slowly come out of posture and repeat it on other foot. This exercise forms correct carriage, develops arms, girdle and back muscles; improves balance.

Posture of armchair: stand upright with feet parted by approximately 40 cm. Stretch arms forward, hands are relaxed, hanging down. Bend legs in knees and squat a little. Imagine that you are sitting in invisible armchair. Keep posture as long as possible. Upper part of legs will be tensed. It is an excellent exercise for legs and back's muscles, as well as for handsome carriage.

Swallow posture: bend forward from main stance. Raise right leg parallel to floor, stretching arms forward. Arms, torso and right leg make straight line. Keep posture for 20-30 seconds and take initial position. Repeat exercise with rising left leg. This exercise trains back muscles as well as muscles of thigh back side and girdle.

Forward bent in sitting position: lie on back, keep feet together. Slowly take sitting position, bend forward as low as possible. Seize ankles. Drop head and relax. Keep posture about 20 seconds. Come out of posture: first sit upright and then, lie on back. Place arms along torso with palms upward. Feet are a little apart.

Cobra posture: lie on abdomen, keep legs together. Place palms on floor at shoulder level. Slowly raise and bend as much as possible head and chest; keep abdomen in contact with floor. Look upwards. Keep posture about 20 sec. Breath normally. Then low slowly first chest and then head. This exercise strengthens back muscles and eliminates shifts in backbone.

Triangle: from main stance part feet wider than shoulders by jump. Raise arms aside at shoulder level with palms downwards. Turn right and left feet to the right – left leg is stretched. Bend torso to the right and touch right ankle with right palm (possible to place right palm on the floor). Stretch left arm upwards. Keep posture for 30-40 seconds. Breathing shall be even and deep. Take initial position and fulfill the exercise to other side. This exercise increase hip joints and backbone's mobility; expands chest.

Forward lunge with arms upwards: From main stance raise arms upwards – palms together. Make deep forward lunge with right leg; raise head and look at palms. Angle in right knee shall be 90°, left leg is stretched. Keep posture for 20-30 seconds. Breathing is free. This exercise increase tonus and strengthen muscles of back, legs and shoulders.

Block "Prophylaxis of flat-footedness" (10 minutes)

Initial position (i.p.) is sitting on gymnastic bench. Seize basketball ball with feet and throw it (12-15 times).

I.p. is sitting on gymnastic bench; rolling of small ball by foot (50-60 sec. by each foot).

I.p. is sitting on gymnastic bench; bending and unbending of feet quickly (20-30 sec.).

I.p. is sitting, resting on floor by hands; rolling of ball by inner feet arches.

I.p. is standing on knees with hands on waist. Sit on heels 10-12 times.

I.p. is standing by gymnastic wall. Walk on the spot highly raising thigh and bending foot in sole.

I.p is standing with hands on waist. Walk on the spot keeping contact of toes with floor (up to 60 sec.).

I.p. is sitting position with hands on floor. Actively bend and unbend feet (by 18-20 times).

Jumps on the spot with little moving forward on tip-toes (up to 1 minute).

Balancing on filled ball – up to 1 minute.

Complex 3

Block "General physical training" (45 minutes)

At first stages of training the quantity of exercises can be reduced; the, with improvement of physical fitness it can be increased.

Run and jumps on the spot; with moving with additional weight (in different directions and with different amplitude, from different initial positions).

Hanging on arms, move forward.

Carrying of moderate loads on back with maximal speed.

Repeated up to 20 meters' run with additional weight and maximal speed.

Outdoor games of power orientation (for example improvised basketball with filled ball).

Chin ups on gymnastic bar.

Squatting with different temp and different initial positions; on one or two feet.

Jumps in depth by method of "strike training".

Long and high jumps from the spot and from run.

Jumps in half squat position in different directions (face, back, right or left side forward).

High jumps with catching hanged objects.

Jumps on one or two feet, moving forward by circle, by "snake", on the spot with turn.

Skipping (or with shortened skipping rope) on the spot and in movement.

Pressing ups in lying position.

Bending of stretched legs in hanging on arms position.

Torso bending in position lying on back, on abdomen.

Jumping down from pedestal of 40-60 cm height.

Exercises on gymnastic bar.

Walking in deep squat.

Shuttle run (5 x 6) with touching floor with hand.

Climbing rope by 2-3 meters' height.

Complex 4

Block "Prophylaxis of cold" (5 minutes)

Exercises for neck consist of three movements:

1. In standing position relax neck and sharply turn head ftp the right and to the left. Repeat 5-25 times;
2. In standing position drop head sharply forward and backward for 5-25 times;
3. In standing position bend head to the right and to the left (5 times). Breathe normally, When bending try to keep shoulders unmovable. After some time you will be able to put ear on shoulder.

This exercise strengthens neck muscles; relaxes in case of tonsillitis, pharyngitis, makes voice louder, eliminates speech defects.

Hatha Yoga exercises (25 minutes):

Triangle: from main stance part feet wider than shoulders by jump. Raise arms aside at shoulder level with palms downwards. Turn right and left feet to the right – left leg is stretched. Bend torso to the right and touch right ankle with right palm (possible to place right palm on the floor). Stretch left arm upwards. Keep posture for 30-40 seconds. Breathing shall be even and deep. Take initial position and fulfill the exercise to other side. This exercise increase hip joints and backbone's mobility; expands chest.

Forward bent from lying position: lie on back, keep feet together. Slowly take sitting position, bend forward as low as possible. Seize ankles. Drop head and relax. Keep posture about 20 seconds. Come out of posture: first sit upright and then, lie on back. Place arms along torso with palms upward. Feet are a little apart. This posture is favorable for back part of legs and abdomen muscles.

Forward bent from standing position: take main stance. Close palms behind back. Raise palms upward up to upper back at blades' level. Put feet wider than shoulders. Bend torso forward to right knee. Keep this posture for 20-30 seconds with normal breathing. Turn to initial stance, removing palms from behind the back. If it is difficult to close hands behind back, it is possible to seize wrist and then continue other movements. This exercise strengthens back and legs' muscles, increase mobility in girdle.

Birch (stand on shoulders): lie on back, arms are along torso with palms down. Raise both straightened in knees legs, until they will be behind head. Bend arms in elbows and place palms on back. The, slowly raise legs, feet towards ceiling. Legs and torso shall make straight line and chin – pressed to chest. Keep this position 15-30 sec. without over tension. Then slowly low legs and place arms on floor, palms down. This exercise is favorable for central nervous system, blood vessels; increases resistance to cold.

Block "psycho-regulation" (15 minutes)

Relaxation lying posture: lie on back with feet at about 40 cm width. Head touches floor, palms – upward and arms are at little distance from torso. Close eyes and relax. Breathe rhythmically. Then breathing will become light and slow. Concentrate on deep and light exhales. Keep this position 3-5 minutes.

Stand on shoulders (birch): Birch (stand on shoulders: lie on back, arms are along torso with palms down. Raise both straightened in knees legs, until they will be behind head. Bend arms in elbows and place palms on back. The, slowly raise legs, feet towards ceiling. Legs and torso shall make straight line and chin – pressed to chest. Keep this position 15-30 sec. without over tension. Then slowly low legs and place arms on floor, palms down. This exercise is favorable for central nervous system, blood vessels; increases resistance to cold.

Stand on one leg: stand upright with feet parted by approximately 40 cm. Stretch arms forward, hands are relaxed, hanging down. Bend legs in knees and squat a little. Imagine that you are sitting in invisible armchair. Keep posture as long as possible. Upper part of legs will be tensed. It is an excellent exercise for legs and back's muscles, as well as for handsome carriage and self-confidence.

Lying rest posture: lie on back with feet at about 40 cm width. Head touches floor, palms – upward and arms are at little distance from torso. Close eyes and relax. Breathe rhythmically. Then breathing will become light and slow. Concentrate on deep and light exhales. Keep this position 3-5 minutes.

Statistical analysis: we used commonly known methods of transformation of questioning empiric data [23]. With the help of logical procedures we revealed correlations of the studied variables and determined mean statistic indicators of boys and girls' physical fitness at the beginning and at the end of academic year. Confidence of differences was determined by Student's t-criterion and significance level (p).

Results

Substantiation of physical education system's effectiveness

Assessment of students' motor fitness

For assessment of effectiveness of the worked out education system' content we fulfilled estimation of main motor qualities. In table 1 we present mean statistic data of students' physical fitness at the beginning and at the end of pedagogic experiment. Data analysis showed that most of the studied indicators witness about increase of results, comparing with initial data ($p < 0.05$). Exclusions were results of 30 meters' run, in which no confident differences were found.

Table 1. Indicators of students' motor fitness at the beginning and at the end of pedagogic experiment (M±m)

Indicators	Testing		Differences	Confidence of differences	
	Initial	Final		t	p
30 meters' run, sec.	7.2 ± 0.14	7.0 ± 0.15	0.2	0.97	> 0.05
Shuttle run 3 x 10 m, sec.	10.65± 0.14	10.2± 0.16	0.45	2.12	< 0.05
Long jump, cm	130.6± 1.95	137± 2.39	6.4	2.07	< 0.05
Chin ups, q-ty of times	10.7 ± 0.27	12.1 ± 0.62	1.4	2.07	< 0.05
Bending, cm	8.9 ± 0.62	11 ± 0.8	2.1	2.07	< 0.05
Run during 6 minutes	1203.2±81.4	1474.4±89.6	271.2	2.24	< 0.05

Assessment of students' physical metric indicators

In table 2 we give mean statistical data of students' physical metric indicators at the beginning and at the end of pedagogic experiment. At the end of pedagogic experiment in the studied indicators we registered statistically confident ($p<0.05$) improvements, comparing with initial data. Exclusions were results of body length and mass, in which no differences were found.

Table 2. Indicators of students' physical metric parameters at the beginning and at the end of pedagogic experiment (M+m)

Indicators	Testing		Differences	Confidence of differences	
	Initial	Final		t	p
Body length, cm	159.0 + 1.23	160.5 + 0.8	1.5	1.02	>0.05
Body mass, cm	57.0 + 0.89	56.9 + 0.89	0.1	0.08	>0.05
Chest circumference, cm	100.8 + 1.12	104.1 + 0.97	3.3	2.23	<0.05
Vital capacity of lungs, l	3300 + 31.67	3398 +28.45	93.0	2.18	<0.05
Right hand dynamometry, kg	47.9 + 0.79	49.9 + 0.53	2	2.1	<0.05
Left hand dynamometry, kg	47.0 + 0.79	49.1 + 0.53	2.1	2.21	<0.05

Assessment of interest to physical culture practicing and formation of healthy life style skills (see table 3).

Table 3. Indicators of students' interest to physical culture practicing and formation of healthy life style skills (points) (M+m)

Indicators	Testing		Differences	Confidence of differences	
	Initial	Final		t	p
Interest to physical culture practicing, points	4.01+0.1	4,.41+0.1	0.40	2.83	< 0.01
Formation of healthy life style skills, conv. un.	8.4 + 0.6	20.9 + 2.8	12.5	4.37	<0.001

After pedagogic experiment we found confident ($p<0.01$) increase of students' interest to physical culture practicing.

Assessment of healthy life style skills' formation resulted in the following: total data showed statistically confident increase ($p<0.001$) of healthy life style skills' formation (see table 3).

Assessment of significant for studying indicators

These indicators were combined as far as we found no statistically confident differences between them (see table 4).

Table 4. Indicators of students' pedagogic characteristics (M+m)

Indicators	Testing		Differences	Confidence of differences	
	Initial	Final		t	p
Interest to studying	2.14 + 0.1	2.47 + 0.1	0.33	2.33	< 0.05
Mental workability	2.25 + 0.1	2.56 + 0.1	0.31	2.19	< 0.05
Aggressiveness	2,.28 + 0.1	2.15 + 0.1	0.13	0.92	> 0.05
Emotional stability	2,.97 + 0.1	3.26 + 0.1	0.29	2.05	< 0.05
Concentration of attention	2,.76 + 0.1	3. 06 + 0.1	0.30	2.12	< 0.05
Diligence	2,.81 + 0.1	3. 11 + 0.1	0.30	2.12	< 0.05

After pedagogic experiment we found that practically all studied indicators were on higher, statistically confident ($p<0.05$) formation level. Exclusion was indicator of aggressiveness, in which differences between groups were not confident.

Assessment of socially significant qualities

Socially significant indicators of different age groups were combined as far as there were found no statistically confident differences between them (see table 5).

Table 5. Socially significant qualities of students (M+m)

Indicators	Testing		Differences	Confidence of differences	
	Initial	Final		t	p
Activity of moral position	3.04 + 0.1	3.36 + 0.1	0.32	2.26	< 0.05
Collectivism	3.16 + 0.1	3.47 + 0.1	0.31	2.19	< 0.05
Civic consciousness	3.24 + 0.1	2.51 + 0.1	0.27	1.91	> 0.05
Diligence	3.30 + 0.1	3.61 + 0.1	0.31	2.19	< 0.05
Creative activity	3.42 + 0.1	3.74 + 0.1	0.32	2.26	< 0.05
Will quality	3.38 + 0.1	3.69 + 0.1	0.31	2.19	< 0.05

At the end of pedagogic experiment most of socially significant qualities (with the exclusion of civic consciousness quality, in which no differences were found) were statistically confident ($p<0.05$) were formed better.

Discussion

Results of our researches supplement the data of other authors about demand in formation of students' healthy life style [13] and their self cognition of their psycho-physical and motor potentials [4]. It should be noted that results of many researches [1, 19] to larger extent are oriented on socialization of students with health problems in conditions of educational medium. Our previous works [15, 27] also point that t is possible to apply the worked out approaches to students of this category.

Significance of students' psycho-physical indicators of health can be one of the most important components in formation of their behavior style in social medium of universities. In this aspect our results are in good agreement with opinion of Gherissi A. Et al. [30] about specificities of realization of national holistic strategy of social constructivist model of students' education. Our previous researches point at worsening of higher educational students' physical, psychic and social moral health [2]. Results of our present research continue solution of this problem. Mc Sharry P. and Timmins F. [38] note significance of behavioral model, which permits for students to master stress control skills. It is especially important for first year students for their successful adaptation to educational medium. Results of our research point that it is possible to strengthen physical, psychic and social-moral health through creation of individualized behavior system.

Analysis of the received results permitted to determine that students indicators before and after pedagogic experiment differ statistically confidently. Effectiveness of the worked out system is proved by the following: confident differences of physical fitness before and after pedagogic experiment, statistically confident advantage by most of physical metric indicators, confident increase of interest to physical culture practicing and formation of healthy life style skills.

It is interesting that change of different personality's features is rather long process, which in some aspects resist to changes. We found statistically confident changes in such parameters as socially significant qualities of person, indicators of pedagogic characteristics. It points at rather adequate and effective means and methods, used in our research. Such approach permits to achieve real positive changes of psychic and social-significant qualities of higher educational establishments' students within one academic year.

Conclusions

Thus, content of additional (health related) physical culture training implies list of knowledge, skills and abilities. Prevailing orientation of such training shall be directed on solution of health related, general developing and recreational tasks. With it, attention of first priority shall be paid to formation of physical, psychic and social-moral health. Application of non traditional health related means, like Hatha Yoga, in physical education system will also be effective. Very important is ability to consciously form healthy life style skills. It permits to strength and deepen professional fitness at the account of activation of creative abilities, releasing of additional time due to rhythmic organization and structuralizing of educational process.

Results of the conducted researches supplement theory and methodic of students' physical education with new ideas about upgrading of educational process. The basis of such process is implementation of personality oriented system of students' physical, psychic and social-moral health strengthening.

References

1. Adyrkhaev SG. Modern technology of physical education of disabled students in conditions of inclusive education. *Pedagogics, psychology, medical-biological problems of physical training and sports*, 2016;1:4-12. doi:10.15561/18189172.2016.0101
2. Ajengar B.K.S. *Pranaiama. Iskusstvo dykhaniia* [Pranayama. The art of breathing]. Kiev: Sofia; 1995. (in Russian)
3. Baskevich OV. Interconnection of students' somatic type with somatic health. *Physical Education of Students*, 2015;6:4-9. doi:10.15561/20755279.2015.0601
4. Bessarabova IuV, Khar'kovskaia EV. Formirovanie psikhofizicheskikh kachestv studentov s ogranichennymi vozmozhnostiami zdorov'ia i invalidov v processe fizicheskogo vospitaniia [Formation of disabled students' psycho-physical qualities in physical education process]. *Istoricheskaia i social'no-obrazovatel'naia mysl'*, 2016;51:23-26. (in Russian)
5. Borisova NIu. Social'noe zdorov'e obshchestva i neobkhodimost' reformirovaniia obrazovaniia [Social health of society and demand in reformation of education]. *IV Vserossijskaia nauchno-prakticheskaia konferenciia "Obrazovanie i zdorov'e" (ss. 48-49)* [4th All Russian scientific-practical conference "Education and health"], Kaluga. 1998. P. 48-49. (in Russian)
6. Vazhenin CA. Koncepciia razvitiia lichnostno orientirovannoj sistemy fizicheskoj kul'tury i sporta v Leningradskoj oblasti [Conception of development of personality-oriented physical culture and sports system in Leningradskaya region]. *Teoriia i praktika fizicheskoj kul'tury*, 2006;3: 12-14. (in Russian)
7. Volkov BS, Volkova NV. *Metody issledovanij v psikhologii* [Methods of researches in psychology]. Moscow: Pedagogical Society of Russia; 2002. (in Russian)
8. Galimov GY, Kuzmin VA, Kudryavtsev MD, Kopylov YuA, Gaskov AV, Strelnikov VA. Peculiarities of formation of students-boxers' socially significant qualities as the basis of their future professional functioning. *The Buryat State University Bulletin,* 2014;13:68–72.
9. Gas'kov AV, Galimov GIa, Kuzmin VA, Kudriavcev MD, Kopylov YuA, Strelnikov VA. Osobennosti formirovaniia social'no znachimykh lichnostnykh kachestv studentov-bokserov kak osnovy budushchej professional'noj deiatel'nosti [Peculiarities of formation of students-boxers' socially significant qualities as the base of future professional functioning]. *The Buryat State University Bulletin,* 2014;1:68-71. (in Russian)

10. Golovina LL, Kopylov YuA, Polianskaia NV. Psikhologo-pedagogicheskie pokazateli uchashchikhsia srednego shkol'nogo vozrasta [Psychological-pedagogic indicators of middle school age pupils]. *Fizicheskaia kul'tura: vospitanie, obrazovanie, trenirovka,* 2009;3:20-22. (in Russian)
11. Zubkov AN, Ochapovskij AP. *Khatkha-joga dlia nachinaiushchikh* [Hatha-Yoga for beginners], Moscow: Medicine; 1991. (in Russian)
12. Ionova OM. Salutogenetic approach to professional training of future teachers. *Pedagogics, psychology, medical-biological problems of physical training and sports*, 2015;2:34–42. doi:10.15561/18189172.2015.0206
13. Ismiianov VV. Zhizneustrojstvo studentov-sirot na osnove formirovaniia psikhofizicheskogo zdorov'ia sredstvami fizicheskogo vospitaniia [Living arrangement of students-orphans on the base of psycho-physical health formation by means of physical education]. *Uchenye zapiski universiteta im. P.F. Lesgafta*, 2015;11(129): 107-110. (in Russian)
14. Kokova EI, Kopylov YuA. Polivariantnye fizkul'turno-ozdorovitel'nye meropriiatiia dlia oslablennykh studentov [Poly-variant health related physical culture measures for weakened students]. *Mezhdunarodnaia nauchno-prakticheskaia konferenciia "Molodaia sportivnaia nauka Belarusi", Minsk, 8–10 apr. 2014 g.* [International scientific-practical conference "Young sport science of Belarus", Minsk, April 8th- 10th, 2014], Minsk: BGUFK; 2014;2: P. 145-146.
15. Kopylov YuA, Jackowska LN, Kudryavtsev MD, Kuzmin VA, Tolstopyatov IA, Iermakov SS. The concept of structure and content of health related trainings for higher educational establishments' students. *Physical Education of Students*, 2015;5:23–30. doi:10.15561/20755279.2015.0504
16. Kuzmin VA, Kudryavtsev MD, Kopylov YuA, Galimov IG, Strelnikov VA. Konceptual'nye osnovy neobkhodimosti obnovleniia dopolnitel'nogo ozdorovitel'nogo fizicheskogo vospitaniia studentov [Conceptual principles of demand in students' health related physical education's renewal]. *Mezhdunarodnaia nauchno-prakticheskaia konferenciia "Molodaia sportivnaia nauka Belarusi", Minsk, 8–10 apr. 2014 g.* [International scientific-practical conference "Young sport science of Belarus", Minsk, April 8th- 10th, 2014], Minsk: BGUFK;.]. 2014; 2 P. 162–165 (in Russian)
17. Kuzmin VA, Kopylov YuA, Kudryavtsev MD, Galimov GY, Iermakov SS. Substantiation of effectiveness of trainings on health related methodic for students with weakened motor fitness. *Physical Education of Students*, 2015;6:43-49. doi:10.15561/20755279.2015.0606
18. Landa BKh. *Metodika kompleksnoj ocenki fizicheskogo razvitiia i fizicheskoj podgotovlennosti* [Methodic of physical condition and physical fitness complex assessment]. Moscow: Soviet sport; 2004 (in Russian)
19. Liashenko VN, Tumanova VN, Hatsko EV. Study of personality's temperament and self-assessment of higher educational establishments' students. *Physical Education of Students*, 2016;2:19-23. doi:10.15561/20755279.2016.0203
20. Motkov IO. *Prakticheskoe rukovodstvo po samoanalizu lichnosti* [Practical guide for personality self analysis]. Moscow; 1993. (in Russian)
21. Opletin AA, Panachev VD. Samorazvitie lichnosti studenta sredstvami pedagogicheskogo autotreninga na zaniatiiakh fizicheskoj kul'turoj [Self development of student's personality by means of pedagogic auto-training at physical culture lessons]. *Pedagogiko-psikhologicheskie i mediko-biologicheskie problemy fizicheskoj kul'tury i sporta,* 2015;2(35): 133-140. (in Russian)
22. Osipov AIu, Pereus OV, Starova OV, Fukalova AO. Povyshenie effektivnosti zdorov'esberegaiushchej deiatel'nosti v vedushchikh universitetakh Krasnoiarskogo kraia [Increase of effectiveness of health related activity in leading universities of Krasnoyarskiy region]. *Problemy sovremennogo pedagogicheskogo obrazovaniia*, 2016;50(3):117-123. (in Russian)
23. Paniotto VI, Maksimenko VS. *Kolichestvennye metody v sociologicheskikh issledovaniiakh* [Quantitative methods in sociological researches], Kiev; 2003. (in Russian)
24. Pichurin VV. Psychological and psycho-physical training as a factor of personal anxiety at students. *Pedagogics, psychology, medical-biological problems of physical training and sports*, 2015;3:46-51. doi:10.15561/18189172.2015.0307
25. Sadov, V.Iu. (2001). *Teoretiko-metodicheskie osnovy zdorovogo obraza zhizni uchashchejsia molodezhi* [Theoretical-methodic principles of students' healthy life style], Sankt Petersburg; Petropolis. (in Russian)
26. Salatenko IO, Dubinskaya OYa. Psycho-physical perfection of economic specialties' girl students under influence of sport-oriented technology, based on prevalence of volleyball practicing. *Pedagogics, psychology, medical-biological problems of physical training and sports*, 2015;12:103-108. doi:10.15561/18189172.2015.12016
27. Skurikhina NV, Kudryavtsev MD, Kuzmin VA, Iermakov SS. Fitness yoga as modern technology of special health groups' girl students' psycho-physical condition and psycho-social health strengthening. *Physical Education of Students*, 2016;2:24-31. doi:10.15561/20755279.2016.0204
28. Bliznevsky A, Kudryavtsev M, Kuzmin V, Tolstopyatov I, Ionova O, & Yermakova T. Influence of personal characteristics of pupils and students on the effectiveness of the relationship to the specific physical activities. *Journal of Physical Education and Sport,* 2016;16(2):424-432. doi:10.7752/jpes.2016.02066
29. Bliznevsky AA, Kudryavtsev MD, Iermakov SS, Jagiełło W. Formation of active-effective attitude of 12–13 years' judo athletes to sports functioning in competition period. *Archives of Budo*, 2016;12:101–115.
30. Gherissi A, Tinsa F, Soussi S, & Benzarti A. Teaching research methodology to student midwives through a socio-constructivist educational model: The experience of the high school for science and health techniques of Tunis. *Special Education Section*, 2016;33:46–48. doi:10.1016/j.midw.2015.10.015
31. Iermakov S, Podrigalo L, Romanenko V, Tropin Y, Boychenko N, Rovnaya O, & Kamaev O. Psycho-physiological features of sportsmen in impact and throwing martial arts. *Journal of Physical Education and Sport,* 2016;16(2): 433-441. doi:10.7752/jpes.2016.02067
32. Ivashchenko O, Khudolii O, Yermakova T, Iermakov S, Nosko M, & Nosko Y. Factorial and discriminant analysis as methodological basis of pedagogic control over motor and functional fitness of 14–16 year old girls. *Journal of Physical Education and Sport,* 2016;16(2): 442-451. doi:10.7752/jpes.2016.02068
33. Kara B, & İşcan B. Predictors of Health Behaviors in Turkish Female Nursing Students. *Asian Nursing Research*, 2016;10(1):75–81. doi:10.1016/j.anr.2015.12.001

34. Khudolii OM, Iermakov SS, & Ananchenko KV. Factorial model of motor fitness of junior forms' boys. *Journal of Physical Education and Sport,* 2015;15(3), 585-591. doi:10.7752/jpes.2015.03088
35. Kozina Z, Repko O, Ionova O, Boychuk Y, & Korobeinik V. Mathematical basis for the integral development of strength, speed and endurance in sports with complex manifestation of physical qualities. *Journal of Physical Education and Sport,* 2016;16(1):70-76. doi:10.7752/jpes.2016.01012
36. Kozina ZL, Iermakov SS, Kuzmin VA, Kudryavtsev MD, & Galimov GJ. Change of cortisol and insulin content in blood under influence of special workability recreation system for students with high motor functioning level. *Research Journal of Pharmaceutical, Biological and Chemical Sciences,* 2016;7(2), 1068–1077.
37. Kuzmin VA, Kopylov YA, Kudryavtsev MD, Tolstopyatov IA, Galimov GY, & Ionova OM. Formation of professionally important qualities of students with weakened motor fitness using a health related and sport-oriented training program. *Journal of Physical Education and Sport,* 2016; 16(1): 136-145. doi:10.7752/jpes.2016.01023
38. Mc Sharry P, & Timmins F. An evaluation of the effectiveness of a dedicated health and well being course on nursing students' health. *Nurse Education Today*, 2016; 44: 26–32. doi:10.1016/j.nedt.2016.05.004
39. Pomeshchikova IP, Shevchenko OO, Yermakova TS, Paievskyi VV, Perevoznyk VI, Koval MV, . . . Moiseienko OK. Influence of exercises and games with ball on coordination abilities of students with disorders of muscular skeletal apparatus. *Journal of Physical Education and Sport,* 2016;16(1), 146-155. doi:10.7752/jpes.2016.01024
40. Pryimakov O, Iermakov S, Kolenkov O, Samokish I, & Juchno J. Monitoring of functional fitness of combat athletes during the precompetitive preparation stage. *Journal of Physical Education and Sport,* 2016;16(2), 551-561. doi:10.7752/jpes.2016.02087

LAW ENFORCERS RECOGNITION LEVEL EMERGING THREATS BASED ON PHYSICAL APPEARANCE AND BEHAVIOR SIGNS THE ENEMY

Radzievskiy R.M., Plisko V.I.
Chernigov National Pedagogical University

Annotation. *Purpose:* examine the effectiveness of the training method of differential approach to the choice of means of influence on the action of law enforcers opponent with different levels of aggressiveness. *Material*: the experiment involved 15 students of the Kyiv National Academy of Internal Affairs and the 15 employees of the State Guard of Ukraine. *Results*: presented curriculum for special physical and tactical training. The program details the conceptual apparatus of THREATS and DANGERS manifestations of different levels of aggressiveness opponent (case analysis of its motor behavior). The study participants underwent 7 day course focused training. The basis of the course is an advanced theoretical base. The base is aimed at developing knowledge and skills of employees in determining the level of danger. Including threats from testing and modeling episodes of extreme situations the options cadets. *Conclusions*: In the simulated collision situations with aggressive opponent to the students significantly improved the adequacy of the response to the threat of execution time and within the legal grounds. Recognition was determined by the level of aggressiveness manifest manners enemy, his emotions, motivation, motor behavior, positional arrangement for 2 - 3 seconds. The program contributed to the development of qualities: attention, orientation, perception, motor lead.
Keywords: law enforcement, enemy, choice of actions, motor behavior, aggression, danger, threat.

Introduction

Analysis of law officers' functioning in condition of fight with adversary showed their relatively weak fitness for such situation. Rather often wrong decisions, incomplete understanding of situation, in respect to different levels of threat result, in law officers' inadequate response that, in its turn, leads to problem of uncompleted conflict.

As a result law officer are often wounded, receive different traumas or, on the contrary, are brought to justice for exceeding limits of physical influence, resulting in legal consequences. The mentioned by us problem shows at importance of its decision because it concerns law officers' resistance to different dangers.

In the course of our research we found the problem of weak self-identification by law officers in such situations and the sense of this problem is that physical education and special-tactic academic programs do not include such directions as mastering of knowledge and skills in recognition of threats, dangers by a number of behavior, external motion signs of adversary.

Analysis of works, fulfilled by specialists in professional training of law officers showed their one-side approach to solution of studied problems. For example, in field of special physical training they are regarded in respect of development of own special, physical and mental qualities, without training of skills in perception and evaluation of external threats and dangers (Anufriyev M.I., Babenko V.G. [9], Bondarenko V.V. [13], Bulachek V.R. [6], Butov S. Ye., Viniarchuk I.S., Gida O.F. [8], Yosypiv Yu.R., Zakorko I.P. [10], Popov O.V., Reshko S.M., Yanko I.V., Belur J. и соавторы [21], Dean G. et al. [22], Heinonen A. et al. [25], Royds D. [26], Ryan B.J. [27], Semukhina O. [28], Thomassen G. [29], Walker S. [30]).

In the same way psychologists (Shoygu Yu.S. [7], Gurenkova T.N., Smirnov B.A., Dolgopolova Ye.V. [11], Yevsiukov O.P. [12], Liefterov O.V. [14]) do not give any estimation of motion responses to danger. Like jurists (Artamanova G.K. [15], Kartashov V.N. [16], Kazakov Yu.N. [17], Derkach A.A., Zazykin V.G. [18], Dmytrenko I.A. [19], Atrekozov V.G. [20]; Dean G., Fahsing I.A., Gottschalk P. [23]; Glomseth R., Gottschalk P., Solli-Sæther H. [24]), give recommendations for already happened situations in compliance with clauses of criminal code.

At the same time the moment of fight with armed (aggressive) adversary is still important for law officer, especially his ability to very quickly (during 2-3 seconds) evaluate situation and take decision what to do. Also it is important to timely respond to adversary with minimal risk for himself and other people, functioning in legal field.

The mentioned requirements can be defined as insufficiently solved problem. That is why it requires new approaches to working out of more perfect methodic for law officers' professional training.

Purpose, tasks of the work, material and methods

The purpose of this article is to analyze law officers' functioning in choosing adequate to danger or threat means.

The tasks:

1. Studying, analyzing and widening of theoretical part of law officers' training for different conditions, connected with threats and danger.

2. To experimentally ground effectiveness of training for determination of threats' motion signs.

Main experiment was carried out with cadets (n – 30 человек) of Kyiv National academy of home affairs as well as with military officers of Governmental security of Ukraine (Kyiv). For testing of data, received in theoretical part we used pedagogic testing and simulation of extreme situation by method of scientific experiment.

Mathematical processing of results of the research permitted to determine a number of indicators, which facilitate strengthening of law officers' fitness.

Results of the research

Training of cadets for positive solution of conflict situations with aggressive adversary requires knowledge about their typical character, multiplicity of variants, conditions, with which they can meet in reality. And in compliance with virtual situation cadets shall be able to compare own abilities to fulfill tasks in conditions of different threats. So it was necessary to form ability to determine the level of sudden threat as quick as possible and adequately respond to it.

Manifestation of sudden threat usually takes from 1 to 3 seconds. It is difficult to train law officers to adequately respond to such threat during so short period and to form their appropriate skills. Every non standard situation has own specific signs of threat. It is necessary to determine these signs by adversary's behavior or movements and create general algorithm with certain deviations with certain parameters. Training process shall not be reduced to seeking of regularities and their determination shall be realized by typical signs of one or another threat considering sense of time.

In working out of modern methodic the newest is formation of skills to determine one or another threat in minimal time with simultaneous responding to it [1].

It should be realized that this methodic does not include threats of natural disasters, fires and so on. In this methodic only subject-to-subject functioning is regarded. With it one should differentiate defense of law officer's safety and defense of human right of a person with, whom law officer comes in contact, fulfilling his duties.

Special course of cadets' training to realize threat or danger is conducted in compliance with corrected program in several stages: 1) mastering of theory; 2) formation of ability to percept situation in the whole; 3) formation of knowledge about motion behavior and other signs of adversary; 4) choosing of actions in conditions of simulated situations. To effectively act in practice it is necessary, first of all, to open sense of main variants of actions, their characteristics [5]. We understand general idea in the following way:

Movements are purposeful and forced manifestation of human motion functioning, conditioned by fulfillment of certain tasks depending on purposes and environment;

Motion functioning – is level of manifestation of motion abilities and skills;

Sense-situational task – is mentally realized and consciously taken decision about fulfillment of purposeful movements in compliance with situation, considering safety of these movements and their efficiency and legal character;

Motion task – is requirement to fulfill certain movements with pre-set bio-mechanical characteristics for achievement of target;

Situational action – is manifestation of sense and motion functioning of a person, directed to seeking of solution of certain situational task;

Control – (informational-psychological structure) is ensured by such functional activity of nervous system, which results in formation of person's motive and target of action. On the base of processing of information about environment operative image of action is constructed (conceptual model), decision is taken, check up of results and correction of functioning is fulfilled.

Threat shall be understood as such behavior of adversary, which, by its characteristics, can bring potential or direct risk for health and life of law officers and other people.

To determine actions by level of threat, level of danger and conditions of their appearing it is necessary to base on general definitions.

Manifestations of levels of threat are as follows: obvious, potential, hidden, spontaneous, absence of threat.

Obvious threat – is registered adversary's physical actions directed against law officer or other person (including action, which can result in irreversible after effects).

Potential threat – is demonstrative aggressive behavior of armed (not armed) adversary without attempts to realize threat in practice. But in case of non-professional behavior of law officer this threat can become obvious (come in previous rank).

Hidden threat: with general tension in subject's behavior aggressiveness is not visible, flexibility is possible. But in specific conditions risk of attack is not excluded.

Indirect threat behavior and actions are not aggressive, but with it they are not controlled. Confusion can be caused by appearing of law officer. Avoiding from contact with law officer is possible.

Spontaneous threat – is uncontrolled behavior of some group, which can cause violation of public order.

Absence of threat is character of situational events between law officers and people, who manifest no threat (though situation is tensed).

Levels of danger are as following: high, middle, low and absence of danger.

High level: situational actions with high dynamic, oriented on traumatizing of vital human organs.

Middle level: physical actions, which can result in serious damage of functionally important human organs.

Low level: physical efforts as a response to external counter action and which can not damage human organs or parts of body.

Absence of danger: in conditions of tensed situation there are no pre conditions to any physical actions or counter actions.

Besides, the trainees were offered main characteristics of preparatory and attacking actions, as well as their analysis:

- Kinds of actions: attacks, counter actions, hidden-aggressive, provoked, neutral.

- Attacks: initial aggressive physical actions with application of different objects, with clear amplitude of movements and which are directed to damaging of certain target.

- Counter actions: physical resistance with different amplitude of movements, with the help and without help of objects in response to actions of "irritator".

- Hidden-aggressive actions, with which amplitude of actions does not point at any aggressiveness. But in favorable conditions of situation there can appear aggressive action directed to achievement of target.

- Provoked actions are motion response to behavior of "irritator" with inadequate manners.

- Neutral actions: actions with character of expectation without any aggressiveness (though in tensed situation).

Means of attack: actions with clear amplitude of movements (straight, from side, from back); actions with hidden amplitude of actions (straight, from side, from back); with different objects and different angles of attack.

Characteristics of attack with clear amplitude of movements are the following: preparatory actions; movements with object (weapon); angle and direction of trajectory of threatening movement by temp, speed, inadequacy, purposefulness. Attack can be from the spot, in walking, frontal or from back, from side. With it direction of adversary's motion can be different.

Characteristics of attacking movements with hidden amplitude: preparatory movements do ot show possible attack, presence of any object in hand or its seizing is not visible, distance to targe6t can be rather short. Movements are fulfilled mainly from the spot in one direction.

After familiarizing with general conceptions on this topic the trainees shall enlarge knowledge on specificity of actions' manifestation, their determination, purposefulness, their legal limits and responsibility. It will permit to evaluate actions themselves in differentiated way.

Constructions of diagrams – models significantly deepen sense order of threats and dangers. It significantly enriches theoretical part of special training course.

For holistic perception of actions in extreme conditions the trainees were offered schematic models, their variant by levels of threat, danger, by means of their realization (see figs. 1, 2).

Analysis of every component in the proposed diagrams give trainees better understanding of interconnections between behavioral characteristics, environment and situational conditions, in compliance with danger's or threat's level.

One of methods of threat's (danger) recognition by law officer is his ability to percept situation. In its base there is working out of certain skills.

Perception of situation is an informational-analytical process, in which system of analyzers and receptors of a person play important role. Such qualities as attention and power of observation help to manifestation of threat even during 1 second. It permits to timely respond to direct threat. With sudden situational threat visual analyzer restricts perception of space; all attention is directed to danger. It substantially hinders from objective and tactic analysis of situation. Adaptation (habit) can be formed in conditions of constant trainings, in which formation of skills goes simultaneously with analysis of threat's level and environment.

It pre conditions further actions of law officer. It is purposeful to train visual analyzer without using of other analyzers (in such conditions visual resource increases). In practice, in conditions of darkness or twilight healing analyzer is engaged to larger extent. . With developed (trained) hearing analyzer there is opportunity to distinguish kind of arm, with which shot was fulfilled, or other sounds (resembling shots).

Undoubtedly, positive result is achieved with ability to be ahead of adversary, resulted from recognition of threat [3]. For this purpose one shall have knowledge about adversary's behavior and act selectively (in the frames of legal field). Acquiring of knowledge of main space-time motion parameters, characteristics and manner of adversary's behavior will permit to accentuate attention on development of qualities, which can ensure motion domination. The acquired motion skills permit to quicker orient in situation by time, to recognize obstacles and prognosticate actions. With respect to adversary's actions behavior can be: motivational, aggressive, forcing, defensive, expressive. In specialists' opinion, there can be no previously planned crimes without motives. But by mentality not every person is able to shoot and kill other person [3].

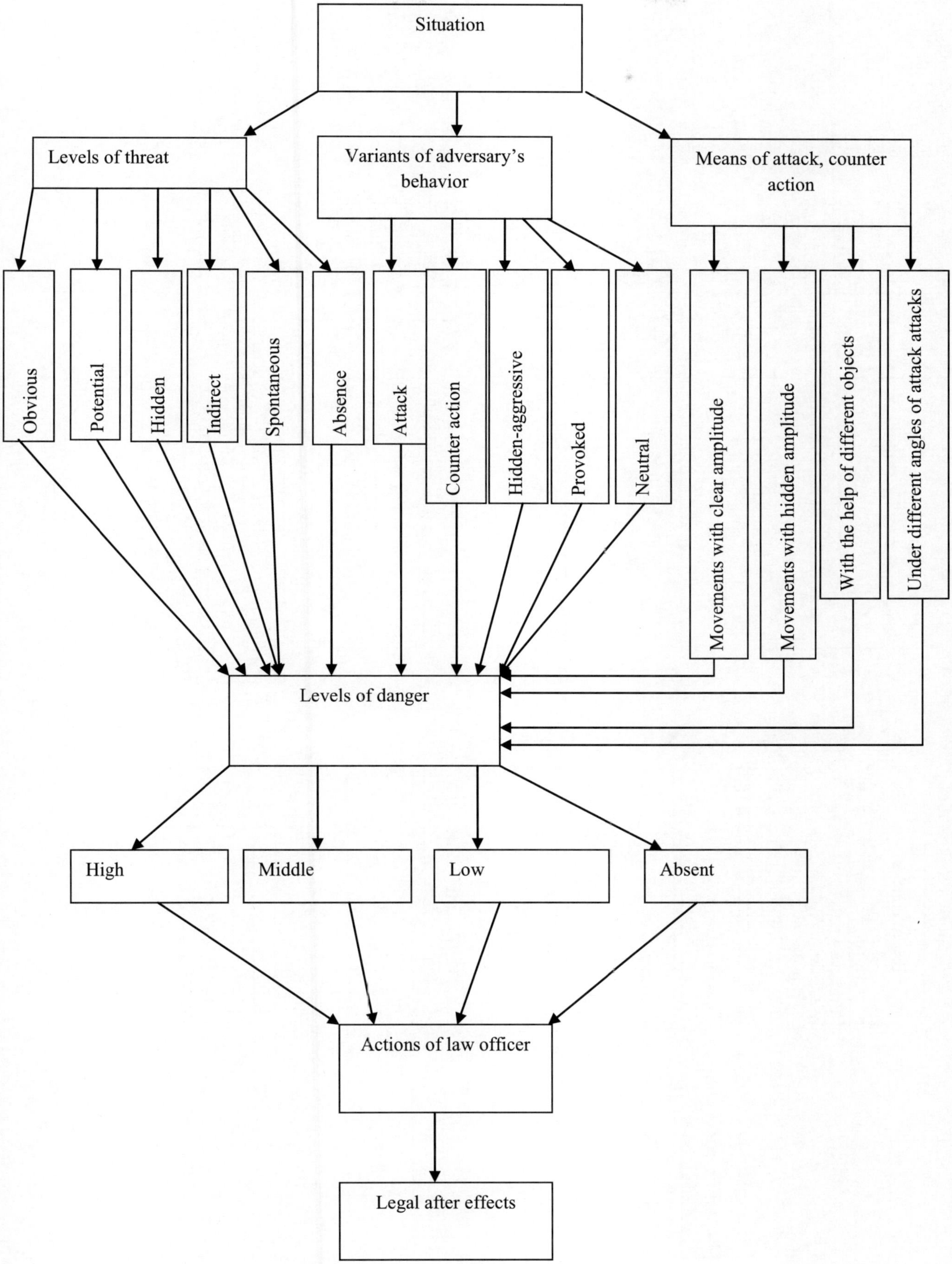

Fig.1 Variants if levels of threat and danger according to situations

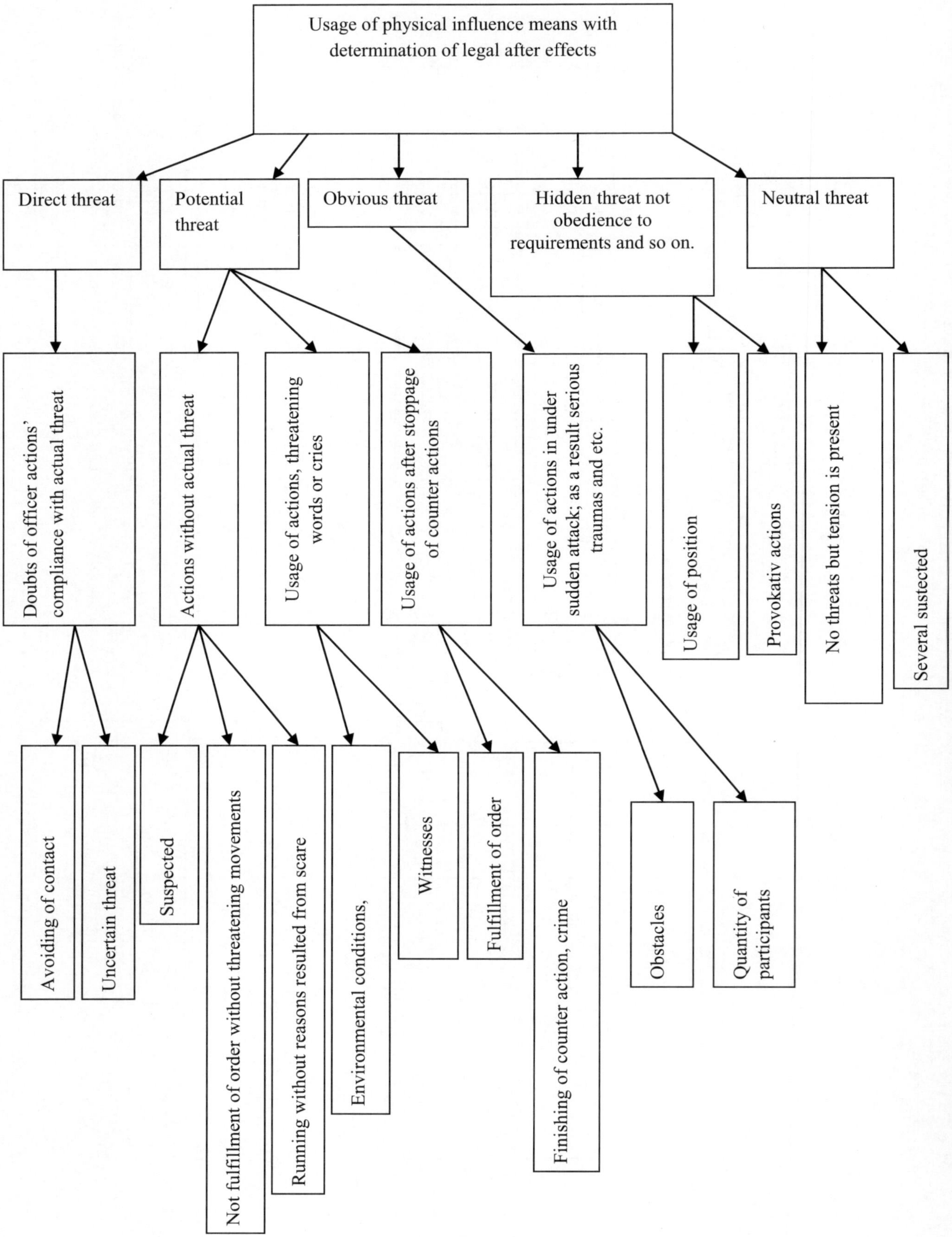

Fig.2. Determination of legal after effects in conditions of danger of different levels

Training based on simulation of situations is a complex process, which stipulates coordination, accordance of actions of all participants. Purpose of simulation shall be compulsory determined. General tasks are set in compliance with this purpose. Then specific functional tasks for every participant are formulated. It should be noted that even insignificant deviation from actual actions' or behavioral criteria (which are simulated) can prevent from achieving of purpose. After simulation of situational episode brief conclusions about achievement of purpose are made. Simulation of situational episodes it is purposeful to conduct in conditions of different threats; it is necessary to create sudden situations with aggressiveness of different level. With it all participants shall not be previously informed about following actions. It can be simultaneous demonstration of situational episode. Besides, changes, in case of trainee's untimely actions, are possible. I.e. there is free transition to other motion action, manners and so on. With simulation of situations it is necessary to avoid excessive fantasy. For simulation situations, which happened in reality, can be used [2].

After seven days special training course we conducted experiment, in which 30 persons participated (control group - CG) and 30 persons – experimental group (EG). The participants were in equal conditions: during period of testing every of them was put three questions. The questions were not repeated; participants had no opportunity to know them beforehand. In total we prepared 90 questions, equal for both groups. With it we used method of pedagogic testing [3].

Simulation of episodes of sudden extreme situations took place in gyms and conference halls. We chose 10 episodes. All they were unknown for participants. Every participant took part only in one episode. With simulation w used method of scientific experiment [4].For example: situations simulated behind curtains. With its opening participant appears. In front of him a person lies; the second bent over him, the third runs away. Participant is offered maximum 3 sec. for solution of this task.

In other case, by composed previously scenario-dialogue (violator and his victim) conflict was played. Deviation from scenario was admitted and at some moment play became "free". But it continued without application of physical force. At the height of dialogue the third party intervened – law officer, who arrived at the place of event. "Victim" obeyed orders of law officer. Behavior of violator was of chaotic character. Participant had to pass situation into peaceful manner. We evaluated: sureness of behavior; tone of speech; tactic techniques; creative approach to the solution of problem (initiative); manner of movements; application of improvised means, position. All ready made combinations of actions started suddenly for participants and order of positions' demonstration was rather variable. With it participant of experiment (or other persons) had to timely respond to the moment of appearing of potential or direct threat. Further progressing of situation was stopped by one of experts.

At the same time trainees put brief characteristics to own actions from the point of adequacy in respect to manifested threat. Criteria of task's fulfillment were: time for perception of situation and threat; time for taking decision; time for taking certain position; correctness of respond to threats; own actions and actions, which could result in certain legal after effects.

Evaluation of correctness of perception and adequacy of analysis was carried out by commission of three experts: two specialists in physical training and tactics and specialists lawyer. Evaluation system includes: 1. Adequacy of actions for taking decision and level of threat; 2. Time of execution; 3. Evaluation of actions in respect to degree of threat; 4. Positional location;, preventing from aggressive adversary's actions, readiness for actions, own safety.; 5. Legal characteristic of every certain moment: what threat can appear in respect to legal field.

Table 1

Level of adequacy of law officers' respond to threats

Tasks	Adequacy (correctness) of motion behavior		Confidence		Emotions manners of behavior and so on.		Confidence		Legal after effects		Confidence	
	CG (n=30), X± m	EG (n=30), X± m	t	P	CG (n=30), X± m	EG (n=30), X± m	t	P	CG (n=30), X± m	EG (n=30), X± m	t	P
Testing (90questions)	13.5± 0.64	64.8± 0.98	43.82 9	<0.00 1	6.3± 0.28	53.1±1. 3	35.1 9	<0.00 1	35.1± 0.92	54.9± 1.1	3.81	<0.00 1
Actions in simulation of extreme situation (30 episodes)	6.9± 0.35	20.1± 0.68	17.26 0	<0.00 1	3.6± 0.26	19.2±0. 57	24.9 0	<0.00 1	12.9± 0.39	19.5± 0.71	8.14 8	<0.00 1

Effectiveness of tasks' solution by EG members in respect to CG is given in table 1.

It should be noted that 10% of participants from EG were not in time with fulfillment of tasks, while in CG – 40%.

Discussion

The worked out by us methodic is a new project in professional training. Scientific novelty is that for the first time we used new algorithm of law officers' training, for formation of knowledge and skills in practical functioning in extreme situations. We proved experimentally effectiveness of actions in time, recognition and perception of threat, choosing of actions and responding to danger.

In experimental group perception time of threat from the moment of its appearing was in average 1.5-2 sec. Time for taking decision - 1-1.5 sec. Time of taking position coincides with time of taking decision and is approximately 1-2 sec. In CG time range was wider – from У КГ 1 to 7 sec. It witnesses about different perception of threatening actions. Some trainees showed certain delay in perceiving of actions' combinations and evaluation. Tim for determination of situation was delayed or excessively accelerated. Such response was registered because of seeking of threat's degree or as too early in respect to event itself (taking position). In experiment it was noted that with every following participation in demonstration of motion and behavioral combinations most of trainees improved their indicators by all items. So, method of fulfillment of experiment, selection of means were approximated to academic process. If during fulfillment of first two-three tasks in EG indicators of effectiveness were 60-65%, in second – (CG) 20 - 23%, then by the end of all tasks indicators significantly improved. Adaptation of participants to experiment's conditions also played important role. At the beginning of test we observed certain psychological tension and there was a trend to reduction of indicators.

Results of the research are in accordance with experts' opinion (V.V. Bondarenko, Yu.V. Denisenko, L.N. Kucheriaviy).

Conclusions:

Our researches showed that effectiveness of cadets' training to special physical and tactic fitness increases significantly with purposeful formation of knowledge and skills in recognitions of different by level threats. At first stage of training cadets (law officers) had to master knowledge about gradations of different situations (typical and not standard), moments of threats' appearing, their consequences, in determination of differentiating factors. Then the mastered knowledge is trained to level of skills. I.e. for short time (in seconds) threat and its after effects are determined. After it, it is necessary to master variants of responding to different threats' manifestations. At second stage of training some cadets simulate different levels of threat and other – respond to them. At third stage sudden threat is simulated, to which it is necessary to adequately respond. Fulfillment is restricted by time.

It was determined that in process of simulated situations of conflict with aggressive adversary cadets substantially increased adequacy of responding to appeared threat during fulfillment (within legal frames). Recognition of aggressiveness level was determined by manifested manners of adversary, his emotions, motivations, motion behavior during 2-3 seconds. Development of attention, ability to orient, to perceive, to be ahead in actions is also important.

References:

1. Belkin R.S. *Teoriia i praktika sledstvennogo eksperimenta* [Theory and practice of investigative experiment], Moscow, Graduate School of the USSR Ministry of Internal Affairs, 1959, 169 p. (In Russian)
2. Plisko V. I., Nosko M. O. *Vikoristannia zakhodiv fizichnogo vplivu z taktichnim osmislenniam situacii vidpovidno do stupenia zagrozi* [The use of physical impact of tactical understanding of the situation according to the degree of threat], Chernihiv, 2010, 284 p. (In Ukrainian)
3. Plisko V.I. *Formirovanie gotovnosti professionala k deiatel'nosti v usloviiakh, opasnykh dlia zhizni: na materialakh sub"ekt-sub"ektnoj deiatel'nosti* [Formation of readiness to professional activity in conditions hazardous to life on the materials the subject of subjective activity], Kiev, Scientific World, 2002, 304 p. (In Russian)
4. Davydov V.V. *Psikhologicheskij slovar'* [Psychological dictionary], Moscow, 1983, pp. 370. (In Russian)
5. Khramovich M.A. *Nauchnyj eksperiment, ego mesto i rol' v poznanii* [Scientific experiment, its place and role in cognition], Minsk, BU V.I. Lenin Publ., 1972, 230 p. (In Russian)
6. Banakh S.M., Bulachek V.R., Viniarchuk I.S., Josipiv Iu.R. *Taktiko-special'na pidgotovka pracivnikiv OVS Ukraini* [Tactical and special training of policemen of Ukraine], Lviv, LvDUVS, 2011, 300 p. (In Ukrainian)
7. Shojgu Iu.S. *Psikhologiia ekstremal'nykh situacij dlia spasatelej i pozharnykh* [Psychology of extreme situations for the rescuers and firefighters], Moscow, Meaning, 2007, 319 p. (In Russian)
8. Anufriiev M. I, Butov S. Ye, Gida O. F., Reshko S. M. *Osnovi special'noi fizichnoi pidgotovki pracivnikiv OVS* [Fundamentals of special physical training police officers], Kiev, 2003, 338 p. (In Ukrainian)
9. Babenko V. G., Popov O. V., Ianko I. V. *Zakhodi fizichnogo vplivu* [Measures of physical restraint], Kiev, 2001, 24 p. (In Ukrainian)
10. Zakorko I. P. *Special'na fizichna pidgotovka u vishchikh navchal'nikh zakladakh MVS Ukraini z urakhuvanniam individual'nikh osoblivostej motoriki kursantiv. Kand.diss*. [Physical training in higher educational establishments of Ukraine, taking into account the individual characteristics of motor cadets. Cand. Diss.], Kiev, 2001, 300 p. (In Ukrainian)
11. Smirnov B.A., Dolgopolova E.V. *Psikhologiia deiatel'nosti v ekstremal'nykh situaciiakh* [Psychology of activity in extreme situations], Kharkov, Humanitarian Center Publ., 2007, 276 p. (In Russian)
12. Yevsiukov O.P. *Ekstremal'na psikhologiia* [Extreme psychology], Kiev, Ltd. "August Trade", 2007, 502 p. (In Ukrainian)
13. Bondarenko V. V. Model' iakostej pracivnika milicii, iaka nadaie jomu perevagu v umovakh nespodivanogo zitknennia z ozbroienim suprotivnikom [Model properties of militia worker, which gives him an advantage in terms of unexpected collision with an armed enemy]. *Visnik Chernigivs'kogo derzhavnogo pedagogichnogo universitetu*, 2010, no.81, pp. 136 – 140. (In Ukrainian)
14. Lefterov V.O. *Osobistisno-profesijnij rozvitok fakhivciv ekstremal'nikh vidiv diial'nosti. Dokt.diss.* [Personally professional development of specialists of extreme activities. Dokt.diss.], Kharkov, 2008, 37 p. (In Ukrainian)
15. Artamanova G.K., Mameeva I.S. Organizacionnye i pravovye formy i metody deiatel'nosti po sozdaniiu normativno-pravovoj bazy v sfere obespecheniia pozharnoj bezopasnosti [Organizational and legal forms and methods of work to create the legal framework in the field of fire safety]. *Vestnik Sankt-Peterburgskogo universiteta GPS MChS Rossii.* 2012, no.2, pp. 97-102. (In Russian)
16. Kartashov V.N. Iuridicheskaia tekhnika, taktika, strategiia i tekhnologiia [Legal technique, tactics, strategy and technology (to the question of the relationship)]. *Problemy iuridicheskoj tekhniki*, 2005, no.1, pp. 111. (In Russian)
17. Kazakov Iu.N. *Psikhologo-akmeologicheskaia sushchnost' ekstremal'nykh situacij v deiatel'nosti municipal'nykh sluzhashchikh* [Psychological akmeological essence of extreme situations in the work of municipal employees], Municipal'naia sluzhba: pravovye voprosy, 2008, no.4, pp. 20-26. (In Russian)
18. Derkach A.A., Zazykin V.G. *Professionalizm deiatel'nosti v osobykh i ekstremal'nykh usloviiakh* [Professionalism activity in special and extreme conditions], Moscow, RAGS, 1998, 178 p. (In Russian)
19. Dmitrenko I.A. *Ekologichne pravo Ukraini* [Environmental Law of Ukraine], Kiev, Inter Yurinkom, 2001, 352 p. (In Ukrainian)
20. Strekozov V.G. *Voennoe pravo* [Military law], Moscow, 2004, 640 p. (In Russian)
21. Belur J., Tilley N., Osrin D., Daruwalla N., Kumar M., Tiwari V. Police investigations: discretion denied yet undeniably exercised. *Policing and Society*. 2014, vol.1, no.24, pp. 45-55. http://dx.doi.org/10.1080/10439463.2013.878343.
22. Dean G., Fahsing I.A., Glomseth R., Gottschalk P. Capturing knowledge of police investigations: towards a research agenda. *Police Practice and Research*. 2008, vol.9, no.4, pp. 341-355. http://dx.doi.org/10.1080/15614260802354650.
23. Dean G., Fahsing I.A., Gottschalk P. Profiling police investigative thinking: A study of police officers in Norway. *International Journal of the Sociology of Law*. 2006, vol.34, no.4, pp. 221-228. http://dx.doi.org/10.1016/j.ijsl.2006.09.002.

24. Glomseth R., Gottschalk P., Solli-Sæther H. Occupational culture as determinant of knowledge sharing and performance in police investigations. *International Journal of the Sociology of Law*. 2007, vol.35, no.2, pp. 96-107. http://dx.doi.org/10.1016/j.ijsl.2007.03.003.
25. Heinonen A., Ellonen N. "Crime or not?" – police officers' perceptions of disciplinary violence, its criminalisation and its investigation. *Policing and Society*. 2014, vol.1, no.19, pp. 56-62. http://dx.doi.org/10.1080/10439463.2014.989151.
26. Royds D. Death Investigation. A Handbook for Police Officers. *Australian Journal of Forensic Sciences*. 2002, vol.34, no.2, pp. 93-94. http://dx.doi.org/10.1080/00450610209410843.
27. Ryan B.J. What the Police are Supposed to Do: Contrasting Expectations of Community Policing in Serbia. *Policing and Society*. 2007, vol.17, no.1, pp. 1-20. http://dx.doi.org/10.1080/10439460601124106.
28. Semukhina O. Public assistance of police during criminal investigations: Russian experience. *Police Practice and Research*. 2014, vol.1, no.20. pp. 67-73. http://dx.doi.org/10.1080/15614263.2014.949263.
29. Thomassen G. Investigating Complaints against the Police in Norway: An Empirical Evaluation. *Policing and Society*. 2002, vol.12, no.3, pp. 201-210. http://dx.doi.org/10.1080/10439460290018445.
30. Walker S. The neglect of police unions: exploring one of the most important areas of American policing. *Police Practice and Research*. 2008, vol.9, no.2, pp. 95-112. http://dx.doi.org/10.1080/15614260802081253.

ANALYSIS OF STUDENTS' NERVOUS SYSTEM'S TYPOLOGICAL PROPERTIES, IN ASPECT OF RESPONSE TO EXTREME SITUATION, WITH THE HELP OF MULTI-DIMENSIONAL ANALYSIS

Kozina Z.L.[1], Iermakov S.S. [2]
[1]H.S. Skovoroda Kharkiv National Pedagogical University
[2]Kazimierz Wielki University in Bydgoszcz

Abstract. *Purpose:* determination of objective and subjective characteristics of students' with different properties of nervous system fear of heights. *Material:* In the research 10 students of 18-19 years old age, who did not practice sports, participated. The students fulfilled one exercises: passing suspended ferriage in hiking. This exercise gives subjective perception of height and creates artificial conditions for appearing of fear. He exercise was fulfilled under all required safety measures and supervised by experienced instructor. Cluster and discriminant analysis were used. *Results:* we have shown that is possible to divide people into groups by indicators of functional changes in extreme situation in combination with indicators of psycho-physiological potentials and properties of nervous system. We have found that the most significant indicators for distribution of students into groups by individual typological properties are speed and accuracy of passing of psycho-physiological tests with different modes of signals' supply as well as functional changes before exercise of extreme character. *Conclusions:* It was determined that students with strong type of nervous system had confidently less heart beats rate before fulfillment of extreme exercise than the students with weak type of nervous system. Subjective feeling of fear before fulfillment of extreme exercise was also confidently less in representatives of strong type of nervous system.
Key words: students, fear, analysis, cluster, discriminant.

Introduction

Modern world often require from person to act effectively in extreme situation [21; 24; 28; 30; 33; 34]. Yu.V. Scherbatykch [21] points at the fact that one of main obstacles for taking correct decisions and realization of effective actions is fear. Fear is accompanied by panic. It blocks adequate perceiving of situation and taking correct decisions for its overcoming [21]. With it, one can assume that people with different types of supreme nervous' functioning [9; 10; 11; 14; 15; 16; 17] respond to extreme situation differently. Understanding of peculiarities of extreme situations' perceiving by people with different types of supreme nervous functioning response to sudden extreme situations will help to work out the methods of fear's overcoming by people with different properties of nervous system. This problem is rather urgent for to-day's youth, with students as the most numerous category [5; 6; 7; 8; 18; 19].

For solution of our tasks it was necessary to conduct researches with students' fulfillment of motor functioning, which can be considered extreme by subjective perceiving. But actually, such kinds of functioning shall not threaten life and health of students. One of such kinds of motor functioning is passing of suspended ferriage over raving of 5 meters depth in hiking [4]. Nowadays technology of this exercise's fulfillment envisages full safety for human life and health with active support of experienced instructor.

Thus, passing of suspended ferriage over raving is completely safe for human life and health. However, this exercise gives subjective perception of height and creates artificial conditions for fear's appearing. In this connection this kind of motor functioning can be used for studying of the mentioned problem.

The urgency of the present research is also connected with need in revelation of individual peculiarities of extreme situations' perceiving for creation of methods for fear's overcoming by students of different psycho-physiological types [37; 38; 40; 41]. Students' age is the most favorable period for development of ability to control emotions [25; 26; 29; 35; 36].

The problem of persons' with different typological properties of supreme nervous functioning response to fear has nearly not been researched. That is why the chosen direction of our researches is actual and urgent..

The hypothesis of the research is an assumption that people with different types of supreme nervous functioning perceive extreme situations differently. It can reflect in different subjective and objective indicators.

Purpose, tasks of the work, material and methods

The purpose of the research: is to determine objective and subjective characteristics of fear of heights' manifestation in students with different properties of nervous systems.

Material and methods: determination of individual typological peculiarities was conducted in convenient for every student time individually with the help of analysis of psycho-physiological indicators (time of simple and complex response to light irritators) in different modes of signal supply. Tests were conducted by program "Psycho-diagnostic" [2; 12; 20]. We registered time and quantity of mistakes in tests for simple and complex responses, indicators of strength and mobility of nervous processes, nervous processes by tests "Complex visual-motor response to signal supply with forced rhythm".

From physiological methods of research we used determination of heart beats rate (HBR) with the help of monitor of HBR continuous registration «Polar» before and after fulfillment of exercise for passing of suspended ferriage in hiking. With registration HBR before exercise students were in rest for 5-10 minutes for HBR stabilization. Then HBR was registered.

The received data (23 indicators) were processed by method of hierarchic cluster analysis and discriminant analysis with obtaining data for every separate case [3]. The received, as a result of multi-dimensional analysis, groups of students were compared between each other by all registered indicators. Besides, we conducted students' questioning for registration of their subjective feelings of fear by non-linear scale of Borg [1; 27] before passing of suspended ferriage. In the research 10 students of 18-19 years old age, who did not practice sports, participated. All students fulfilled exercise "passing suspended ferriage" for the first time.

Results of the research

For determination of groups of students, who distinguish by individual typological features, different methods can be used [3]. For example, we can divide students into groups, having built Sigma scale by registered indicators. Then, it is necessary to choose the most significant indicator and divide students into groups by it. This method is suitable in case if there is present one the most significant indicators from all registered in research. In our case all registered indicators were significant for determination of students' individual features. In this connection it is necessary to analyze all complex of indicators. For this purpose method of multi-dimensional analysis is used: factorial, cluster, discriminant [3]. As far as in our research main task is connected with students' distribution into groups, we do not use factorial analysis. In our case the most informative for students' distribution into groups by properties of nervous system is cluster analysis.

Cluster analysis permits to receive groups of the tested as a result of generalization of all tests' results [3]. It conditions application of complex approach to revelation of individual features of the tested.

For substantiation of optimal quantity of clusters we used cluster coefficients, which reflect step-by-step process of students' combining into clusters. It is considered that key step of combining of the tested in clusters is the step of beginning of non-linear increasing of clustering coefficients [3]. In our case it is step 7 (see table 1). Exactly on seventh step increasing of cluster coefficient sharply exceeds values of its increasing on previous steps. On the next stage, for determination of clusters' optimal quantity it is necessary to deduct quantity of steps of smooth cluster coefficients' increasing from quantity of the tested [3]. In our case from 10 tested we deduct 7 steps; we receive 3 clusters.

Then, in order of combining in clusters (see table 1) and by dendogram of cluster analysis (see fig.1) we can determine belonging of every tested to cluster. At first step tested number 3 and 5 combined. At second stem number 4 joined to them (see table 1, fig.1). At third step tested number 7 and 1- combined with this cluster. At forth step tested No.1 joined (see table 1, fig.1). At fifth step second cluster started to form: tested number 2 and 8 combined (see table 1 and fig.1). At sixth step combining inside first cluster continued; tested 7 combined with tested 1 (see table 1, fig.1).

The sevenths step is rather special in process of students' combining in clusters: just from it non-linear increase of cluster coefficients starts. In this case the tested, joining at this and at further steps significantly differ from the previous by integral assessment of indicators. At this step tested number 6 combined. That is why he can be related both to the first cluster and to the second. On the other hand, it can be specified into third cluster. More over, optimal quantity of clusters, according to start of non-linear cluster coefficients' increase, is 3. On dendogram (fig.1) this tested is shown nearer to the first cluster.

At eighth step combining of second cluster continued: tested with conventional number 2 and 9 combined (see table 1, fig.1). At last step tested of two clusters combined. As we can see in table 1 and fig.1 conventional distance (cluster coefficient) between integrated indicators of testing of these groups' members dozens times exceed previous cluster coefficients. From it, it is followed that combined at the last stage tested belong to different clusters.

Table 1

Process of students' combining in clusters (groups) with the help of cluster analysis by values of heart beats rate (HBR) in situation of fear of heights' overcoming and by psycho-physiological indicators

Agglomeration Schedule			
Stage	Cluster Combined 2 Clusters		Coefficients
	Case №	Case №	
1	3	5	2339
2	3	4	4738
3	7	10	7774
4	1	3	9234
5	2	8	10767
6	1	7	12775
7	1	6	24137
8	2	9	27064
9	1	2	80628

Thus, cluster analysis of testing indicators of 10 tested resulted in the following: students are divided into 2 groups (see table 2, fig.1). The first group includes students under conventional numbers 3,5,4,1,7,10 by degree of similarity of testing results (see table 2, fig.1); the second group includes students numbered 2,8,9 (see table 2, fig.1). Tested number 6 can form separate cluster, intermediate in respect to the first two ones. He can also be related both to the first and to the second clusters. According to dendogram he bends more to the first cluster (see fig.1).

Discriminant analysis permits to specify belonging of the tested to groups with producing of statistic for every case [3; 27]. With it, belonging of other tested to groups is unknown. In our research, when conducting discriminant analysis, we assumed that tested under numbers 3, 4 belonged to group 1 and tested 2 and 8 – to group 2. To group 1 we related tested number 6 as well (see table 3).

Discriminant analysis confirmed belonging of tested 3, 4, 2 and 8 to the mentioned groups. Besides, the tested whose belonging to groups was not shown, were distributed by discriminant analysis analogous to results of cluster analysis. Exclusion was tested number 6: as a result of discriminant analysis he was characterized as "wrongly classified case" and related to group 2 with probability of 0.583 (see table 3). This value of probability (close to 0.50) reflects little preponderance (by 0.083 conv.un.) in favor of second group.

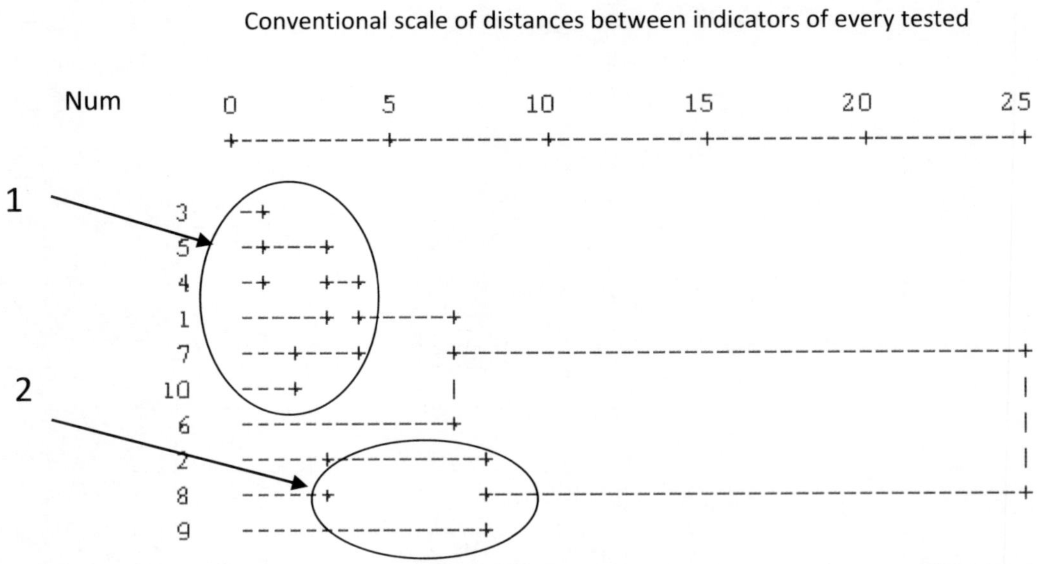

Fig.1. Dendogram of cluster analysis of students' distribution into groups by heart beats rate (HBR) values in situation of fear of heights' overcoming and by psycho-physiological indicators:

Num (by vertical axis) -= conventional number of the tested;

Horizontal upper scale – standardized "scale of distances" between testing indicators of the tested;

1, 2 – groups of the tested, formed as a result of cluster analysis.

Table 2

Students' belonging to clusters by heart beats rate (HBR) values in situation of fear of heights' overcoming and by psycho-physiological indicators

Conventional number of the tested	Belonging to cluster
1	1
2	2
3	1
4	1
5	1
6	1**
7	1
8	2
9	2
10	1

Notes:** - belonging to other cluster is possible

Thus, cluster analysis resulted in students' distribution in two groups. Belonging to cluster was specified with discriminant analysis.

Таблица 3

Students' distribution into groups with discriminant analysis by heart beats rate (HBR) values in situation of fear of heights' overcoming and by psycho-physiological indicators

Case №	Actual Group	Highest Group	
		Predicted Group	P
1	Ungrouped	1	0,997
2	2	2	0,935
3	1	1	0,975
4	1	1	0,841
5	Ungrouped	1	0,635
6	1	2**	0,583
7	Ungrouped	2	0,920
8	2	2	0,661
9	Ungrouped	2	0,920
10	Ungrouped	1	0,752

Notes:** - misclassifies case

For clarification of the question, which indicators influenced on formation of clusters most of all, we compared the received samples by all testing indicators with the help of non parametrical statistic's methods [3] (in connection with relatively small samples). We found out confident differences between groups by HBR indicator before passing of suspended ferriage: in first group this indicator was 68.50±16. b.p.m. $^{-1}$, in second – 86.50±5.45 b.p.m. $^{-1}$ (p=0.039). Besides, confident differences were found between groups by psycho-physiological indicators. For example, time of complex visual-motor response in first group was 435.33±43.27 m.sec.; in the second group – 559.00±31. m.sec. (p=0.000). Also, quantity of mistakes in complex visual-motor response is less in first group, comparing with the second:11.7±1.60 in first group and 13.25±1.50 in second (p=0.038).

We detected confident differences also in tests, which are specific for determination of nervous system's properties: "complex visual-motor response with feedback, time" (358.50 18.50 m.sec. in first group and 439.50±65.74 m.se. in second group, p=0.018); "complex visual-motor response with feedback, quantity of mistakes" 19.50±2.95 in first group and 23.50±1.73 in second, p=0,041); "complex visual-motor response with feedback, minimal time of signal exposure" (320.00±30.33 m.sec. in first group and 365.00±41.23 m.sec. in second, p=0.040); "complex visual-motor response with forced rhythm of signal supply, time" (404.50±16.55 m.sec. in first group and 511.25±60.92 m.sec. in second group, p=0.000). Besides, quantity of mistakes in complex visual motor response with forced rhythm of signal supply is confidently less in the first group than in the second at first, second, third and fifth stages (p=0.009-0.037).

It is known [14; 15; 16; 17], that in tests for complex visual0-motor response with feedback and with forced rhythm if signal supply quantity of mistakes indirectly characterizes power of nervous processes, while time of reaching of signal's minimal exposure in tests for complex visual-motor response with feedback – characterizes mobility of nervous processes. In our research quantity of mistakes and time of signal's minimal exposure are confidently less in the first group. This fact permits to conclude that first group consists of students with greater power and mobility of nervous processes in comparison with the second group.

Basing on analysis of the received data, we named first group "and second – "participants with weak type of nervous system". It should be noted that in the first group (i.e. participants with strong and moderate type of nervous system) HBR was confidently less before passing of suspended ferriage. It witnesses that they are less anxious in comparison with participants with weak type of nervous system.

Subjective feeling of fear was registered by Borg's scale [1; 23; 31]. This scale was offered for registration of subjective feelings during fulfillment of physical wok [23]. Numerous researches showed informative character of subjective feelings and their high interconnection with physiological processes [1; 13; 23; 31]. That is why we applied Borg's scale for registration of students' subjective feelings of fear before passing of suspended ferriage. In group of students with strong nervous system mean value of feeling of fear was 0.51±0.05 points (very-very weak, nearly not felt). In group of students with weak nervous system mean value of subjective feelings of fear was 4.06±1.08 points (p=0.000) (above middle). Thus, subjective feelings of fear were confidently higher in students with weak type of nervous system.

The received data of subjective feelings are comparable with heart beats rate values before fulfillment of exercise. Students with strong type of nervous system have confidently less HBR in comparison with representatives of weak nervous system's type.

Discussion

Our research closely overlaps with conception of fear as one of human emotion, which results from extreme situation. In psychology [21] it is considered that fear is negatively painted basic emotion. It is called basic as far as it can not be divided into components, but, at the same time, it can be the basis for other emotions.

Fear is sometimes called emotional process. It is not only manifested, it causes organism's reaction. Fear is transmitted to brain by neuro mediators. From there answer is supplied: which actions shall be undertaken in the situation [21].

Under influence of fear human organism starts to intensively excrete hormones. In skeletal muscles hormones facilitate emitting of energy. It happens for a person to be able either to defend against danger or to run away. It should also be noted that there are internal and external fear manifestations. External – is appearance of the person. Internal are physiological processes, which occur in organism [21].

Just, as a result of these processes fear is called negative emotion, because it influences on all organism. Besides, strong fear is considered to be toxic emotion, as far as it facilitates progressing of different diseases, including cancer, throat diseases, diabetes [21; 32; 39; 42]. That is why studying of individual features, manifesting in overcoming of extreme situations, is rather important task.

We conducted analysis of response to extreme situation of representatives with strong and weak types of nervous system. In this context is would be pertinently to conclude that definitions "strength" and "weakness" of nervous system are rather conventional at present. In opinion of modern researchers [15; 16], this indicator characterizes ability to perceive information per unit of time. Representatives of the so-called strong nervous system perceive less information per unit of time and that is why they are less sensitive to external and internal impacts. Hence, they are more resistant in respect to external and internal irritators. Representatives of the so called weak nervous system perceive more information per unit of time. They are more sensitive to external and internal irritators and get tired quicker. Thus, different people have different nervous system's mechanisms of adaptation to life. These mechanisms are equal by significance from the point of view of evolution and survival.

However, as our research illustrated, preparation from action in unknown situation is different for representatives of different nervous system's types. With the help of questioning we determined, that students with weaker strength and mobility of nervous processes spend more time to thinking over details of the fulfilled exercise; they try to clear up all difficult moments, maximally reduce to algorithms the process of complex exercise's fulfillment. Students with strong type of nervous system are more bent to take decisions directly in the process of exercise's fulfillment.

Thus, as a result of our researches we supplemented the data of G.V. Korobeynikov [14; 15], V.S. Lizogub [16], N.I. Makarenko [17] about presence of confident difference between representatives of strong and weak nervous system by psycho-physiological indicators.

It is purposeful to apply the received data when training specialists, whose work will be connected with danger for life as well as for physical education of students for their over coming fear in different life situations in the future. Полученные данные целесообразно применять при подготовке специалистов, работа которых связана с риском для жизни. Further working out of methodic of individual psychological training for extreme situations is of great practical significance. Such methodic shall envisage consideration of perceiving of extreme situation, specific features of life settings of people with different types of nervous system, understanding of different aspects of extreme situations' overcoming, safety measures and general state of mood.

The conducted research also showed that for distribution of the tested in groups by properties of nervous system and responses to extreme situation the most adequate are methods of multi-dimensional analysis [3; 22; 27].

Conclusions:

1. We have shown that it is possible to divide people by indicators of functional changes in extreme situation together with psycho-physiological indicators and nervous system's properties into groups with the help of multi-dimensional analysis.

2. We have conducted analysis of subjective perceiving of extreme situation and functional changes in such situations of people with different types of nervous system on example of passing of suspended ferriage in hiking. We found out that there are confident differences between participants with strong and weak types of nervous system by HBR indicator before fulfillment of exercise, analogous to extreme situation (people with strong type of nervous system have confidently less HBR indicators than people with weak nervous system). Subjective feelings of fear also are confidently less in representatives of strong nervous system.

The prospects of further researches imply working out of methodic of fear's overcoming for people with different types of nervous system.

Acknowledgement

The authors acknowledge students, who participated in the researches and collection of experimental material.

The research has been conducted in compliance with:

- "Combined plan of scientific research works in sphere of physical culture and sports for 2011-2015" by topic 2.4 "Theoretical-methodic principles of individualization in physical education and sports" (state registration number 0112U002001);
- Scientific-research work, financed by Ministry of education and science of Ukraine for 2013-2014 "theoretical-methodic principles of application of informational, pedagogic and medical-biological technologies for formation of healthy life style" (state registration number 0113U002003)
- Scientific-research work, financed by Ministry of education and science of Ukraine for 2015-2016 "Theoretical-methodic principles of application of informational, pedagogic, medical-biological orientation for motor and mental progress and formation of healthy life style" (state registration number 0113U002003).

Conflict of interests

The authors declare that there is no conflict of interest.

References:

1. Alekseev VM, Ruzhinskaia ZhL. Sub"ektivnaia i fiziologicheskaia ocenka napriazhennosti global'noj i regional'noj fizicheskoj nagruzki [Subjective and physiological assessment of tension of global and regional physical load]. *Sbornik trudov uchenykh RGAFK* 1998;4:148-151. (in Russian)
2. Kozina ZhL, Baribina LM, Korobiejnikov GV, Mishchenko DI, Cikunov OA, Kozin OV. *Komp'iuterna programa «Psikhodiagnostika»* [Computer program "Psycho-diagnostic"]. Patent UA, no. 39679; 2011. (in Ukrainian)
3. Biuiul' Akhim, Efel' Peter. *SPSS: iskusstvo obrabotki informacii* [SPSS: [Atr of processing of information], Sankt Petersburg: DiaSoftYuP; 2001. (in Russian)
4. Kozina ZhL, Kozin SV, Antonov OV, Grin' LV. Verevochnye parki kak sredstvo povysheniia dvigatel'noj aktivnosti uchashchejsia molodezhi [Rope Parks as mean of increasing of students' motor functioning]. *Physical education of students* 2011;6:40-45. (in Russian)
5. Iermakov SS. Informacionnye aspekty zdorov'ia i zdorovogo obraza zhizni v elektronnom nauchnom prostranstve [Informational aspects of health and healthy life style in electronic scientific space]. *Valeologiia: suchasnij stan, napriamki ta perspektivi rozvitku* [Valueology: modern status, directions and prospects of development]. 2006;2:59-65. (in Russian)
6. Iermakov SS. Informacionnoe obespechenie prepodavaniia lechebnoj fizicheskoj kul'tury v gumanitarnykh vuzakh [Informational provisioning of teaching of therapeutic physical culture in humanitarian HEEs].

Mezhdunarodnaia nauchno-metodicheskaia konferenciia "Rol' fizicheskoj kul'tury, sporta i zdorov'ezberegaiushchikh tekhnologij v podgotovke specialistov", Belgorod, BGTU [International scientific-methodic conference "Role of physical culture, sports and health related technologies in training of specialists", Belgorod, BSTU], 2006. p. 100-106. (in Russian)

7. Zajcev VP, Prusik Kristof, Iermakov SS. Fizicheskaia rekreaciia v strukture aktivnogo otdykha studentov [Physical recreation in structure of students' active leisure]. *Physical education of students* 2011;1:68-77. (in Russian)
8. Kashuba VA, Futornyj CM, Andreeva EV. Sovremennye podkhody k zdorov'esberezheniiu studentov v processe fizicheskogo vospitaniia [Modern approaches to students' health-preservation in process of physical education]. *Physical education of students* 2012;7:50-58. (in Russian)
9. Kozina ZhL. Analiz i obobshchenie rezul'tatov prakticheskoj realizacii koncepcii individual'nogo podkhoda v trenirovochnom processe v sportivnykh igrakh [Analysis and generalization of results of practical realization of individual approach conception in trainings of sport games]. *Fizicheskoe vospitanie studentov tvorcheskikh special'nostej* 2009;2:34-47. (in Russian)
10. Kozina ZhL. Nauchno-metodicheskie puti individualizacii uchebno-trenirovochnogo processa v sportivnykh igrakh [Scientific-methodic ways of individualization of training process in sport games]. In: Iermakov SS (editor) *Problemy i perspektivy razvitiia sportivnykh igr i edinoborstv v vysshikh uchebnykh zavedeniiakh* [Problems and prospects of development of sport games and martial arts in higher educational establishments].]. Kharkov: KSADA; 2005:188-191. (in Russian)
11. Kozina ZhL. *Sistema individualizacii podgotovki sportsmenov v igrovykh vidakh sporta* [System of individualization of sportsmen's training in game kinds of sports], Lambret Academic Publishing Russia; 2011. (in Russian)
12. Kozina ZhL. Metodologicheskie osnovy vzaimointegracii nauchnykh znanij v oblasti fizicheskogo vospitaniia i sporta i smezhnykh nauk [Methodological principles of scientific knowledge inter-integration in field of physical education, sports and allied Sciences]. *Physical education of students* 2012;2:41-46. (in Russian)
13. Kozina ZhL. Vzaimosviaz' sub"ektivnykh i ob"ektivnykh parametrov fizicheskoj nagruzki v basketbole [Interconnection of subjective and objective parameters of physical load in basketball]. *Pedagogics, psychology, medical-biological problems of physical training and sports* 2000;7:43-46. (in Russian)
14. Korobejnikov GV, Koniaieva LD, Rossokha GV. Osoblivosti funkcional'nikh staniv nervovoi sistemi u sportsmenok - gandbolistok visokoi kvalifikacii [Peculiarities of nervous system's functional states in sportswomen – elite handball players]. *Pedagogics, psychology, medical-biological problems of physical training and sports* 2004;24:22-31. (in Ukrainian)
15. Korobejnikov GV. *Psikhofiziologicheskie mekhanizmy umstvennoj deiatel'nosti cheloveka* [Psycho-physiological mechanisms of human mental functioning], Kiev; 2002. (in Russian)
16. Lizogub VS. Individual'ni psikhofiziologichni osoblivosti liudini ta profesijna diial'nist' [Human individual psycho-physiological features and professional functioning]. *Fiziologichnij zhurnal* 2010;56(1):148 - 151. (in Ukrainian)
17. Makarenko NV. Metodika provedennia obstezhen' ta ocinki individual'nikh nejrodinamichnikh vlastivostej vishchoi nervovoi diial'nosti liudini [Methodic of examinations and assessment of individual neuro-dynamic properties of human supreme nervous functioning]. *Fiziologichnij zhurnal* 1999;45(4):125–131. (in Ukrainian)
18. Nosko MO, Iermakov SS, Garkusha SV. Teoretiko-metodichni aspekti zmicnennia fizichnogo zdorov'ia uchnivs'koi ta students'koi molodi [Theoretical and methodological aspects of strengthening physical health of pupils and students]. *Visnik Chernigivs'kogo nacional'nogo pedagogichnogo universitetu* 2010;76:243-247. (in Ukrainian)
19. Prusik Krzysztof, Prusik Katarzyna, Kozina ZhL, Iermakov SS. Features of physical development, physical preparedness and functional state of boys and girls - students of Polish higher educational establishments. *Physical Education of Students* 2013;1:54-61. doi:10.6084/m9.figshare.96415
20. Kozina ZhL, Barybina LN, Mishchenko DI, Kozin AV. Programma «Psikhodiagnostika» kak sredstvo opredeleniia psikhofiziologicheskikh osobennostej i funkcional'nogo sostoianiia v fizicheskom vospitanii studentov [Program "Psycho-diagnostic" as mean of determination of students' psycho-physiological

characteristics and physical condition in physical education]. *Physical education of students* 2011;3:56-60. (in Russian)

21. Shcherbatykh IuV. *Psikhologiia strakha* [Psychology of fear], Moscow: Eksmo – Press; 2001. (in Russian)
22. Volodymyr Adashevsky, Sergii Iermakov, Krzystof Prusik, Katarzyna Prusik, Karol Gorner. *Biomechanics: theory and practice*. Gdansk: Zdrowie-Projekt; 2012.
23. Borg G. Psychophysical bases of percieved exertion. *Medicine and Science in Sports and Exercise* 1982;14:377-381.
24. Chao-Chien Chen, Shih-Yen Lin. The impact of rope jumping exercise on physical fitness of visually impaired students. *Research in Developmental Disabilities* 2011;32(1):25-29.
25. Cieślicka M, Napierała M, Zukow W. State building somatic and motor abilities in kids practicing tennis on prebasic training. In: Hagner-Derengowska M, Zukow W. (red.) *Health - the proper functioning of man in all spheres of life*, School of Bydgoszcz, Bydgoszcz; 2012.
26. Cieślicka M, Napierała M. The somatic build of lightweight rowers. *Medical and Biological Sciences* 2009;23(3):33 – 38.
27. Ivashchenko OV, Yermakova TS, Cieślicka M, Zukowska H. Discriminant analysis in classification of motor fitness of 9-11 forms' juniors. *Journal of Physical Education and Sport* 2015;15(2):238 - 244.
28. Forzoni R. 'Personal motivational videos: so where's the downside. *The Sport and Exercise Scientist* 2006;7:10–11.
29. Frank Hookin Fu, Linxuan Guo, Yanpeng Zang. An overview of health fitness studies of Hong Kong residents from 2005 to 2011. *Journal of Exercise Science & Fitness* 2012;10(2):45-63.
30. Gonzalez SP, Metzler JN, Newton M. The influence of simulated 'pep talk' on athlete inspiration, situational motivation, and emotion'. *International Journal of Sports Science and Coaching* 2011;6(3):445–459.
31. Kovářová Lenka, Pánek David, Kovář Karel, Hlinčík Zdeněk. Relationship between subjectively perceived exertion and objective loading in trained athletes and non-athletes. *Journal of Physical Education and Sport* 2015;15(2):186 - 193.
32. Loewenstein VR. *Handbook of Sensor Physiology. Principles of Receptor Physiology*. Berlin-Heidelberg-New York, Springer; 1992.
33. Loren L, Toussaint Mary O, Whipple Lana L, Abboud Ann Vincent, Dietlind L, Wahner-Roedler. A Mind-Body Technique for Symptoms Related to Fibromyalgia and Chronic Fatigue. *EXPLORE: The Journal of Science and Healing* 2012;8(2):92-98.
34. Mikael Bäckström, Mats Tinnsten, Andrey Koptyug, Lars-Erik Rännar, Peter Carlsson, Jonas Danvind, Håkan Wiklund. Sports Technology Education at Mid Sweden University. *Procedia Engineering* 2013;60:214-219.
35. Hribovska Iryna, Danylevych Myroslava, Ivanochko Victoria, Shchur Lydia. Organizational conditions of healthy lifestyle promotion for arts students. *Journal of Physical Education and Sport* 2015;15(2):218 - 224.
36. Paul R Medwell, Laura A Brooks, Barry S Medwell. Analysis of the Lawn Bowl Trajectory as a teaching tool for Sports Engineering: development of a graphical user-interface. *Procedia Engineering* 2011;13:531-537.
37. Paul R Medwell, Paul N Grimshaw, Will S Robertson, Richard M Kelso. Developing sports engineering education in Australia. *Procedia Engineering* 2012;34:260-265.
38. Prusik Katarzyna Iermakov SS, Kozina ZhL. Indexes of physical development, physical preparedness and functional state of polish students. *Pedagogics, psychology, medical-biological problems of physical training and sports* 2012;12:113-122.
39. Reginald Xi Wang. *Self-determination and framing. An Interactionist Perspective on Self-Determination Theory: Place for Framing in AutonomySupport*. New York University; 2013.
40. Shiloh S, Salton E, Sharabi D. Individual differences in rational and intuitive thinking styles as predictors of heuristic responses and framing effects. *Personality and Individual Differences* 2002;32:415-429.
41. Thomas AK, Millar PR. Reducing the framing effect in older and younger adults by encouraging analytic processing. *The Journals of Gerontolog* 2012;67(2):139-149.
42. Vargas TM, Short SE. Athletes' perceptions of the psychological emotional, and performance effects of coaches' pre-game speeches'. *International Journal of Coaching Science* 2011;5(1):27–43.

COORDINATION TRAINING OF SPORTSMEN, SPECIALIZING IN SPORT KINDS OF GYMNASTIC

Tereshchenko I.A., Otsupok A.P., Krupenya S.V., Liauchuk T.M., Boloban V.N.
National University of Physical Education and Sport of Ukraine

Abstract. _Purpose:_ experimental substantiation of effectiveness of coordination training program, worked out for sportsmen, specializing in sport kinds of gymnastic. _Material:_ In the research first year students (21 persons: 14 girls and 7 boys of age 17-18 years) participated. All they specialized in sport kinds of gymnastic. From them there were 15 masters of sports and 6 candidate masters of sports. _Results:_ students' sensor motor coordination was confidently increased by means of realization of program of exercises for perfection of static-dynamic and static-kinetic stability. _Conclusions:_ we recommend new direction of specific exercises' realization; exercise, developing and improving static-dynamic and static-kinetic body balance. Coordination training of sportsmen, specializing in sport gymnastic shall take one of priority places in system of physical education and sport training means.
Key words: student, physical education, gymnastic, sensor motor, coordination, tests, practice.

Introduction

Trainees of sport gymnastic, calisthenics, sport acrobatic, jumping on trampoline, jumping on acrobatic track (i.e. sport kinds of gymnastic) fulfill exercises in complex conditions of static-dynamic and static-kinetic (vestibular) balance (in complex conditions of sensor-motor coordination). In process of exercises' fulfillment sportsmen execute motor tasks of body postures' control, body positions, coordination accuracy of motor actions in phase structure of sport exercises. As practical experience [3, 4, 10, 16] and scientific-methodic researches show sensor-motor coordination is not sufficiently effective in sportsmen's demonstration of gymnastic, acrobatic exercises in training and competitions' conditions [1, 5, 8]. It is manifested as body imbalance, disordering of space-time orientation on support and without support, temp-rhythm, differentiation of motor parameters, practically all elements of motor coordination structure [7].

Purpose, tasks of the work, material and methods

The purpose: experimental substantiation of effectiveness of coordination training program, worked out for sportsmen, specializing in sport kinds of gymnastic.

The tasks: 1. Research level of first year students' (NUPESU), who specialize in sport kinds of gymnastic, sensor motor coordination.

2. To work out coordination training program for first year students, specializing in sport kinds of gymnastic as well as to test its effectiveness in practical training.

Material, methods and organization of the researches: In the research first year students (21 persons: 14 girls and 7 boys of age 17-18 years) participated. All they were from NUPESU and specialized in sport kinds of gymnastic. From them there were 15 masters of sports and 6 candidate masters of sports.

The methods: analysis of literature sources (theoretical-methodic review of literature, devoted to this problem); pedagogic testing; successive pedagogic experiment, fulfilled with technique of one group; experts' assessment. The researches' results were processed by method s of mathematical statistic (MO Excel, Statistika).

Pedagogic testing (detail description of tests is given in works [1, 2, 8, 9]:

Test1 – balance on one leg: assessment of static balance on one leg, other is bent aside with sole placed on thigh of supporting leg, arms are at level and width of shoulders; fingers are parted. Time – 5 seconds with open eyes and 15 seconds with closed eyes. Marks: "very good", if the tested keeps balance with closed eyes during 14-15 seconds. "Good" – balance is kept during period from 11 to 13 seconds; 8-10 seconds – "satisfactory".

Test 2 – Biriuk's test: assessment of body static balance when standing on tip toes with closed eyes.

Test 3 – Barany's test: assessment of static-dynamic body stability after 10 rotations in Barany's armchair.

Test 4 – five forward rolls in tuck: assessment of static-kinetic body balance after loading of vestibular analyzer.

Test 5 – coordination: assessment of coordination in complex conditions.

Test 6 – hanging on bent legs: assessment of proprioceptive sensitivity in changed conditions of haemo-dynamic and irritation of otolith analyzer (hanging with head downward press dynamometer with hand of convenient arm with strength of 200 N for boys and 100 N for girls).

Test 7 – travel along perimeter of polygon: assessment of dynamic balance with passing of polygon's five perimeters for 20 seconds. Coefficients of tests' reliability are 0.490–0.990 [1, 7].

Testing was conducted in three stages. At fist stage (September 2014) we measured level of sensor-motor coordination of first year students, specializing in sport kinds of gymnastic (initial measurements of successive pedagogic experiment) At second stage (October-December 2014) students fulfilled practical material from program on specialization and on general gymnastic in compliance with curriculum (three times a week) as well as exercises from the worked out by us coordination training program.

At the end of the second stage (December 2014) we carried out intermediate study for assessment of offered by us exercises' effectiveness, oriented on development of sensor-motor coordination (intermediate measurements of successive pedagogic experiment). At third stage (duration – five months: January – May 2015) students fulfilled exercises with objects for general development, vaults, acrobatic exercises, hanging and pressing up exercises as well as improved (after intermediate measurements) exercises of coordination training program. At the end of the third stage we conducted final measurements of indicators of successive pedagogic experiment.

Results of the researches

Initial indicators of first year students, specializing in sport kinds of gymnastic, sensor-motor coordination are given in tables 1-3.

Table 1

Initial indicators of sensor-motor coordination of first year girl students (NUPESU), specializing in calisthenics (n=7)

The tested	Sport grade	Motor tests							
		Test 1 – balance	Test 2-Biriuk's text	Test 3-Barany's test	Test 4- test 5 forward rolls	Test 5-Coordination test	Test 6-hanging on bent legs	Test 7-walking along perimeter	
								Quantity of walked facets	Spent time
B - a	M/S	12	12	31	25	9.5	13	4	26
D - ch	M/S	14	12	35	20	9.6	13	2	10
Zh - o	M/S	11	14	28	25	9.5	12	3	18
I - a	CMS	14	9	27	25	9.1	13	2	22
S - k	CMS	13	8	25	18	9.2	14	1.5	11
S - a	M/S	15	14	30	21	9.7	11	1.5	11
Sh - a	M/S	14	14	30	25	9.3	13	2	15
$\overline{x}$		13.29	11.86	29.43	22.71	9.41	12.71	2.29	16.14
S		1.38	2.48	3.21	2.98	0,22	0.95	0.91	6.15
m		0.56	1.01	1.30	1.21	0.09	0.38	0.37	2.51
V%		10.39	20.90	10.90	13.14	2.33	7.48	39.65	38.09

Notes: MS – master of sports; CMS – candidate master of sports.

Table 2

Initial indicators of sensor-motor coordination of first year girl students (NUPESU), specializing in sport gymnastic (n=7)

The tested	Sport grade	Motor tests							
		Test 1 – balance	Test 2-Biriuk's text	Test 3-Barani's test	Test 4- test 5 forward rolls	Test 5-Coordination test	Test 6-hanging on bent legs	Test 7-walking along perimeter	
								Quantity of walked facets	Spent time
Z - a	M/S	13	10	35	20	9.5	11	4	25
S - o	M/S	11	9	35	22	9.4	13	5	28
B - a	M/S	12	10	21	17	9.5	12	4	23
V - a	M/S	15	12	25	21	9.8	12	5	28
К - a	CMS	10	7	30	25	9.0	13	5	27
К - va	M/S	14	9	25	16	9.3	11	5	25
A - o	CMS	12	8	35	20	9.0	13	5	30
$\overline{x}$		12.43	9.29	29.43	20.14	9.36	12.14	4.71	26.57
S		1.72	1.60	5.83	3.02	0.29	0.90	0.49	2.37
m		0.70	0.65	2.37	1.23	0.11	0.36	0.19	0.96
V%		13.82	17.27	19.80	15.01	3.08	7.41	10.35	8.92

Table 3

Initial indicators of sensor-motor coordination of first year students (NUPESU), specializing in sport gymnastic (n=7)

The tested	Sport grade	Motor tests							
		Test 1 – balance	Test 2-Biriuk's text	Test 3-Barany's test	Test 4- test 5 forward rolls	Test 5-Coordination test	Test 6-hanging on bent legs	Test 7-walking along perimeter	
								Quantity of walked facets	Spent time
L - к	M/S	10	8	20	20	9.0	30	4	23
P - o	M/S	13	11	15	25	8.5	22	5	20
P - к	M/S	10	11	30	20	9.5	24	5	33
R – y	M/S	12	9	27	23	9.2	22	5	25
Ye – n	M/S	15	7	16	18	9.0	26	5	23
L - a	CMS	12	10	35	18	9.1	23	4	25
K - r	CMS	13	8	30	30	8.9	29	5	35

$\overline{X}$	12.14	9.14	24.71	22.0	9.03	25.14	4.71	26.29
S	1.77	1.57	7.74	4.36	0.30	3.29	0.49	5.56
m	0.72	0.64	3.16	1.78	0.12	1.34	0.19	2.27
V%	14.60	17.21	31.32	19.81	3.27	13.08	10.35	21.15

Fulfillment of test balancing on one leg (test 1) showed: most of the tested (14 persons– 66%) demonstrated trembling of arms, oscillations of body and lost of balance (shifting from spot of supporting leg) on 10th second, after closing eyes. Girl-students, specializing in calisthenics demonstrated a little better results ($\overline{X}$ =13.29; 1.38 sec.).

In Biriuk's test (test 2) the tested keep static body balance insufficiently. Their motor skill was formed with technical mistakes. In the test they keep balance with the help of arms' movements, make body movements and keep balance insufficient time (especially girl students, specializing in sport gymnastic) (11.86; 2.48 sec.). It is explained by the fact that position "standing on half tip toes" is their main working posture when fulfilling sport exercises.

Results of vestibular balance research by indicators of dynamic balance (Barany's test, test 3) witness that after rotations in Barany's armchair 12 tested (57.1%) demonstrated weakened coordination of vertical body position from axial line by 20 – 35 cm. After one or two steps some of the tested demonstrated rough loss of balance. The better indicators belonged to girl students (24.71; 7.74 cm).

Vestibular load – five forward rolls for 5 sec. (test 4) significantly worsened dynamic stability of body. It resulted in the fact that after rolls part of the tested (8 persons - 38%) could not fulfill 10 jumps in the center of graduated circle, jumping out of its limits. The worst indicators were registered in those, who specialized in calisthenics (22.71; 2.98 cm.) and in students, specializing in sport gymnastic (22. 0; 4.35 cm).

Coordination (test 5): was tested with jumps on both legs with successive movements of arms: on waist, to shoulders, upward and back-downward. The test was easy for those, who specialized in sport kinds of gymnastic and did not show any differences in indicators. In this connection we replaced it with more difficult, videlicet: initial position (IP) stance – legs apart, arms directed to sides.

1. Turn to the left in stand on left leg, right one is back on tip toe, right arm is directed by arch forward-downward, left arm is directed backward.
2. Forward wave of right leg, right arm – backward, left arm – forward.
3. Forward wave of right leg, right arm –forward, left leg – backward on tip toe.
4. Turn to the right in stand – legs apart, right leg goes by arch downwards; arms are directed to sides (IP).

5 – 8. The same but with turn to the right.

Coordination level of the tested (fulfilling complicated test for coordination) is characterized as middle and above middle. It coincides with results of Polish specialists' researches [10]. Marks for test's fulfillment were 9.0; 0.29 – 9.36; 0.28 points. Better coordination was registered in girl students, specializing in calisthenics (9.41; 0.21 points).

Indicators of proprioceptive sensitivity in changed conditions of haemo-dynamic and irritation of otlith analyzer (test 6) witness that the tested in most cases demonstrated muscular efforts with over estimation or under estimation of the required value. For example among girl students over estimation of muscular efforts was 2.71; 0.95 N. Boy students demonstrated over estimation of 5.14; 3.28 from initial values (100 N; 200 N). Better results were registered in students, specializing in sport gymnastic (2.14; 0.90 N).

Assessment of dynamic body balance with passing of polygon's facets in conditions of restricted support (test 7) witnesses the tested have not got sufficient dynamic balance. For example, from the planned fives travels along polygon's perimeter for 20 seconds the tested passed in average 2.5 – 4.5 of perimeter for 26.57; 2.37 sec. The worst results of dynamic balance were registered in girl-students, specializing in calisthenics (2.29; 0.9 of perimeter for 16.14; 6.14 sec.).

On the base of the received results we can say that sensor-motor coordination of persons, specialized in sport gymnastic has certain reserve for perfection. In this connection we worked out coordination training program for persons, specializing in sport kinds of gymnastic. It consists of two parts, structurally and functionally interconnected. Part 1 – Training of static-dynamic balance. Part 2 – Vestibular training.

When training of the program's exercises and fulfilling them it is extremely important to master required elements of working posture. Working posture shall become a firm skill. It permits to control sensing of body postures, body positions on support and without support. Yu.K. Gaverdovskiy [4], S.V. Veldiayev [3], Yu.A. Maximova [6] conventionally mark out types of postures in positions: lying, standing, hanging, rest.

1. *Closed posture* – head is bent with chin touching chest, insignificant bending in shoulder and hip joints. It is convenient for fulfillment of exercises on bar, rings, at the beginning of downward-backward declines. Also it can be used as mean, which helps to sense possibilities of movements' control.

2. *Half-closed posture* head is between arms, shoulders are clamped. It is close by characteristics to previous one, but also is convenient for keeping strictly upright body position.

3. *Half open posture* – head is half raised above arms. It leaves possibility for rather convenient keeping of straightened, stretched position with good visual control, but does not exclude possibility of sportsman's body bending.

4. *Open posture* – head is raised. Angle in shoulder joints is possible. It is used rather rarely because it is connected with ostentatiously tensed movements in shoulder joints and danger of too strong body bending.

5. *Bent posture* – head is slightly bent downward to chest, body is in bent position, angle between axes of torso front and legs is within 35 – 45°. Specificity of physical and sport exercises and resulting from them solved motor tasks determine also other borders. For example, when jumping in water (body position – bent in fulfillment of double forward rotation) – it is dense fold of body (example from gymnastic is also possible).

6. *Posture in half tuck* – vertical position of body with legs, bent in knee and hip joints with drawn out toes, bent and pressed to body arms; head is insignificantly dropped on chest.

7. *Posture in tuck* is a position, in which torso is maximally rounded with head dropped to chest; arms embrace shins in the middle; elbows are pressed to torso.

8. *Dynamic posture* – is multiplication of postures and body positions in phase structure of sport exercise. For example "working posture in tuck" and its multiplication in double back flip in tuck are regarded as dynamic posture [1].

For fulfillment of exercises from our program's parts we applied up-to-date pedagogic technologies of their mastering and perfection: functional pedagogic equation (FPE), which has the following form (V.N. Boloban) [1]):

$$P \rightarrow DP \rightarrow DR \rightarrow MT \rightarrow MTr \rightarrow MFOT \rightarrow RC \leftrightarrows RT,$$

Where:

P – purpose and tasks;

DP – didactic principles (individualization, strength, conjugated impact);

DR – didactic rules (train energetically, go from simple to complex, from easy to difficult, compare, repeat, consolidate, perfect coordination, strive for balance);

MT – methods of training (practical, programming, competitions);

MTr – means of training – exercises from parts of coordination training program;

MFOT – methods and forms of organization of trainees (frontal, group, individual);

RC –regulation and control of training process (quantity of training sessions, exercises, repetitions, time of program's fulfillment, control tests;

RT – result of training (fulfillment of control tests with high marks of static-dynamic and static-kinetic body balance).

General algorithm of functional pedagogic equation's action is as follows: as per planned result of sportsmen's training to exercise (in formula – it is right part of equation, RT,, which is a pedagogic directive – to teach to sport exercise, i.e. to achieve the desired result) didactic programming is carried out as well as structuring of knowledge formation's process, motor skills of the trained exercise. I.e. the most adequate and effective didactic elements are selected (in formula – it is left part of equation).

Functional pedagogic equation is mentioned in connection with dynamic character of training and teaching process, creative search of the most effective elements of training, where main condition is level of sportsmen's fitness. It pre-determined formulation of the tasks of program material's mastering, means of trainees' organization, elements of regulation, control and correction with the help of biological feedback.

Table 4

Exercises of program "Coordination training" of first year students of NUPESU, specializing in sport gymnastic

Part 1 Training of static-dynamic balance

Task: perfection of static and dynamic balances with fulfillment of exercises for dynamic posture and durable keeping of balance (4–32 sec.) in different positions of body and in motion.

Control: Biriuk's test (fixing of position for 15–20 sec.)

№	Description of exercises, regulation	Methodic recommendations
	Exercises for perfection of skill in keeping dynamic balance on support	
1	Initial position (i.p.): lying on back, arms directed upward. Insignificant bent in hip joints (closed posture). Keep position 3-5 seconds, then turn to the left in position lying on abdomen, straightened (open posture) and keep this position again 3-5 seconds. Repeat exercise 4-8 times, making turns to the left – to the right. The same do with closed eyes.	During turning bend slightly hip joints as in half-open position
2	I.p. lying on back, arms directed upward. 1. Sit in angle (bent posture). Unbending torso 2-4 times quickly turn to the left by 360° in initial position. Repeat exercise 3-4 times to both sides.	When unbending, in turn try to keep vertical position of body with closed legs and arms above
3	I.p. lying on back, arms directed upward. 1. Sit in angle (bent posture). Unbending torso 2-4 times quickly turn to the left by 360° in position of sitting in angle with bent torso. Repeat exercise 3-4 times to both sides.	When unbending, in turn try to keep vertical position of body with closed legs
4	I.p. lying on abdomen (open posture). 1 – 2. Turn to the left by 360°. 3 – 4. Turn to the left by 180°. 5. Sit in angle, arms directed forward (bent posture). 6 – 7 unbending torso make quick turn to the left by 360° in position sitting in angle, bending. 8. I.p. repeat exercise 2-4 times to both sides.	When unbending, in turn (body is elastic-rigid) try to keep vertical position of body with closed legs
5	I.p. lying. 1. Turn to the left to rest on arm, lying by left side; right arm is raised upward. 2 – 3. Keep this position. 4. But with turn by I.p. Repeat exercise 2 – 4 times by right and left sides. The same exercise but with turn by 180° into back rest on arms and again in front rest on arms.	При поворотах сохранять полуоткрытую осанку
	Exercises for perfection of skill of dynamic posture keeping in unsupported position	
1	Jumping from height of 1 meter 20 cm (jumping table). I.p. main stance – with waving arms – jump forward-upward, straightening (half-closed posture); arms go upward-outside, then balanced landing in position of half-squat, with arms forward-downward (position of pre-jump). Fulfill 2-3 times.	Accent is on straightened position of body in upper point of jump and on balanced landing
2	I.p. – main stance - with waving arms – jump forward-upward, touching chest with knees; head is dropped on chest; arms directed forward-downward – outside (half-tuck posture). Then legs actively unbend and balance landing occurs in position of pre-jump. Fulfill 2-3 times.	Attention to half-tuck in upper point of jump and on balanced landing
3	I.p. main stance - with waving arms – jump forward-upward, in tuck (tuck posture), followed by active straightening of torso and steady landing in position of pre-jump. Fulfill 2-3 times.	Active tuck in upper point of jump and balanced landing
4	I.p. main stance - with waving arms – jump forward-upward, bending with legs apart, arms forward-outside (bending posture), followed by active unbending and balanced landing in pre-jump position. Fulfill 3-4times.	Accent of fulfillment of fold only in ascending part and balanced landing
5	I.p. main stance - with waving arms – jump forward-upward, straightening with turn by 180 degrees; arms go upward-outside (half-open posture), followed by landing in balanced position of pre-jump. Fulfill 2-3 times with turn to both sides.	Accurate turn in ascending part of jump and balanced landing

6	I.p. main stance - with waving arms – jump forward-upward, straightening with turn by 360, and 540 degrees; arms go upward-outside (half-open posture), followed by landing in balanced position of pre-jump. Fulfill 2-3 times with turn to both sides.	Vertical posture without twisting in hip joints
Exercises for static dynamic balance in different positions of body		
1	I.p. – hands are on waist. Walking on tip toes with turns by 360° to the left and to the right, followed by stops and fixation of vertical posture with arms upward. Fix posture for 4 seconds. Fulfill the same with turns by 90° in jumps. Repeat exercise 3 – 4 times to both sides.	Attention to keeping of vertical posture without twisting in hip joints; jumps shall be fulfilled with waving arms
2	I.p. – closed stance with hands on waist. 1. Bent with arching – arms are directed outside. 2. Back bent with arms upward – outside. 3. High balance on left leg – right one is directed backward; left arm – upward – right arm is directed to side. 4 – 7.Keep posture. 8. I.p. Repeat exercise 3 – 4 times on left and right legs. The same in stance on tip toes with closed eyes.	High balance shall be fulfilled on half tip toes, with head kept straight; body shall be rigid-elastic and maximally
3	I.p. Stance on right leg with left one directed aside on tip toe. 1 – 2. Wave to the left, wave to the right. 3 – 4. Side balance on right leg, left one – aside with right arm directed upward and left one – behind the back. 5 – 7. Keep posture. 8. I.p. The same on left leg. Repeat exercise 4 – 6 times. The same on tip toe with closed eyes.	When waving stand on tip toes keeping balance. Attention to functioning of torso and legs' muscles.
4	I.p. Stance on tip-toes with hands directed aside. 1. Bend to the left, arms – upward. 2. I.p. 3. Bend to the right, arms – upward. 4. I.p. 5. Back step with right leg; back balance on right leg, left one is directed forward-upward; arms – upward-aside. 6 – 7. Keep the posture. 8. I.p. Fulfill exercise 2 times on left and 2 times on right legs. Repeat exercise, increasing time of posture's keeping up to 6-8 sec.	Keep balance on high half tip toes; the same with closed eyes. Pay attention to functioning of legs and torso's muscles.
5	I.p. Stance on tip-toes with hands directed aside. 1. Jump on left leg, forward wave with right leg; left arm goes forward, right one – backward. 2. I.p. 3. Jump on right leg, forward wave with left leg; right arm goes forward, left one – backward. 4. I.p. 5. Jump on left leg in high balance by "ring" of right leg; arms are directed upward-outside. 6 – 7. Keep position. 8. I.p. Fulfill exercise 2 times on both legs, keeping balance by "ring" up to 8 – 10sec. Do the same with closed eyes.	Attention to ability to keep position of leap in flight and balance in high balance by "ring".
6	I.p. Stance on tip toes; arms are directed aside. 1. Wave with right leg forward-upward; left arm is directed forward, right arm – backward. 2. I.p. 3. Wave with right leg backward; left arm is directed backward, right – forward; forward bend in position balanced split with capture of shin by hands. 4 – 7. Keep the posture. 8. I.p. Do the same with left leg with closed eyes. Repeat exercise 2 – 4 times, keeping balance in split 6 – 8 sec.	Keep balance when fulfilling waves forward-backward and in balanced split.
Exercises for dynamic balance (moving on low and standard balance beam)		
1	I.p. Stance on tip toes at end of low balance beam. Walking on tip toes with arms aside – walking with back forward and arms aside; walking with crossed steps (left step – right step) with arms aside; jumps on both legs with arms upward; run by "gallop" from left (right" legs; run on tip toes to the end of balance beam and dismount downward in straighten position of torso. Repeat combination 1 – 2 times.	Accent on tension of muscles and vertical carriage on high half tip toes; on change of kinds of movement at the end of balance beam
2	I.p. Main stance at the end of balance beam. Back balance (keep 3-3 sec.); then two "gallop" steps from left leg and two – from right leg with unlike circles made by arms inside; turn by 360 degrees on left (right) leg with right leg bent forward and arms directed upward; turn by 180 degrees on both legs with arms – upward; jumps on both legs with arms aside; the same with changing of legs (arms – aside); run up to the end of balance beam with arms aside and dismount straightening. Repeat combination 1-2 times.	When turning exclude any torso movements. When jumping keep vertical posture; change of kinds of movements shall be at the end of balance beam.
3	I.p. Main stance at the end of balance beam. Walking on tip toes, waving legs forward-upward at every step with arms aside; turn by 180 degrees by left	When waving and jumping pay attention to

	(right) leg with other leg bent forward and arms directed upward; turn by180 degrees with forward waving of one leg; forward jumps from left to right legs (and vice versa), arms – aside; forward balance on left (right) leg; run up to the end of balance beam and dismount straightening. Repeat combination 1-2 times.	verticality of posture without extra body movements; change of kinds of movements shall be at the end of balance beam.
4	I.p. Stance on tip toes at end of balance beam, arms - aside. Moving forward with different combinations of two, three jumps; keep balance for 4 – 8 sec.; alternation of jumps, legs' waving and turns to different sides. Repeat exercise 3 – 4 times, without dismounting from the beam.	Increase amplitude of legs' waving, keep balance; change of kinds of movements shall be at the end of balance beam..
5	I.p. Stance on tip toes; arms are directed aside. Three steps, starting from left leg; back waving with right leg with turn around, arms are directed upward and stance on tip toes; turn around in i.p. Repeat combination 2 times from right and 2 time from left legs. Fulfill 3-4 attempts.	When turning keep steady balance and carriage; accurate position of arms, directed upward and aside.
6	I.p. squat with left leg ahead and arms – aside. Make three steps in squat position and turn by 180° to the right, the turn by 180° to the left. Repeat combination 2 times from right and 2 times from left legs. Fulfill 3-4 attempts.	When turning keep vertical posture and accurate position of arms, directed upward and aside.
Exercises for keeping of dynamic posture (jumps on trampoline)		
1	Fulfill 4-8 temp jumps.	Keep verticality of body with arms dropped down
2	3 – 4 temp jumps: make high jump in tuck (keeping carriage in tuck) with following quick opening in ascending part of jump and landing with stop. Repeat 2 – 4 times.	Attention to rounded back, dropped head, hands' capture of shins with elbows pressed to torso
3	2 – 3 temp jumps: jump on knees and jump upward with turn by 180° and landing with stop. Repeat combination 2 – 4 times with turning to both sides..	When landing on knees, do not admit any angle in hip joints
4	2 – 3 temp jumps: jump in sitting position and jump upward with turn by 180° and landing with stop. Repeat combination 2 – 4 times with turning o both sides.	When landing in sitting position pay attention to upright position of torso and head with arms bent back on support
5	3 – 4 temp jumps: jump upward with turn by 180°; jump upward with turn by 360° and landing with stop. с приземлением в остановку. Repeat combination 2 – 4 times with turning o both sides, also applying turns by 180° and 540°.	Turn shall be fulfilled in ascending part of jump, with vertical posture and arms pressed to body

Part 2. Vestibular training

The task: perfection of static-kinetic body balance with the help of exercises, oriented on progressing of stability and sensitivity of vestibular analyzer.

Control: Barany's test (deviation of body to the left-right from vertical line in passing of 5 meter' segment of width not more than 15-20 cm.

№	Description of exercises. Regulation	Methodic recommendations
Acrobatic exercises on track (mat) for static-kinetic balance		
1	I.p. Hands on floor in squat position. Forward roll; jump upward with turn by 360° with landing in squat (hands on floor; two back rolls, jump upward with landing in half squat position and arms forward-downward-aside (pre-jump position). Fulfill exercise 2 times in one attempt, keeping pre-jump position up to 5 sec. Repeat exercise 3-4 times.	Jump upward shall be fulfilled with energetic wave of arms upward; when turning keep vertical carriage; keep balance when landing

2	I.p. Main stance. Step with one leg; temp jump (valset); turnover with turn (rondat); jump with turn around and arms upward; jump with turn by 360° in pre jump position. Fulfill combination 2 times in one attempt. Repeat exercise 3-4 times, fulfilling turns to both sides.	When turning keep verticality of body; keep balance when landing
3	I.p. Hands on floor in squat position. Forward roll; long forward roll; temp jump and forward turnover on one; forward turnover on two with landing in pre-jump position. Fulfill combination 2 times. Repeat exercise 3-4 times, fulfilling turns to both sides.	Accent on straightened body in temp jump and keep balance when landing
4	I.p. Main stance. Step with one leg; temp jump; forward turnover on two; upward jump straightening; long forward roll; upward jump bending with legs apart and arms forward-aside; landing in pre-jump position. Fulfill combination 2 times. Repeat exercise 3 – 4 times.	Jump transition from turnover to roll; horizontal legs' position (bent posture) in jump
5	I.p. Main stance with arms directed upward. Step with left leg and back wave with right one; left overturn in stance with legs apart and arms aside; step with right leg with turn to the left in stance "legs apart"; turnover to the right. Fulfill combination 3 times. Fulfill 3-4 attempts.	Attention to keeping flatness when fulfilling turnovers
6	I.p. Arms are directed upward. Back roll, bending in front arms and turn by 180° (front arms shall be kept 3 sec.) – forward roll bending and jump upward with turn by 360 degrees; landing in pre-jump position. ° – приземление в положение доскока. Fulfill combination 2 times in one attempt. Repeat exercise 3 – 4 times turning to both sides.	Attention to straightened body when turning; do not admit more then two over stepping in front arms
Exercises on trampoline for static-kinetic balance		
1	Temp jumps; jump in sitting position; upward jump; jump on knees; upward jump with arms upward and turn around in sitting position; upward jump and turn around on knees; upward jump and landing with stop. Repeat combination 3-4 times with turning to both sides.	Attention to vertical position of body when ascending and in turns; in sitting positions arms are slightly bent behind the back. Knees are closed and tightly pressed to each other.
2	Temp jumps; jump in sitting position; upward jump with arms directed upward and turn to the left by 180 degrees in sitting position; upward jump and turn to the right by 180 degrees in sitting position; upward jump and landing with stop. Repeat combination 3-4 times with turning to both sides.	Attention to vertical body position when ascending and in turn
3	Temp jumps; upward jump with right turn by 180degrees in sitting position; jump on legs; back jump on back in tuck; upward jump with turn by 180degrees; upward jump and stop. Repeat combination 3-4 times with turning to both sides.	Attention to vertical body position when ascending and in turn
4	Temp jumps; jump on knees; jump on hands in kneeled position; upward jump with turn around in sitting position; upward jump with turn around in kneeled position, on hands; upward jump with turn by 360 degrees in kneeled position, on hands; upward jump and stop. Repeat combination 3-4 times.	Keep vertical body position when turning, legs shall be in close contact
5	Temp jumps; jump in kneeled position, on hands; forward jump, bending, on back; upward jump with turn by 360 degrees; jump and stop. Repeat combination 3-4 times to both sides.	Arms are dropped head is on chest (half closed posture). When unbending from bacl press arms tightly to torso
6	Temp jumps; back flip in tuck; forward flip bending with turn by 180 degrees; half jump and jump with stop. Repeat combination 3-4 times to both sides.	Attention to position of arms directed upward and half closed posture

Table 5

Algorithm of exercises' fulfillment o coordination training program for persons, specializing in sport kinds of gymnastic

№	Description of parts and number of exercise	Days of week		
		Monday	**Tuesday**	**Friday**
Part1. Training of static-dynamic balance on support				
1	Exercises for skill in keeping dynamic posture in lying position			

	Exercises 1, 2, 3, 4, 5	3, 4	1, 2	5
2	Exercises for skill in keeping dynamic posture in unsupported position			
	Exercises 1, 2, 3, 4, 5	3, 4	1, 2	5, 6
3	Exercises for static-dynamic balance in different positions of body			
	Exercises 1, 2, 3, 4, 5,6	3, 4	1, 2	5, 6
4	Exercises for dynamic balance when moving on low ans standard balance beam			
	Exercises 1, 2, 3, 4, 5,6	3, 6	1, 2	4, 5
5	Exercises for dynamic posture when jumping on trampoline			
	Exercises 1, 2, 3, 4, 5	3, 4	1	5
	Part 2. Vestibular training			
1	Acrobatic exercises on acrobatic track (mat) for static-kinetic balance			
	Exercises 1, 2, 3, 4, 5,6	3, 4	1, 2	5, 6
2	Exercises on trampoline for static-kinetic balance			
	Exercises 1, 2, 3, 4, 5,6	3, 4	1, 2	5, 6

At the end of the second stage of successive pedagogic experiment we conducted additional testing of static-dynamic and static-kinetic balance of persons, practicing sport kinds of gymnastic.

Results of the research witness that there are no confident differences between indicators of sensor motor coordination. We observed only tendency for improvement of tests' indicators. That is why we inserted some changes in our program. They concern, mainly, part 2 "Vestibular training". New variants of exercises are given in table 4.

The third stage (duration 5 months, January – May 2015) was characterized by fulfillment of curriculum exercises in course of general gymnastic. The latter envisaged mastering of applied, general, acrobatic exercises, exercises on gymnastic apparatuses, vaults. The trainees also fulfilled exercises from our program of improvement of body static-dynamic and static-kinetic balance. Final indicators are given in table 6-8.

Table 6

Final indicators of static-dynamic and static –kinetic balance of first year girl students of NUPESU, who specialize in calisthenics (n=7)

The tested	Sport grade	Motor tests							
		Test 1 – balance	Test 2-Biriuk's text	Test 3-Barani's test	Test 4- test 5 forward rolls	Test 5-Coordination test	Test 6-hanging on bent legs	Test 7-walking along perimeter	
								Quantity of walked facets	Spent time
B - a	M/S	14	22	20	17	9,6	12	4	27
D - ch	M/S	15	14	25	16	9,8	11	3	13
Zh - o	M/S	15	10	22	15	9,7	12	4	20
I - a	CMS	14	20	23	20	9,7	9	4	25
S - k	CMS	15	17	25	15	9,5	12	2	12
S - a	M/S	15	22	22	12	9,6	10	3	21
Sh - a	M/S	14	12	20	15	9,9	9	3	18
$\overline{x}$		14.57	16.71	22.43	15.71	9.69	10.71	3.29	19.43
S		0.53	4.86	2.07	2.43	0.13	1.38	0.76	5.62
m		0.21	1.98	0.84	0.99	0.05	0.56	0.30	2.29
V%		3.67	29.05	9.23	15.46	1.39	12.88	23.01	28.94
p		$p<0.05$	$p<0.05$	$p<0.05$	$p<0.05$	$p<0.05$	$p<0.05$	$p>0.05$	$p>0.05$

Table 7

Final indicators of sensor-motor coordination of first year girl students (NUPESU), specializing in sport gymnastic (n=7)

The tested	Sport grade	Motor tests							
		Test 1 – balance	Test 2-Biriuk's text	Test 3-Barani's test	Test 4- test 5 forward rolls	Test 5-Coordination test	Test 6-hanging on bent legs	Test 7-walking along perimeter	
								Quantity of walked facets	Spent time
Z - a	M/S	14	16	25	12	10	9	4	24
S - o	M/S	13	10	25	15	9,9	10	5	25
B - a	M/S	14	14	20	13	9,6	12	4	22
	A-a CMS	15	15	21	16	10	11	5	27
V - a	M/S	15	13	25	18	9,7	12	4	25
K - a	CMS	15	17	20	10	9,7	10	5	23
K - va	M/S	14	14	25	17	9,9	9	5	25
$\overline{x}$		14.29	14.14	23.0	14.43	9.83	10.43	4.57	24,43
S		0.76	2.27	2.52	2.88	0.16	1.27	0.53	1.62
m		0.30	0.92	1.02	1.17	0.06	0.51	0.21	0.66
V%		5.29	16.03	10.94	19.95	1.63	12.20	11.69	6.62
p		$p<0.05$	$p<0.05$	$p<0.05$	$p<0.05$	$p<0.05$	$p<0.05$	$p>0.05$	$p<0.05$

Table 8

Initial indicators of sensor-motor coordination of first year students (NUPESU), specializing in sport gymnastic (n=7)

The tested	Sport grade	Motor tests							
		Test 1 – balance	Test 2-Biriuk's text	Test 3-Barani's test	Test 4- test 5 forward rolls	Test 5-Coordination test	Test 6-hanging on bent legs	Test 7-walking along perimeter	
								Quantity of walked facets	Spent time
L - к	M/S	15	15	12	15	9,5	21	4	22
P - o	M/S	15	19	15	10	9,8	22	5	19
P - к	M/S	14	17	20	16	9,7	21	5	23
R – y	M/S	12	10	20	17	9,5	19	5	24
Ye – n	M/S	15	10	15	18	9,5	22	5	22
L - a	CMS	13	11	25	15	9,6	23	4	21
K - r	CMS	14	9	20	15	9,4	22	5	25
$\overline{x}$		14.0	13.00	18.14	15.14	9.57	21.43	4.71	22.29
S		1.15	3.96	4.38	2.54	0.14	1.27	0.49	1.98

m	0.47	1.61	1.78	1.03	0.05	0.51	0.19	0.80
V%	8.25	30. 45	24.12	16.81	1.44	5.94	10.35	8.87
p	p<0.05	p<0.05	p>0.05	p<0.05	p<0.05	p<0.05	p>0.05	p>0.05

On finishing the course of general gymnastic and fulfilling program "Coordination training", designed for perfection of organism's sensor systems, we registered confident improvement of indicators of static-dynamic and static-kinetic body balance. For example in tests 1,2 the tested became confidently longer keep balance with closed eyes, standing on one keg and on high half tip toes, accordingly 14.57; 0.53 sec. and 16.71; 4.86 sec. ($p<0.05$). Vestibular balance, in passing 5 meters' segment (test 3) also improved. Deviations from axial line reduced and became more stable, being within admissible tolerance from 18.14; 4.37 cm for boy students and см up to 22.43; 2.07 cm for girl students ($p<0.05$). Quantity of tested, who fulfilled high jumps within graduated circle (test 4) increased. For example from 21 tested 13 persons (62%) yimproved their indicators in average by 5.5 cm, comparing with initial indicators and were 14.43; 2.87 cm of girl students and 15.14; 2.54 cm of boy students ($p<0.05$). Indicators of coordination in complicated conditions (test 5) increased up to 9.83; 0.16 points by the end of experiment. Indicators of space orientation and proprioceptive sensitivity (test 6) improved and reached to the set conditions: girl students: 10.57; 1.27 and boy students accordingly: 21.43; 1.27 N ($p<0.05$). Indicators of dynamic body balance in passing of polygon's perimeter (test 7) in conditions of restricted support improved, in average, by 3 sec., comparing with initial time. For example, boy students showed time of passing of five polygon's perimeters for 20 second – 22.29; 1.97sec.; girl students a little worse: 24.43; 1.61 sec.

Persons, specializing in calisthenics improved quantity of perimeters' passing up to 3.29; 0.75 perimeters.

Thus, as a result of realization of academic programs on specialization, on general gymnastic and as a result of fulfillment of coordination training exercises, considering variation coefficients, the tested confidently ($p<0.05$) increased static-dynamic and static-kinetic body balance, comparing with initial indicators. Results of the research agree with tendency of sport science and practice, in which great attention is paid to development and perfection of static-dynamic body balance. In the world [5, 7, 11, 12, 13, 14, 15] there are successfully worked out and realized local programs of exercises, video-materials with application of such new technical means as SportKat, step-platforms, Body – Balance (exercises on mobile platforms), semi-spheres BOSU Balance Training and other fitness systems (for example like Sokker) [www.soccer.pm4]. Sportsmen have opportunity to develop surface muscles and deep muscles. For this purpose they fulfill different by structure exercises: twisting and bends of torso, arching of body, supporting by ball; long fixation of balance on mobile, narrowed and high platforms; they can train vestibular sensor system.

The prospects: perfection of methods and means of coordination training of those, who practice sport kinds of gymnastic in training process at all stages of sport perfection.

Conclusions:

1. In process of practical training of general gymnastic we registered insufficient level of NUPESU first year students' sensor motor coordination (students specialized in sport kinds of gymnastic).

2. We worked out program of coordination training for persons, specializing in sport kinds of gymnastic. This program consists of two parts. The first part is training of static-dynamic balance; the second part – vestibular training. The implemented in academic process program of exercises confidently improved sensor-motor coordination of persons, specializing in sport kinds of gymnastic ($p<0,05$).

3. Coordination training of persons, specializing in sport kinds of gymnastic (as new direction of realization of specific and preparatory exercises, developing and improvinf static-dynamic and static-kinetic balance) shall take one of priority places in physical education system and sport training.

Acknowledgement

The researches have been fulfilled in compliance with "Combined plan of scientific-research works in sphere of physical culture and sports for 2011-2015" of Ministry of Ukraine of family, youth and sports by topic 2.15 "Control of static-dynamic balance of sportsman's body and bodies' systems in sports with complex coordination" (state registration number 0111U001726). Scientific supervisor of the topic – doctor of pedagogic sciences, professor V.N. Boloban.

Conflict of interests

The authors declare that there is no conflict of interests.

References:

1 Boloban VN. *Reguliaciia pozy tela sportsmena* [Regulation of sportsman's body posture], Kiev: Olympic Literature; 2013. (in Russian)

2 Boloban VN. Sensomotornaia koordinaciia kak osnova tekhnicheskoj podgotovki [Sensor-motor coordination as the basis of technical fitness]. *Nauka v olimpijskom sporte* 2006;2:96 – 102. (in Russian)

3 Vel'diaev SV. *Metodika obucheniia rabochim osankam v uprazhneniiakh na perekladine. Cand. Diss.* [Methodic of training to working postures in exercises on horizontal bar Cand. Diss.], Volgograd; 1999. (in Russian)

4 Gaverdovskij IuK. *Teoriia i metodika sportivnoj trenirovki* [Theory and methodic of sport training], Moscow: Soviet sport; 2014. (in Russian)

5 Litvinenko Iu, Sadovski E, Nizhnikovski T, Boloban V. Biomekhanicheskaia kharakteristika statodinamicheskoj ustojchivosti sportsmenov vysokoj kvalifikacii [Bio-mechanical characteristic of elite sportsmen's balance]. *Nauka v olimpijskom sporte* 2014;4:74–78. (in Russian)

6 Maksimova IuA. *Profilaktika funkcional'nykh narushenij pozvonochnika iunykh akrobatov. Cand. Diss.* [Profilaktika funkcional'nykh narushenij pozvonochnika iunykh akrobatov], Kiev; 2013. (in Russian)

7 Platonov VN. *Sistema podgotovki sportsmenov v olimpijskom sporte* [System of sportsmen's training in Olympic sports], Kiev: Olympic Literature; 2004. (in Russian)

8 Tereschenko IA, Otsupok AP, Krupenio SV, Levchuk TM, Boloban VN. Evaluation of freshmen coordination abilities on practical training in gymnastics. *Physical Education of Students* 2013;3:60-71. http://dx.doi.org/10.6084/m9.figshare.663628

9 Tereshchenko IA, Otsupok AP, Krupenya SV, Liauchuk TM, Boloban VN. Sensomotor coordination, theoretical and physical (motor) preparedness of first year students of higher educational institutions of physical education and sport. *Physical Education of Students* 2013;6:88-95. http://dx.doi.org/10.6084/m9.figshare.840509

10 Bołoban W, Kuśmierczyk P, Szyper M. Sensor-motor coordination as indicator of students motor functioning's perfection at practical trainings [Sensomotoryczna koordynacja jako czynnik ukierunkowanych dzialań ruchowych studentów w zajęciach praktycznych]. *Pedagogics, psychology, medical – biological problems of physical training and sports* 2007;7:160–168. (in Polish)

11 Hoffman Jay R. *NSCA/s Guide to Program Design.* Human Kinetics; 2012.

12 Hrysomallis C, McLaughlin P, Goodman C. Relationship between statics and dynamic balance test among elite Australian footballers. *J. Sci. Med. Sport.* 2006;9(4):288–291.

13 Hrysomallis C. Relationship between Balance Ability, Training and Sports Lnjury Risk. *Sports Med.*2007;37(6):547–556.

14 Myer GD. The effect of plyometric versus dynamic stabilization and balance training on lower extremity biomechanics.*Am J. Sport Med.* 2006;34(3):445–455.

15 Sarabon N. Balance and Stability Training. In: Hoffman Jay R. *NSCA/s Guide to Program Design.* Human Kinetics; 2012.

16 Sadowski J, Boloban V, Wisniowski W. Equilibrium regulation by youth acrobats during selected exercises execution. *4th International Scientific Conference on kinesiology. "Science and Proffesion – Challenge for Future".* Zagreb, Croatia; 2005.

PHYSICAL CULTURE IN LIFE OF EASTERN-EUROPEAN REGION STUDENTS: MODERN STATE AND PROSPECTS OF DEVELOPMENT

Iermakov S.S., Cieślicka Mirosława, Muszkieta Radosław
Kazimierz Wielki University in Bydgoszcz, Poland

Abstract. *Purpose:* analysis of researches on physical culture problems among students in countries of Easter-European region (2013–2015). *Material:* As sources of information we chose data base of Russia, Poland and Ukraine. Besides, we used sites of the most known journals of Easter-European region. When choosing journals we based on rating of Russia (RISC), Poland (Index Copernicus) and Ukraine (bibliometryka of Ukrainian science) data bases. *Results:* thematic focus of researches on different physical education, sports and students health aspects was determined. The promising directions of researches are as follows: re-organization of system of students' physical education; interconnection of life quality and organism's resistance to environmental impacts; dependence of students' motor functioning on bad habits' presence; determination of factors, facilitating motivation for sport games in system of students' health related trainings; perceiving of life quality by disabled students; competence and professional skillfulness of specialists in physical culture and sports. *Conclusions:* it is recommended to use new, attractive forms of students' motor functioning. It is necessary to regulate students' motor functioning, considering motivation for success and for avoiding failures as well as to increase students' psycho-physiological stresses' resistance and to form students' culture of health.
Key words: student, health, physical culture, motivation, physical education.

Introduction

Practical realization of different scientific projects is important direction of physical culture and sports development in educational establishments. Some of such projects are implemented with governmental financial support. But main part of the projects is realized as initiative of educational establishments' teachers. All these, taken together, create certain scientific-research medium, which facilitates progress of physical culture – sports activity in educational establishments. Searching of ways to improve students' health, development of some kinds of sports, creation of favorable conditions for formation of youth's positive attitude to healthy life style, training of professional-applied skills of future specialists and other can be considered to be the main purpose of such researches. Demand in such works is conditioned by negative tendencies to worsening of students' health. Such tendencies are characteristic for all countries of Eastern-European region. Even in more developed countries of the region (for example in Poland) there is observed the same trend to worsening of students' health. Alongside with it, the countries of this region have many common problems, which concern development of physical culture and sports in youth medium.

It is necessary to note that countries of Eastern-European region (Ukraine, Poland, Russia, Belarus and Moldova) have equal climatic and geographic conditions. More than half of Ukrainian and Belarus territory, northern-eastern part of Poland and western part of Russia are still polluted with radiation, resulted from the accident on nuclear power plant (Ukraine, Chernobyl, 1986). This accident's after-effects have being continued to negatively influence on youth's health that requires consolidation of these countries' scientific researches in this direction. It pre-determines demand in coordination of appropriate scientific researches of scientists of these countries. All these, taken together, mark out Eastern-European countries from other countries of Europe.

Sports' development in students' medium of these countries takes place in close regional frontier cooperation of universities, institutes and academies. Characteristic feature of this region is presence of physical education departments in structure of higher educational establishments (with staff from 5 to 70 workers): approximately 300 departments in Ukraine, Poland, Russia and a little less in Belarus and Moldova. These educational establishments have discipline "Physical education" in their curriculums. In most of educational establishments this discipline is compulsory (2-4 hours a week). Now there appears a trend to making this discipline an optional one (Poland, Ukraine, Moldova and partially in Russia and Belarus). Besides, distinctive peculiarity of this region's countries is practice to conduct physical education classes, depending on students' health and their division into three health groups:

1) Main health group (consists of students, having no health problems);
2) Preparatory health group (students with insignificant health disorders); Подготовительная группа (студенты с незначительными отклонениями в уровне здоровья);
3) Special health group, consisting of students with disorders of health. From this group, the group of therapeutic physical culture is formed for students with pathologies and disabled students.

The countries of Eastern-European region have approximately equal system of coaches and teachers' training. This training if mainly conducted at faculties (or institutes) of physical education of pedagogic universities (approximately 15 in every country) and in specialized educational establishments of physical culture profile (approximately 6 in every country).The largest technical universities in these countries also deal with training of coaches, physical culture instructors and teachers (approximately 5 in every country). In sport competitions these educational establishments seriously compete with specialized physical culture educational establishments. Distinctive feature of this region's countries is two-step preparation of scientific staff: candidate of sciences (PhD) and doctor of sciences (PhD professor).

Finally, countries of Eastern-European region have the same problems in students' physical education, in protection and improvement of heir health, development of sports, training of scientific staff and other. Increased radiation pollution forces the scientists of these countries to search solution of problem of students' health improvement and protection. Scientific researches in these directions often duplicate each other. It results in unjustified financial losses and ineffective researchers' work in this countries. It should be noted that in this region Russian language is used: to large extent in Russia, Belarus and Ukraine and to less extent in Poland. It permits for most of scientists to communicate and present their works in easy to understand for them language. In this region there appear positive tendencies to use English in scientific sphere of educational establishments. That is why demand in concentration and coordination of scientific results of Easter-European scientists in solution of physical culture and sports problems in students' medium is evident.

Recent years researches, dealt with students' life quality and health, development of physical culture and sports in educational establishments, have been being oriented more on solution of applied tasks. Analysis of thematic focus of the researches witnesses about presence of same problems in countries of Eastern-European region in educational establishments' physical culture – sport functioning: Russia [51, 54, 55, 78, 82, 88, 100, 182 et al.); Ukraine (2–4, 86, 87, 103, 142–146, 152, 162, 189–191 и другие); Польша (65–67, 130, 147–149, 151, 157, 159–161 и другие); Belarus (50, 101, 111 et al.). It can be added with researches of scientists from neighboring countries: Lithuania (211). The authors researched wide circle of problems, which are characteristic for educational establishments of their countries and for all Eastern-European region. Most of information is concentrated in several data bases: Index Copernicus (Poland) RISC (Russia), National library of Ukraine (Ukraine). The other portion is elucidated in journals of these countries. Such distribution of information resources about scientific researches requires analysis of recent researches on physical culture and sports problems in students' medium. It will permit to mark out promising directions of these topics' development.

Purpose, tasks of the work, material and methods

The purpose of the work is analysis of researches on physical culture problems among students in countries of Easter-European region (2013–2015).

As sources of information we chose data base of Russia, Poland and Ukraine. Besides, we used sites of the most known journals of Easter-European region.

Results of the researches

The most interesting for analysis was journal "Physical education of students" (http://www.sportedu.org.ua), which is in the data base of Russia (RISC), Poland (Index Copernicus) and Ukraine (bibliometryka of Ukrainian science) (see tables 1,2,3). This journal to the largest extent presents researches' results, devoted to problems of students'; physical culture and sports. The journal takes leading positions by citation. In rating Index Copernicus the journal goes just after publications, which have impact factor.

Table 1. Rating of journals in RISC data base (Physical culture and sports; 64 journals in total) for 2014 by indicator SCIENCE INDEX (http://elibrary.ru)

№	Name of journal	Indicator
1.	Equine and horse riding	0,195
2.	Sports; economic, law, management	0,178
3.	Theory and Practice of Physical Culture	0,177
4.	Bulletin of sport science	0,133
5.	Physical culture: cultivation, education, training	0,132
6.	**Physical Education of Students**	**0,127**

Table 2. Rating of journals in Index Copernicus data base (Sciences about sports; in total 27 journals were indexed; other have no indices) for 2013 by indicator ICV (http://www.indexcopernicus.com)

№№	Journal	ISNN	Country	ICV 2013
1.	Archives of Budo	1643-8698	Poland	16.04
2.	Biology of Sport	0860-021X	Poland	13.74
3.	**Physical Education of Students**	**2308-7250**	**Ukraine**	**7.60**

Table 3. Rating of journals in data base "Bibliometryka of Ukrainian science" (TOP 200, all sciences) for 2010–2014 by indicator h5 (http://nbuviap.gov.ua)

Item number	Journal	Index h5
10	Theory and methodic of physical education	14
14	**Physical Education of Students**	**13**
23	Pedagogics, psychology, medical-biological problems of physical training and sports	11

The researches for 2013–2015 are presented by Ukrainian authors (70%) and by authors from other countries (30%). Thematic focus of the researches is presented by articles about different aspects of physical education, sports, and students' health. Topics cover also adjacent areas: bio-mechanics, kinesiology, medicine, psychology, sociology, technology of sport equipment. Besides, topics include researches of effectiveness of trainings and sport selection, workability, health protection and other interdisciplinary directions (see fig. 1).

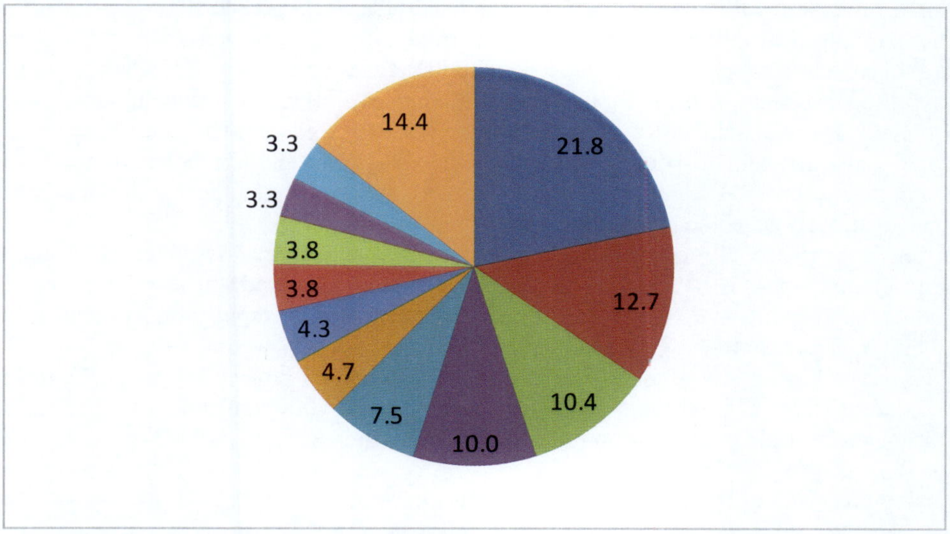

Fig.1. Topics of scientific researches of students' physical culture and sports problems, %:
1–Health and life quality, 21.8%; 2–Physical education, 12.7%; 3–Sport games, 10.4%; 4–Martial arts, 10.0%; 5–Acrobatic, gymnastic, kinds of aerobics, 7.5%; 6–Power kinds of sports, 4.7%; 7–Biomechanics, 4.3%; 8–Psychological problems, 3.8%; 9–Water and winter kinds of sports, 3.8%; 10–Cadets' training, 3.3%; 11–Teachers' training, 3.3%; 12–The rest, 14.4%.

The highest quantity of researches is presented in direction "Health and life quality" (21.8%). Authors determined general and specific components of health: motor functioning [111, 114, 123, 197–199, 207, 208]; motivation [57, 64, 68]; morphological-functional state [29]; psychological state [69, 91]; self-assessment [28, 99, 112, 163, 118–121, 135] and etc. The authors render specific recommendations on increasing of health and life quality indicators [52, 53, 56, 58].

Among above listed works there are works, characterizing modern students:

1) Absolute majority of students have resilience indicators high or within norm [140];
2) Dynamic of students' physical workability depends on period of student's studying in university. During all academic week physical condition changes are typical for first and second year students. Concerning third year students, the curve of dynamic workability has descending character. In senior students it has ascending – descending character [156];
3) Alternation and equal correlation of motor elements and sport game elements increase general level of somatic health, cardio-vascular system's functional state, self-feeling, activity and emotional state of students [82];
4) Possibility of students' division into groups by indicators of functional shifts in extreme situations is shown. The most important indicators are quickness and accuracy of psycho-physiological tests passing with different modes of signal supply as well as functional shifts before fulfillment of exercise of extreme character [87].

Among other works we can mark out researches, oriented on increasing of life quality indicators [158, 165–170, 172].

The promising direction of further researches in this direction we can consider the works, which pay attention to the following:

–Changes in social-economic way of students' life [148];
– Re-organization of students' physical education system;
– Interconnection of life quality and organism's resistance to external impacts [123];

– Interconnection of parameters of subjective life quality assessment and the factors of its formation depending on specialization; revelation of negative tendencies to reduction of students' life quality; dependence between motor functioning, positive attitude to own life quality and presence of bad habits, irrational eating, psychic overloads on students' organism [90];

– Application of new, attractive forms of physical functioning: sailing [160], rock-climbing [85, 164], hiking [34, 194]; cheer dance [155], cheer leading [108, 117], shaping [179], aerobic [15, 28, 186, 188], aqua fitness [139], sport and ballroom dances [134, 183]; some kinds of sport martial arts [13, 72, 111, 201].

In general structure of the researches "Physical education" took 12.7%.

Authors give recommendations on the following problems of students' physical education:

1) Motor functioning directly influences on students' educational progress and morbidity. Original technology of regulation of students' motor functioning on the base of control over their independent physical trainings is offered. It is recommended to practice independent training for not less than 15 minutes a day (in the morning, day and in the evening) with periodicity of not less than 3-4 times a week [55];
2) Motivation for physical culture practicing results from different demands: demand in motion, demand in fulfillment of student's obligations, demand in competition functioning. It is offered to use game and competition methods: setting of certain, feasible for a student, training tasks; usage of sufficient number of sport equipment of proper quality; urge of students to independent physical exercises through system if encouragement [39];
3) It is offered to use a system of specific forms of trainings' organization, which would meet humanistic principle "to urge but not to force". The function of such methods shall imply reconstruction of students' motivational sphere and adequately accepted by them purpose of functioning [78];
4) It was found that specially organized elective trainings on three disciplines (Pedagogic anthropology, Personality-oriented physical education, Creative valueology) formed sufficient volume of knowledge in undergraduate students. Some problems of innovative technologies' application in students' theoretical and practical trainings were outlined [17–19];

Among other researches we can note the following works: training of power abilities [171], pedagogic control of students' physical condition [11, 12], formation of personalities' physical culture of students [16, 131], individualization of physical education process [14], optimization of physical education [76, 77, 124–126, 129, 136], sport-oriented physical education [35, 133].

The promising direction of further researches in this direction we can consider the works, which pay attention to the following:

– Changes of students', having bad habits, functional indicators [141];

– Regulation of students' motor functioning, considering motivation for success and avoiding failures [49];

– Personality-oriented approach [18].

Direction of trainings "Sport games" took 10.4% in total structure of the researches.

Authors give recommendations on increasing of students' sportsmanship: basketball [27, 86, 150, 176, 180, 181]; baseball [6]; volleyball [36, 210]; handball [47]; tennis [43, 65, 83, 173]; football [1, 20, 59, 113, 200]; hockey [89]. The authors accentuate attention on consideration of peculiarities of different sides of students-sportsmen's training, considering specificities of educational environment in educational establishment, specific features of students' competitions (Universiades, students' leagues on kinds of sport games).

The authors render the following recommendations on students' sport games:

1) Analysis of basketball throws' accuracy, basketball players' logical thinking and depth of perception. It was found that ability to think logically and certain depth of perception were two main variables. These variables influence on deviations in basketball players' throw accuracy [176].
2) It was shown that the offered simulation methods permit to form optimal orientation of training process with application of specialized means at different stages of year cycle of volleyball players' training [36].
3) Analysis of different qualification female handball players' selection through interconnection of psycho-physical parameters showed that elite sportswomen are characterized by average and high degree of dependence of competition functioning successfulness on space perception indicators, on logical and space thinking [47].
4) The researches permitted to find the following correlation of rugby players' special physical training: September – special endurance is accentuated (100% of training time); October – special endurance (70%), power endurance (20%), training of strength (10%); November – accordingly 50, 30, 20%; December – 30, 40, 30% [137].

The promising direction of further researches in this direction we can consider the works, which pay attention to the following:

– Inviting of sportsmen to educational establishments;

– Mechanisms of educational establishment's interest in development of students' sports;

– Creation of conditions for combination of academic studies with trainings of sportsmen;

– Determination of factors, facilitating motivation for sport games in system of students' health related trainings [59].

Among other researches we can note the works, devoted to practicing of sport games by disabled students [180]. It should be added with researches of problems of women football teams' training [60], students' involvement in refereeing of sport games' competitions [20,113].

Direction "Martial arts took 10 % in total structure of the researches.

The authors render the following recommendations on improvement of students' sportsmanship in the following kinds of martial arts: arm wrestling [142–146, 204], boxing [7, 73, 74, 114, 115], freestyle wrestling [25], Greco-Roman wrestling [195], Judo [66], Kick boxing [177], Thae quan do [67, 132], fencing [26, 105], other kinds [95–97].

The authors note that it is necessary to attract students to different kinds of martial arts and underline health related significance of sport martial arts.

Among the most interesting researches we would like to mark out solution of the following problems:

1) Working out of system of sportsmen's training individualization. In this case system is simulated as combination of elements and subsystems, which mutually, in controlled way, facilitate revelation, formation, development and perfection of personal martial art style [98].
2) It was found that hand dynamometry is an important and informative criterion, which determines arm wrestling training. Such criterion is characterized by maximal system-formation contribution [114].
3) It was shown that increase of sportsmanship reflects in rising of blows' density in duel. Innovations in competitions rules resulted in high intensity of combat actions in boxing. Attacking actions are fulfilled with rater higher quickness [115].
4) It was found that final part of competitions is the most informative for assessment of wrestlers' technical tactic abilities. It is determined by efficiency, effectiveness, quantity of attacks, technical arsenal. It was shown that wrestlers shall conduct duel at rapid rate. It is recommended to use movements, pulls, pushes as well as to make 1-2 actual attempts to fulfill definite technique [196].

The promising direction of further researches in this direction we can consider the works, which pay attention to the following:

1) Substantiation of approaches to development of future specialists' assertiveness by martial arts' means (sambo and judo). Means of sport martial arts are described as tools of personality's qualities training in future specialists. Potentials of assertiveness formation by martial arts' means are determined [72].
2) Analysis of different aspects of students' resistance to psycho-physiological stresses at martial arts trainings is presented. Specificity of individual psychologically-oriented methodology in modern system of martial arts is elucidated as well as its usage at physical education trainings. It is noted that the most destructive factors are excessive psychogenic stresses, caused by unfavorable psychological factors. Psychogenic stress influence in the most destructive way on health. It is the main reason of students' morbidity. Authors recommend didactically literally worked out methodic of prophylaxis [201].
3) Authors give analysis of cadets' endurance and workability rising by means of martial arts. As exercises for special endurance they recommend: throws of partner with high intensity; throws in average temp; training duels [8, 9].

"Acrobatic, gymnastic, different kinds of aerobics" took 7.5% [10, 84, 109, 110].

The authors give recommendations on the following problems:

1) Influence of health related aerobics on girls' motor fitness [175].
2) Dozing of physical loads at girl students' aerobic trainings [15].
3) Assessment of pedagogical HEEs girl students' communicative skills resulted from aerobic trainings [188].
4) Application of highly intensive training means at health related aerobic trainings [28].
5) Training of girl students' physical condition at extra curriculum cheer dance sessions [155].
6) Development of pedagogic college girl students' quickness and endurance under influence of cheer leading [117].
7) Interconnection of general and special physical fitness indicators of students cheer leaders at stage of specialized basic training [108].

The authors note high motivation of girls for health related trainings with dance exercises. Such authors' position is a **perspective direction** of organization of girl students' different motor functioning kinds.

Other researches are presented in the following directions:

1) Power kinds of sports (4.7%) [42, 102, 153, 154, 178, 185, 202, 203, 209];
2) Bio-mechanics (4.3%) [127, 128];
3) Psychological problems (3.8%) [21, 45, 46];
4) Water and winter kinds of sports (3.8%) [174];
5) Training of cadets (3.3%) [33, 44, 94];
6) Training of teacher (3.3%) [62, 63, 187];
7) Other researches (14.4%) [22, 24, 70, 71, 104, 106, 107, 116, 192, 193];

Among them researchers, devoted to protection and strengthening of students' health [29-32, 37, 48, 75, 122], and training of physical condition [79–81, 92, 93, 184, 205] can be marked out.

The promising directions in this case can be solution of the following problems with the help of modern means of health bio mechanical indicators' registration:

1) It was found that 63,3% with normal posture were in risk zone. Students with worsened posture's bio-geometric profile (scoliosis posture - 43,33%; round back– 23, 33%; slouching back– 22, 73%) got in the so-called pre-morbid state of muscular skeletal apparatus [38].
2) Quantitative indicators of bio-dynamic and coordination structure of motor qualities during aerobic training are determined. Bio-mechanical models are offered for control of motor fitness and prognostication of results [186].
3) It was found that there is objective demand in studying of bio-mechanical characteristics of free style wrestlers' technique. Such approach is required for further development of technology of athletes' sport technique formation at stage of initial basic training [206].

Ensuring of disabled students' life quality shall be considered to be **promising direction of researches:**

1) The researches proved that practicing of sports by disabled persons influence positively on their life quality. Research of aspect of life quality perception is a complex problem, but it deserves proper attention and appropriate efforts [23, 138].
2) Also organizational-methodic priorities of disabled students' physical education and sports were revealed. Application of physical education model permits their complete integration in students' medium. Students feel themselves more comfortable. They change their attitude to themselves. It is reflected in adequate perception, in finding certain masking of disability, in self presentation. The authors showed effectiveness of didactic technology of disabled students' physical education in pedagogic process [5].

Training of future teachers is not less important as well as their physical condition. In this aspect we can mark out the following problems:

1) Formation of future teacher's culture of health [61];
2) Emotional competence of future physical culture teachers [161];
3) Methodological requirements of competence approach in hiking education of future teachers [40, 41];
4) Competence and professional skillfulness of specialists in physical culture [182].

Discussion

Analysis of publications on problems of physical culture and sports in students' medium shows that most of scientists' recommendations remain out of higher educational teachers' and coaches' attention. There can be several reasons to this fact:

1) Level and quality of trainings of teachers themselves as well as their unwillingness to use modern technologies of students' health improvement in their practice.
2) Students' low motivation for physical culture and sports practicing in their every day life.
3) Insufficient material-technical provisioning of training sites as well as insufficient financing of physical culture and sports.
4) Students' overloading in week academic program. Transition from 36 hours' week to 30 hours' did not influence noticeably on students' activity.
5) Changes in higher educational establishments' curriculums, in which discipline "Physical culture" became an optional one.

The situation can be changed by proper organization of students' military patriotic education, application of more attractive physical functioning forms, usage of motivation approaches, implementation of encouragement and rating system in functioning of teachers and student.

It should be noted that it is necessary to use the above mentioned promising researches in scientific work of higher educational establishments. All these, taken together, will facilitate formation of teachers' positive attitude to their works and students' – to their health.

Conclusions

We can relate the following works to possible promising in the future researches:

1) Re-organization of students' physical education system.
2) New attractive forms of students' physical functioning.
3) Regulation of students' physical functioning, considering motivation for success and avoiding failures.
4) Inviting of students-sportsmen in educational establishments.
5) Mechanisms of educational establishments' interest in development of students' sports.
6) Creation of conditions for combination of academic classes with sport trainings for sportsmen.
7) Determination of factors, facilitating increasing of motivation for sport games in system of students' health related trainings.
8) Strengthening of students' resistance to psycho-physiological stresses.
9) Perception of life quality by disabled students.

10) Formation of student's culture of health.
11) Competence and professionalism of specialists in sphere of physical culture and sports.

Conflict of interests

The authors declare that there is no conflict of interests.

References:

1. Abdula AB, Lebedev SI. Features of physiological responses on organism of football players aged 10–12 years in exercise using different training methods. *Physical education of students*, 2014;1:3–8.
2. Adashevskiy VM, Iermakov SS, Firsova IuIu. Physical mathematical modelling of difficult elements of acrobatic rock-and-roll. *Physical education of students*, 2013;3:3–11.
3. Adashevskiy VM, Iermakov SS, Korzh NV, Muszkieta Radoslaw, Prusik Krzysztof, Cieslicka Miroslawa. Biomechanical study athletes' movement techniques in the hurdles (on example of phase of flight). *Physical education of students*, 2014;4:3–12.
4. Adashevskiy VM, Iermakov SS, Marchenko AA. Biomechanics aspects of technique of high jump. *Physical education of students*, 2013;2:11–18.
5. Adyrkhaev SG. Optimization of physical education and sports of students with disabilities throughout the entire period of study at the university. *Physical education of students*, 2013;6:3–8.
6. Agapov DV, Krovykov VF, Boyko UG, Hodorchenko VM. Method of estimation of technical preparedness level of baseballs aged 12–14 years. *Physical education of students*, 2013;2:3–11.
7. Aksutin VV, Korobeynikov GV. Study of special capacity in boxers with different styles of fight. *Physical education of students*, 2014;5:3–7. http://dx.doi.org/10.15561/20755279.2014.0501
8. Alekseev NA, Kutergin NB, Kulinichev AN, Gorbatenko AV. Integrated method development of general and special students stamina involved in the fight. *Physical education of students*, 2014;3:3–9.
9. Alekseev NA, Kutergin NB, Kulinichev AN. Perfection of physical training of students and listeners of educational establishments of Ministry of Internal Affairs of Russia. *Physical education of students*, 2013;1:3–7.
10. Bachinskaya NV. Features of construction of structures in long-term training acrobatics at the modern stage. *Physical education of students*, 2015;1:3–10. http://dx.doi.org/10.15561/20755279.2015.0101
11. Balamutova NM, Shyryaeva SV . Study of special performance and volume training loadings at swimmers in the year preparation. *Physical education of students*, 2014;1:8–13.
12. Balamutova NM. Pedagogical control of students' physical state after research results of cardiovascular system functional indicators. *Physical education of students*, 2013;1:7–12.
13. Baljinder Singh Bal. Impact of short-term Bhastrika Pranayama on respiratory parameters: an ancient practice with contemporary significance. *Physical education of students*, 2015;3:66–73. http://dx.doi.org/10.15561/20755279.2015.0308
14. Barybina LN, Kolomiec NA, Komotskaja VA. The application of the algorithm of the individualization of students' physical education process. *Physical education of students*, 2014;6:3–7. http://dx.doi.org/10.15561/20755279.2014.0601
15. Beliak YuI, Zinchenko NM. Dosing method of physical activity in aerobics classes for students. *Physical education of students*, 2014;5:8–13. http://dx.doi.org/10.15561/20755279.2014.0502
16. Belykh SI, Chernigovskaia SA. About forming of personality physical culture of students in the process of physical education (in aspect of athletic activity). *Physical education of students*, 2013;2:18–25.
17. Belykh SI. Estimation of efficiency of experimental model of optimization of teaching of students of faculty of physical education. *Physical education of students*, 2013;5:3–13.
18. Belykh SI. Methodological foundations of individually oriented approaches to ground of physical education unprofessional university students. *Physical education of students*, 2013;3:11–18.
19. Belykh SI. Structure of the concept of personality oriented physical education university students. *Physical education of students*, 2013;4:3–10.
20. Berezka SM, Chopilko TG. An investigation of individual functionality football referees qualifications. *Physical education of students*, 2014;6:8–12. http://dx.doi.org/10.15561/20755279.2014.0602
21. Bilichenko EA. Gender aspects of personal and motivational sphere of students to physical education and sport. *Physical education of students*, 2013;6:8–15.
22. Bobrovnik VI, Tykhonenko YP. Improvement of strength capacities of middle-distance runners as the major factor of achieving high sports results at the stage of maximal realization of individual capabilities. *Physical education of students*, 2014;3:9–18.
23. Bolach Bartosz, Prystupa Tetyana. Evaluation of perception of quality of life of disabled athletes. *Physical education of students*, 2014;1:13–17.
24. Bondar TS. Classification of physical education of adolescent by subjects of pedagogical influence. *Physical education of students*, 2013;3:18–22.

25. Boyko VF, Malinsky II, Andriitsev VA, Yaremenko VV. Competitive activity of highly skilled freestyle wrestlers at the present stage. *Physical education of students*, 2014;4:13–19.
26. Briskin YA, Pityn MP, Zadorozhnaya OR. Structure and content of fencers' theoretical training. *Physical education of students*, 2013;4:10–15.
27. Brynzak SS, Krasnov VP . Role of force training in physical training of student basketball team players. *Physical education of students*, 2013;5:13–18.
28. Bryukhanova NA, Bulgakova OV, Mokrova TI, Bogashchenko YA. Determination of possibilities of the use of high-intensive trainings facilities on lessons health aerobics. *Physical education of students*, 2013;2:25–30.
29. Bukov UA, Georgieva NG. The ways of teaching process optimization in physical education of the students' special medical group. *Physical education of students*, 2013;3:22–26.
30. Cherednychenko MA, Artemieva GP. Special physical preparation of athletes in motor sport during testing methods basic training level of preparedness for competitive athlete load. *Physical education of students*, 2014;2:46–50.
31. Chernenko S A. Description of how the specialization influences the dynamics of the functional and motor abilities among the third to fifth year male student. *Physical education of students*, 2014;1:50–56.
32. Chovgan RYa, Ivanishyn IM, Prezliata AV. Level of development of the physical components of social activity schoolchildren 10–11 years children summer camp. *Physical education of students*, 2014;2:50–56.
33. Danylchenko VA, Khabinets TA. Typical mistakes, made by the cadets, mastering the submission locks, of the higher educational establishments of the Ministry of Internal Affairs of Ukraine. *Physical education of students*, 2014;4:20–25.
34. Denisenko IA. The peculiarities of functional state changes of cardiovascular system of girls at the age 18–19 years in the process of practicing sport and health tourism. *Physical education of students*, 2013;5:32–37.
35. Dolinnyj UA, Olejnik ON, Sorokin US, Homenko AA. Physical education of students from sports-oriented technologies. *Physical education of students*, 2013;5:37–41.
36. Doroshenko EIu. Model parameters of technical and tactical actions in the competitive activities of volleyball players. *Physical education of students*, 2013;5:41–46.
37. Drogomeretsky VV, Kondakov VL, Gorelov AA. Application of improving swimming to the correction of joint and ligament students. *Physical education of students*, 2013;5:46–55.
38. Dudko MV. Characteristic of bio-geometric profile of students' posture and physical fitness in process of physical education. *Physical education of students*, 2015;4:10–16. http://dx.doi.org/10.15561/20755279.2015.0402
39. Dudnyk IO. Formation of positive motivation as the basis of students will qualities' perfection in physical culture practicing. *Physical education of students*, 2015;3:3–9. http://dx.doi.org/10.15561/20755279.2015.0301
40. Dudorova LJ. Conceptual approaches to vocational and tourism training of teachers in higher education institutions. *Physical education of students*, 2013;4:19–23.
41. Dudorova LJ. Methodological requirements of the competitive approach in tourist formation of the future teachers. *Physical education of students*, 2014;2:13–18.
42. Dzhym VYu. Peculiarities of perfection of training process of the qualified bodybuilder in the competitive period.. *Physical education of students*, 2015;1:11–16. http://dx.doi.org/10.15561/20755279.2015.0102
43. Emshanova YO. Comparative analysis of individual peculiarities for tennis players of different qualification. *Physical education of students*, 2013;4:23–27.
44. Evtushov FM. Features of organization and extra-curricular classes on the subject "Special physical education" with the cadets of higher educational establishments of Ministry of Internal Affairs of Ukraine. *Physical education of students*, 2013;1:27–30.
45. Fatemeh Eloon Kashkuli, Mehrdad Moharramzadeh, Sohrab Ghalehgir. The role of advertisement factors in development of sport tourism industry of fars province . *Physical education of students*, 2014;3:61–67.
46. Feuerman VV. Influence of socio-philosophical and spiritual values on the formation of social orientation and physical health specialists the sphere of physical culture and sports. *Physical education of students*, 2014;2:41–46.
47. Frolova LS, Glazirin ID, Petrenko YO, Suprunovich VO, Menshikh EE, Kharchenko IA, Pivnenko AO. Effect of psychophysical state on different qualification's handball players on their preparedness. *Physical education of students*, 2013;3:72–75.
48. Futornyi SM. Problem of shortage of motor activity students. *Physical education of students*, 2013;3:75–80.
49. Gavrishova EV, Gorelov AA. On the regulation of motor activity of students with the motivation to achieve success and avoid failure. *Physical education of students*, 2013;5:18–25.
50. Gerasevich AN, Shytov LA, Shytova EM, Bokovets VS, Schenovsky YI, Gmir TA, Parkhots EG. Comparative characteristics of the separate morphological and functional state indicators of the organism of modern students (Part 1). *Physical education of students*, 2013;5:25–32.
51. Goginava SE, Rumba OG. On improving effect combining aerobic and anaerobic loads of character in the classroom for physical training in universities. *Physical education of students*, 2014;3:18–30.

52. Gordieieva MV. Perfection of hoe-type motions of sportswomen specialized in synchronous swimming in base positions of compulsory exercise. *Physical education of students*, 2013;2:30–35.
53. Gordienko YV. Theoretical training in physical education of higher educational establishments' girl students. *Physical education of students*, 2015;4:3–9. http://dx.doi.org/10.15561/20755279.2015.0401
54. Gorelov AA, Kondakov VL, Belikova ZhA. About necessity of use of Hatha Yoga exercises for correction of deformation of students' spine of special medical groups with violations of posture. *Physical education of students*, 2013;2:35–45.
55. Gorelov AA, Kondakov VL, Usatov AN. To the question about the use of independent physical training in educational space of modern higher institute. *Physical education of students*, 2013;1:17–27.
56. Grad Rafal. Physical activity and leisure time among 13–15-year-old teenagers living in Biala Podlaska. *Physical education of students*, 2013;2:74–80.
57. Grygus IM, Kucher TV. Optimizing the level of the physical health of the students with a glance of the type of autonomic nervous system. *Physical education of students*, 2013;3:26–31.
58. Hamid Mohebbi, Abdulbaset Maroofi, Nazanin Anasri, Aboozar Jorbonian. The effects of stretching exercise on hemodynamic responses and post-exercise hypotension in normotensive women students. *Physical education of students*, 2014;5:53–58. http://dx.doi.org/10.15561/20755279.2014.0510
59. Hotenceva EV, Shpichka TA. The motivation for playing football among students. *Physical education of students*, 2013;3:80–84.
60. Huzar VN, Shalar OG, Norik AO. Relationship as an aspect of psychological climate of women's soccer team. *Physical education of students*, 2014;2:8–13.
61. Iermakova TS. Forming a health culture of future teachers in Polish educational establishments. *Physical education of students*, 2014;5:14–19. http://dx.doi.org/10.15561/20755279.2014.0503
62. Ilnitskaya AS, Kozina ZhL, Barybina LN, Kolomiez NA, Cieslicka Miroslawa, Stankiewicz Blazej, Pilewska Wieslawa. Author's internet blog as information and communication technologies in the educational space within the physical education students. *Physical education of students*, 2014;1:22–27.
63. Ilnitskaya AS, Kozina ZhL, Lakhno E G, Ilnitskaya LV, Cieslicka, Miroslawa, Stankiewicz Blazej, Pilewska Wieslawa. Students' attitude to the possibility of applying modern information and communication technologies in the educational process in physical education. *Physical education of students*, 2014;2:18–25.
64. Ivaskiene VP, Skyriene VV, Markevicius VZ. Comparative analysis of prestart condition of students girls in Olympic and non-Olympic kinds of sport. *Physical education of students*, 2013;4:27–31.
65. Jagiello M, Jagiello W. Final preparations to the girls' tennis Europe junior masters. *Physical education of students*, 2014;5:59–64. http://dx.doi.org/10.15561/20755279.2014.0511
66. Jagiello Wladyslaw, Dornowski Marcin, Wolska Beata. Basic technical skills (throws) in 17–19-year-old judokas. *Physical education of students*, 2014;6:77–80. http://dx.doi.org/10.15561/20755279.2014.0615
67. Jagiello Wladyslaw, Kozina ZhL, Jagiello Marina. Somatic aspects of sports championship in taekwon-do ITF. *Physical education of students*, 2015;4:51–55. http://dx.doi.org/10.15561/20755279.2015.0408
68. Kazem Sotoode, Bahman Mirzaei, Farhad Rahmani-Nia. Influence of upper-body exercise order on muscle damage in untrained men. *Physical education of students*, 2013;5:100–108.
69. Kazem Sotoodeh, Aliakbar Alizadeh, Bahman Mirzaei. The comparison of three type of exercise sequence on maximum strength in untrained young men. *Physical education of students*, 2014;5:65–69. http://dx.doi.org/10.15561/20755279.2014.0512
70. Kedrovskiy BG, Shalar OG, Grinevich AV . Understanding of coaches with young athletes. *Physical education of students*, 2013;4:31–35.
71. Kholodova OS. Modeling of competitive activity of skilled athletes specialized at 1500 m distance on short-track skating. *Physical education of students*, 2013;5:93–100.
72. Khripunova LD. To the question of the formation of personal qualities of future doctors by means of combat sports. *Physical education of students*, 2014;5:43–47. http://dx.doi.org/10.15561/20755279.2014.0508
73. Kiprych SV, Donets AV, Makhdi Omar Ali. Improvement of management by training process of boxers at a stage of direct preparation for competitions. *Physical education of students*, 2013;6:20–25.
74. Kiprych SV. Control system improvement of qualified boxers based assessment system change reaction cardiorespiratory during the immediate preparation for competition. *Physical education of students*, 2014;4:26–31.
75. Klimatskaya L G. Physical activity students and university professors as leaders of health. *Physical education of students*, 2013;3:31–35.
76. Kolokoltsev MM, Ambartsumyan RA. Improving physical health international students enrolled in a technical college in Baikal region. *Physical education of students*, 2014;1:34–39.
77. Kolokoltsev MM, Cieslicka Miroslawa, Muszkieta Radoslaw. Optimization of physical training of students of high school with regard to quantitative features muscular components of their bodies. *Physical education of students*, 2015;1:17–21. http://dx.doi.org/10.15561/20755279.2015.0103

78. Kondakov VL, Kopeikina EN, Balysheva NV, Usatov AN, Skrug DA. Causes of declining interest of students to employment physical education and sports. *Physical education of students*, 2015;1:22–30. http://dx.doi.org/10.15561/20755279.2015.0104
79. Konovalov VV, Kirpenko VN, Marakushyn AI, Poddubny AG. Grounds of optimum level of development of basic physical qualities which provide high level the functional state of students in the period of flying training. *Physical education of students*, 2013;5:55–60.
80. Korobeynikov GV, Drojjin VU. The prevention programs of physical rehabilitation for chernobyl disaster survivors. *Physical education of students*, 2013;1:78–82.
81. Kovalenko SO, Nechyporenko DL. Application of biological feedback for estimation of anaerobic performance in jumping test. *Physical education of students*, 2014;5:20–24. http://dx.doi.org/10.15561/20755279.2014.0504
82. Kovaleva MV, Rumba OG. Active games in physical education students of special medical group with limited capacity of cardiovascular system. *Physical education of students*, 2013;4:35–46.
83. Kozak A M, Ibraimova M V. Construction of training process of tennis players aged 5–6 years, taking into account the specifics of the development and control of their coordination skills. *Physical education of students*, 2014;6:17–23. http://dx.doi.org/10.15561/20755279.2014.0604
84. Kozhanova OS. Compatibility of sportswomen at selection in commands on group exercises of artistic gymnastics accounting their functional condition. *Physical education of students*, 2013;1:33–37.
85. Kozina Zh, Ryepko OA, Prusik Krzysztof, Prusik Katarzyna, Cieslicka Miroslawa. Theoretical-methodological study of development of power-speed in climbing. *Physical education of students*, 2014;1:27–34.
86. Kozina ZhL, Sobko IN, Prokopenko AI, Guba AV, Iermakov SS, Prusik Krzysztof, Cieslicka Miroslawa. Methods of technical and tactical training basketball players with hearing impairments using innovative technologies. *Physical education of students*, 2014;3:30–40.
87. Kozina ZL, Iermakov SS. Analysis of students' nervous system's typological properties, in aspect of response to extreme situation, with the help of multi-dimensional analysis. *Physical education of students*, 2015;3:10–19. http://dx.doi.org/10.15561/20755279.2015.0302
88. Kramida I E. Exercises for students of different medical groups as factors of the weakening bad habits at students. *Physical education of students*, 2013;4:46–51.
89. Kugayevskiy SO. Innovative ways of special endurance of skaters in the competition period. *Physical education of students*, 2013;4:51–55.
90. Kulthickiy ZI, Kurko YaV. Analysis of the main parameters of quality of students' life of different specialties. *Physical education of students*, 2013;6:25–30.
91. Kurmaeva EV. Fitness - programs as mean of forming of personality physical culture of students. *Physical education of students*, 2013;1:37–40.
92. Kutek TB. Application of hardwares in the process of training of skilled sportswomen. *Physical education of students*, 2013;5:60–65.
93. Kutek TB. Features special physical readiness of the qualified jumpers from the takeoff. *Physical education of students*, 2015;2:3–7. http://dx.doi.org/10.15561/20755279.2015.0201
94. Kutergin NB, Tkachenko AI, Kulinichev AN. Physical perfection of students of educational institutions law enforcement by means of outdoor games. *Physical education of students*, 2013;6:30–34.
95. Latyshev SV, Korobeynikov GV. Approach of the systems to problem of individualization of training of fighters. *Physical education of students*, 2013;5:65–69.
96. Latyshev SV. Individualization program training in freestyle wrestling. *Physical education of students*, 2013;6:34–38.
97. Latyshev SV. The development of assessment scales of physical training of wrestlers at the stage of basic specialized training. *Physical education of students*, 2013;4:55–59.
98. Latyshev SV. Theoretical bases of individualization of training in wrestling. *Physical education of students*, 2013;2:45–49.
99. Lazarenko MG. Pedagogical aspects of effective use of simulator "Straps with ring" during the formation motor skills of pupils of 10 classes during the skiing training in the lessons of physical culture. *Physical education of students*, 2014;6:24–28. http://dx.doi.org/10.15561/20755279.2014.0605
100. Leyfa AV. The social basis of the development of physical activity of students in terms of their quality of life. *Physical education of students*, 2013;3:35–42.
101. Lisowski VO, Mihuta IYu. Importance of coordination skills essential psychophysical demonstrated competencies as a military specialists. *Physical education of students*, 2013;6:38–43.
102. Litvinenko AM. Efficiency of application of means of sports preparation of combat sportsmen in physical training of students of technical high school. *Physical education of students*, 2013;2:49–54.

103. Litvinenko YV, Niznikowski Tomasz, Boloban VN. Evaluation of the kinematic structure of indicators key elements of sports equipment exercise by postural orientation movements. *Physical education of students*, 2014;6:29–36. http://dx.doi.org/10.15561/20755279.2014.0606
104. Liu Yong Qiang. Operative correction of judoists' training loads on the base of on-line monitoring of heart beats rate. *Physical education of students*, 2015;2:13–21. http://dx.doi.org/10.15561/20755279.2015.0203
105. Lopatenko GO, Tumanova VN, Gatsko EV. Application of mobilizing extra-training means in process of pre-start martial arts sportsmen's training (on example of fencing). *Physical education of students*, 2015;2:8–12. http://dx.doi.org/10.15561/20755279.2015.0202
106. Lotfali Bolboli, Navid Lotfi, Mostafa Bagheri, Ali Rajabi. Evaluation and comparison of VO2max assessment models in high school students. *Physical education of students*, 2013;2:80–83.
107. Lutovinov IuA, Martin VD, Oleshko VG, Lisenko VN, Tkachenko KV. Physical development, the level of physical and technical preparedness of 14 – 15 year old young weightlifters of different weight categories groups. *Physical education of students*, 2014;5:25–29. http://dx.doi.org/10.15561/20755279.2014.0505
108. Lutsenko LS, Bodrenkova IA. Correlation of general and special physical training of athletes cheerleaders at the stage the specialized training base. *Physical education of students*, 2013;6:43–50.
109. Lyulina NV, Zakharova LV, Vetrova IV. Effect of complex acrobatic elements in the development of physical skills of preschool children. *Physical education of students*, 2013;4:59–63.
110. Makarova OV. Quantitative estimation of the state of vault feet gymnasts on the different stages of the long-term training. *Physical education of students*, 2013;5:69–73.
111. Maksimuk OV, Vrublevskiy EP, Lin Wang. Students' motivation to study Chinese recreational gymnastics classes wushu. *Physical education of students*, 2014;3:40–44.
112. Malakhov VA, Puhach YaI, Serebrjakov AM, Bakanova AF, Druz VA. Influence of the emotional state on behavior in extreme conditions of competitive sports activities. *Physical education of students*, 2014;2:25–33.
113. Manilo YV. Locomotor activity of professional football referees. *Physical education of students*, 2014;6:37–40. http://dx.doi.org/10.15561/20755279.2014.0607
114. Martsiv VP. Comparative analysis of competitive activity parameters of amateur boxers high qualification. *Physical education of students*, 2014;6:41–44. http://dx.doi.org/10.15561/20755279.2014.0608
115. Martsiv VP. Model characteristics of average skill boxers' competition functioning. *Physical education of students*, 2015;4:17–23. http://dx.doi.org/10.15561/20755279.2015.0403
116. Martyniuk OV, Vilyanskiy VN. Assessment of students' health condition by indicators of adaptation potential, biological age and bio-energetic reserves of organism. *Physical education of students*, 2015;3:20–28. http://dx.doi.org/10.15561/20755279.2015.0303
117. Masliak IP. Quickness and endurance fitness of pedagogic college girl students under influence of cheer-leading. *Physical education of students*, 2015;4:24–30. http://dx.doi.org/10.15561/20755279.2015.0404
118. Mehran Azarian, Robab Yadollahzadeh, Mehrdad Hefzollesan, Mehrdad Moharramzadeh, Sohrab Ghalehgir. Order in the chaos in sports organizations. *Physical education of students*, 2014;4:49–54.
119. Mehrdad Hefzollesan, Sohrab Ghalegir. Study of postural abnormalities of male students of Sahand University of Technology. *Physical education of students*, 2013;2:83–87.
120. Mehrdad Hefzollesan, Sohrab Ghalehgir, Mostafa Ekrami. The effect of 36 hours sleep deprivation on dribbling skills of soccer players. *Physical education of students*, 2013;4:97–101.
121. Mehrzad Shabani, Saeid Shakerian, Rouholah Fatemi. Study of body mass index (BMI), body fat percent (%BF), and waist to hip ratio (WHR) in male physical education students. *Physical education of students*, 2015;3:74–78. http://dx.doi.org/10.15561/20755279.2015.0309
122. Menshikh EE. The peculiarities of physical development of pupils and students. *Physical education of students*, 2013;6:50–55.
123. Michael Chia, Marcus Lee. Relationship between quality of life and resilience among sport-active Singaporean youth. *Physical education of students*, 2015;2:29–36. http://dx.doi.org/10.15561/20755279.2015.0205
124. Michuda YP, Zhuliaiev VN. Features of financing of mass sports in Europe at the beginning of XXI century. *Physical education of students*, 2013;1:40–45.
125. Mikhnov AP. Rationale set of indicators and prioritize relevant to assess competitive activity of hockey players of high qualification of different roles. *Physical education of students*, 2015;1:31–35. http://dx.doi.org/10.15561/20755279.2015.0105
126. Mukhamediarov NN. The theoretical basis of formation mental health of students on physical education. *Physical education of students*, 2013;3:42–46.
127. Muntian VS. Definition of biomechanical parameters of technical actions in the martial arts. *Physical education of students*, 2013;4:63–68.
128. Muntian VS. Theory of safety needs (about the theory of arise of physical education). *Physical education of students*, 2014;6:45–48. http://dx.doi.org/10.15561/20755279.2014.0609

129. Mysiv V M. Physical readiness and performance of adolescents of different somatotype. *Physical education of students*, 2014;2:33–37.
130. Niewiadomska Monika. Agility as a modern form of recreation. *Physical education of students*, 2013;3:84–87.
131. Nooshing Benar, Ayoub Behrozi, Manizheh Mansor Sadeghi, Mahdi Mohammadi, Maryam Yosefi. The consideration of attitude and motives relative to leisure time activities in students of Guilan University, Iran. *Physical education of students*, 2013;4:101–107.
132. Ohromiy G V, Makarova NU, Kasyuha AM. Psychophysiological methods and criteria for the selection of individual metered loads in athletes of taekwondo section. *Physical education of students*, 2014;6:54–62. http://dx.doi.org/10.15561/20755279.2014.0611
133. Olkhovy OM, Petrenko YM, Temchenko VA, Timchenko AN. Model of students' sport-oriented physical education with application of information technologies. *Physical education of students*, 2015;3:29–37. http://dx.doi.org/10.15561/20755279.2015.0304
134. Omelyanenko VI. Complex integrated method of improvement of sports ballroom dance performance. *Physical education of students*, 2014;6:49–53. http://dx.doi.org/10.15561/20755279.2014.0610
135. Omelyanenko VI. Express-method of sportsmen's psychological tune-up. *Physical education of students*, 2014;3:44–49.
136. Pashkevich LP. A structure of morbidity and prevalence of illnesses of the respiratory system in Ukraine. *Physical education of students*, 2013;4:68–72.
137. Pasko VV. Perfection of educational-training process on the basis of account of parameters special physical preparedness of rugby-players. *Physical education of students*, 2014;3:49–56.
138. Perederiy AV. The structure of the ensuring of the functioning of Special Olympics' program. *Physical education of students*, 2013;5:73–79.
139. Petrenko N V, Loza T A. Model of recreational and training sessions based on the use of funds aqua professionally applied in the preparation of students of economics. *Physical education of students*, 2014;4:32–36.
140. Pichurin VV. Resilience of students and their readiness for professional functioning. *Physical education of students*, 2015;3:38–43. http://dx.doi.org/10.15561/20755279.2015.0305
141. Pidpomoga AY. Dynamic of functional indicators' changes of students having harmful habits (on example of smoking) under influence of organized motion functioning. *Physical education of students*, 2015;2:22–28. http://dx.doi.org/10.15561/20755279.2015.0204
142. Podrigalo L V, Galashko M N, Galashko N I. Study of specificities of arm wrestlers' psychological status in competition period. *Physical education of students*, 2015;3:44–51. http://dx.doi.org/10.15561/20755279.2015.0306
143. Podrigalo LV, Galashko MN, Galashko NI . Goniometric researches of armwrestling sportsmen. *Physical education of students*, 2013;1:45–49.
144. Podrigalo LV, Galashko MN, Galashko NI, Prusik Krzysztof, Cieslicka, Miroslawa. Research of hands' strength and endurance indications of arm sport athletes having different levels of skills. *Physical education of students*, 2014;2:37–41.
145. Podrigalo LV, Galashko MN, Galashko NI. Study and evaluation of indicators of relationships motor analyzer sportsmen of armsport. *Physical education of students*, 2013;3:46–50.
146. Podrigalo LV, Platonova AG, Cieslicka M. Comparative analysis of vitamin status of schoolchildren in recreational period. *Physical education of students*, 2013;5:79–83.
147. Podstawski Robert , Boryslawski Krzysztof. Influence of pe teachers' qualifications on the motor abilities of early school-age children. *Physical education of students*, 2014;1:56–64.
148. Podstawski Robert, Boryslawski Krzysztof, Urbanska-Gizinska Renata. Physical and motor development of the students enrolled at the University of Warmia & Mazury in Olsztyn, Poland, in relation to their financial and urbanization status. *Physical education of students*, 2014;6:81–89. http://dx.doi.org/10.15561/20755279.2014.0616
149. Podstawski Robert, Omelan Aneta, Zapert Monika, Zurek Piotr. School and out-of-school physical activity of children in rural areas. *Physical education of students*, 2014;4:55–60.
150. Pomeschskova IP, Kycherenko AS, Yevtushenko IM. Analysis of the performance of the Ukrainian women's team at the European Basketball Championship 2012. *Physical education of students*, 2013;1:49–54.
151. Prosvirina LN, Kolokoltsev MM, Kolchanova MA, Cieslicka Miroslawa, Stankiewicz Blazej. The characteristic of the engine qualities of the students of technical institute of III functional health group (special medical group). *Physical education of students*, 2015;1:43–49. http://dx.doi.org/10.15561/20755279.2015.0107
152. Prusik Krzysztof, Prusik Katarzyna, Kozina ZhL, Iermakov SS. Features of physical development, physical preparedness and functional state of boys and girls – students of Polish higher educational establishments. *Physical education of students*, 2013;1:54–62.
153. Pryimakov AA, Eider E, Omelchuk EV . Stability of equilibrium in upright stance and voluntary motion control in athletes-shooters in the process of ready position and target shooting. *Physical education of students*, 2015;1:36–42. http://dx.doi.org/10.15561/20755279.2015.0106

154. Prystupa TD. Effect of partial sports massage on blood pressure and heart rate. *Physical education of students*, 2013;6:55–60.
155. Pyatnickaya DV. Development of girl-students' physical qualities at extracurricular cheer-dance classes (cheer-dance show). *Physical education of students*, 2015;4:31–38. http://dx.doi.org/10.15561/20755279.2015.0405
156. Pyatnychuk GO. Assessment of speed and power abilities of the students during the weekly training cycles. *Physical education of students*, 2014;1:39–44.
157. Radzievskiy RM, Plisko VI. Law enforcers recognition level emerging threats based on physical appearance and behavior signs the enemy. *Physical education of students*, 2015;1:50–59. http://dx.doi.org/10.15561/20755279.2015.0108
158. Rastegar Hoseini, Fatemeh Ghasemi, Mahri Hoseini. Effect of 8 weeks of aerobic or resistance training on blood pressure in non-physical education male students. *Physical education of students*, 2014;1:64–68.
159. Robert Podstawski, Danuta Zwolinska, Renata Urbanska-Gizinska, Danuta Nowosielska-Swadzba. The effect of learning environment factors on biological development of first year students. *Physical education of students*, 2013;6:103–108.
160. Romanowska-Tolloczko Anna, Piwowarczyk Piotr. The assessment of difficulty of yacht sailing classes and students' global self-esteem. *Physical education of students*, 2015;3:79–83. http://dx.doi.org/10.15561/20755279.2015.0310
161. Romanowska-Tolloczko Anna. Emotional competencies of the forthcoming physiotherapists and physical education teachers. *Physical education of students*, 2014;5:70–73. http://dx.doi.org/10.15561/20755279.2014.0513
162. Roters T T. Physical improvement of students during interactive physical and aesthetic education. *Physical education of students*, 2013;4:72–77.
163. Rovniy AS, Lastochkin VM. Mechanisms of adaptation to intensive loads of 400 meters' hurdles runners at stage of initial basic training. *Physical education of students*, 2015;4:39–43. http://dx.doi.org/10.15561/20755279.2015.0406
164. Ryepko OA. Features and functionality of speed and power capabilities of elite climbers and various types of rock climbing. *Physical education of students*, 2013;6:60–66.
165. Saeed Jamshidi Far, Mirza Hossein Norouzi Kamareh. The effect of sleep deprivation on serum igg responses to aerobic activity in college student athletes. *Physical education of students*, 2014;6:90–95. http://dx.doi.org/10.15561/20755279.2014.0617
166. Sedova OO. The investigation of the level of preschool children with eyesight problems functional state. *Physical education of students*, 2013;2:54–59.
167. Semanychyn TM, Popel' SL. Professional portrait of future instructors for physical education of preschool. *Physical education of students*, 2015;1:60–66. http://dx.doi.org/10.15561/20755279.2015.0109
168. Sergienko VN. Complex estimation of development of power capabilities of students of higher educational establishments. *Physical education of students*, 2013;5:83–88.
169. Sergienko VN. Evaluation of integrated testing the maximum force of students aged 17–20 years. *Physical education of students*, 2013;4:77–82.
170. Sergienko VN. Morphological indicators of the female students of the 17–20 age group. *Physical education of students*, 2013;6:73–78.
171. Sergienko YP, Andreianov AM. Models of professional readiness of students of higher military schools of the Armed Forces of Ukraine. *Physical education of students*, 2013;6:66–73.
172. Shahram Gholamrezai, Mina Zali, Ramin Shabani, Rastegar Hoseini. Effect of 8 weeks of aerobic on body composition and blood pressure in postmenopausal women. *Physical education of students*, 2014;5:74–78. http://dx.doi.org/10.15561/20755279.2014.0514
173. Shalar OG, Strikalenko EA, Ivaschenko AN. Individual properties of personality as criterion of choice of style of game of tennis players. *Physical education of students*, 2013;2:69–74.
174. Shul'ga LM, Rudkovskaya TI. Estimation of competitive activity in synchronized swimming. *Physical education of students*, 2013;1:82–87.
175. Shypulo I P. Influence employment by improving aerobics on motor readiness of girls. *Physical education of students*, 2015;1:67–71. http://dx.doi.org/10.15561/20755279.2015.0110
176. Singh Virendra Kumar, Agashe Chandrakant D. Effect of information processing and depth perception upon throwing accuracy of basketball players. *Physical education of students*, 2015;2:37–42. http://dx.doi.org/10.15561/20755279.2015.0206
177. Skyrta OS. Conditional duel, as methodical reception of perfection to technical tactical preparedness in kickboxing, and its classification. *Physical education of students*, 2013;1:62–68.
178. Slavityak OS. The problem of search safe and effective method in reducing injuries in bodybuilding stage of specialized basic training. *Physical education of students*, 2014;6:63–68. http://dx.doi.org/10.15561/20755279.2014.0612
179. Smaylova SA. Evaluation of correction in shaping body mass women first adulthood with different personal features. *Physical education of students*, 2013;3:50–55.

180. Sobko I N. Characteristics of competitive activity of qualified basketball with hearing impairment compare to qualified healthy basketball player. *Physical education of students*, 2013;4:82–87.
181. Sobko IN. The preparation for the year main competition teams in basketball with hearing impairments with innovative technologies. *Physical education of students*, 2014;5:30–37. http://dx.doi.org/10.15561/20755279.2014.0506
182. Sobyanin FI, Dudkina SG. About a competence and professional trade of specialists in the field of physical culture. *Physical education of students*, 2013;1:68–74.
183. Soronovich IM, Chaikovsky EV, Pilevskaya V. Features of functional support of competitive activity in sports dance given the differences prepared by partners. *Physical education of students*, 2013;6:78–88.
184. Sovenko SP, Budkevych HB, Lytvynchuk TV. Technical specifications of qualified sportswomen who specialize in race walking for 10 km. *Physical education of students*, 2014;4:37–41.
185. Stetsenko AI. The highest achievements of Ukrainian powerlifting at international events during its origin and formation. *Physical education of students*, 2014;1:44–50.
186. Supilo IP. Biomechanical modeling of the physical training of girls during aerobic activities in non-school educational institutions. *Physical education of students*, 2014;6:73–76. http://dx.doi.org/10.15561/20755279.2014.0614
187. Surovov AA. Specialized Internet resources as interactive technology in the training of future teachers of physical training. *Physical education of students*, 2013;3:55–60.
188. Synytsya S V, Shesterova L E, Synytsya T O. Assessment of communicative abilities of students of pedagogical universities on the results of primary instruction on improving aerobics. *Physical education of students*, 2014;3:56–61.
189. Tereschenko IA, Otsupok AP, Krupenio SV, Levchuk TM, Boloban VN. Evaluation of freshmen coordination abilities on practical training in gymnastics. *Physical education of students*, 2013;3:60–72.
190. Tereshchenko IA, Otsupok AP, Krupenya SV, Liauchuk TM, Boloban VN. Coordination training of sportsmen, specializing in sport kinds of gymnastic. *Physical education of students*, 2015;3:52–65. http://dx.doi.org/10.15561/20755279.2015.0307
191. Tereshchenko IA, Otsupok AP, Krupenya SV, Liauchuk TM, Boloban VN . Sensomotor coordination, theoretical and physical (motor) preparedness of first year students of higher educational institutions of physical education and sport. *Physical education of students*, 2013;6:88–96.
192. Tereshchuk MV. The system of world golf ranking among amateur players – WAGR. *Physical education of students*, 2014;6:69–72. http://dx.doi.org/10.15561/20755279.2014.0613
193. Tikhonova NV. Sale leisure activities of children and youth in out of school educational establishments of physical culture and sports destinations. *Physical education of students*, 2014;5:38–42. http://dx.doi.org/10.15561/20755279.2014.0507
194. Toporkov AN. The preparation of tourists to the ski sports tours in a limited time in order to prevent injuries and accidents. *Physical education of students*, 2014;4:42–48.
195. Tropin YM. Analysis of technical tactical training of highly skilled fighters of Greco-Roman wrestling. *Physical education of students*, 2013;2:59–63.
196. Tropin YM. Comparative analysis of technical and tactical preparedness Greco-Roman style wrestler at the Olympic Games-2008 and the Olympic Games-2012. *Physical education of students*, 2013;4:92–97.
197. Tsybul'ska VV. Self-appraisal adequacy of students' physical abilities of pedagogical specialties involved in various forms of education. *Physical education of students*, 2014;5:48–52. http://dx.doi.org/10.15561/20755279.2014.0509
198. Tsyganenko OI, Persheguba YaV, Paladina OL, Sklyarova NA, Oksamytnaya LF. Problem of inadequate food conduct of persons, engaged in fitness and during physical rehabilitation as a component of health-improvement – fitness programs, way of its decision. *Physical education of students*, 2013;2:63–69.
199. Tyshchenko VA. Research of the role of self-consciousness on the efficiency of sportsmen rehabilitation. *Physical education of students*, 2013;4:87–92.
200. Usakovsky YO, Bova NI. Comparative analysis of motive activity with a ball and without in training of different playing lines of young footballers aged 11–15 years. *Physical education of students*, 2013;1:74–78.
201. Uskov SV. Formation of stress students in the process of notions of martial arts in high school. *Physical education of students*, 2013;5:88–93.
202. Vasilios Giovanis, Kiriakos Amoutzas, Efstathios Vasileiou, Efstathia Ramadani, Efthimios Badas. The diet of skiers with regard to the frequency of dinners. *Physical education of students*, 2013;6:96–103.
203. Vorfolomeeva LA. Individualization of training process as a leading construction of skiers' training component in preparation for higher achievements. *Physical education of students*, 2013;4:15–19.
204. Voronkov AV, Nikulin IN, Sobyanin FI. On the improvement of the control force readiness students engaged arm sport. *Physical education of students*, 2014;2:3–8.

205. Wang Lihua, Zhang Wei Shou. Study results on estimation of non-specialized physical training university students in Hunan Province. *Physical education of students*, 2013;1:12–17.
206. Yaremenko WW. Research of kinematic characteristics of basic attacking technical action young wrestlers freestyle. *Physical education of students*, 2014;2:56–59.
207. Yurchyshyn YV. Modern information tools: their place in students' extra-curriculum and involvement of them in motor activity of health related orientation. *Physical education of students*, 2015;4:44–50. http://dx.doi.org/10.15561/20755279.2015.0407
208. Zaharova LV, Lyulina NV. Basis of integrated approach to sports and recreational activities of students of special medical groups. *Physical education of students*, 2014;1:17–22.
209. Zakorko IP. Use of employments on swimming in pulling in and restoration microcycles in the training process of the highly skilled sportsmen of the highly skilled heavy weight sambo wrestlers. *Physical education of students*, 2013;1:30–33.
210. Zhula VP. Development of motive skills of students while making underarm pass during playing volleyball. *Physical education of students*, 2014;6:13–16. http://dx.doi.org/10.15561/20755279.2014.0603
211. Zuoziene IJ. Peculiarities of physical fitness and body composition of students engaged and not engaged in sports. *Physical education of students*, 2013;6:15–20.

PECULIARITIES OF SPECIAL PHYSICAL FITNESS OF ELITE HIGH JUMPERS FROM RUN

Kutek T.B.
Zhytomyr Ivan Franko State University

Abstract. _Purpose:_ analysis of special physical fitness features of elite high jumpers from run, considering main competition exercise's specificities. _Material:_ experiments covered 87 sportsmen. As a result of known coaches' questioning tests for special physical fitness were selected. _Results:_ we outlined the test, which permits to determine prevailing of components of power, speed or speed-power character in sportsman's physical fitness. The most important condition of determination of training programs' content shall be components of speed-power fitness. _Conclusions:_ the offered test meets requirements to informative character and reliability and can be used in practical work for assessment of elite high jumpers' from run special physical fitness and correction of training process at different stages of many years' sport perfection.
Key words: test, control, fitness, correction, jump, informative, reliability, program.

Introduction

Effectiveness of sportsmen's training depends on determination of their condition on the basis of objective criteria of special physical fitness, followed by correction of training process's components [8; 10; 11].

Controlling such complex dynamic system as sport training, it is necessary to consider all main laws of administrating. In this case coach is a controlling system and sportsman – a controlled one. Multifaceted, often variable under influence of different factors sportsman's condition shall be constantly monitored by introducing changes in trainings program. This task shall be solved on principle of feedback. According to this principle, controlling system shall receive information about effect of influencing on controlled object [1; 16; 17].

The used in training process methods of sportsman readiness assessment do not permit their application as objective criteria at different stages of training. At the same time trend to intensification of training process implies optimizing of controlling system, which is realized in systemic character and with prognostication. For this purpose, informative and reliable pedagogic tests of sportsman's specific motor functioning are used [2; 9; 12; 14; 15].

In many kinds of sports orientation of sport training depends on prevalence of power, speed or speed-power components of sportsmen's special physical fitness [1; 3; 4; 18]. As on to-day, various pedagogic tests permitting assessment of these components have been offered [2; 7; 8]. Analysis of scientific literature proves that many tests for assessment of high jumpers' components do not meet requirements of reliability and informative [8; 16; 20-23].

Specialists could not determine degree of reliability for Cooper's test (12 minutes' run on track). That is why it is used only by some sportsmen and only one time (in first half of October). Besides, for jumper this test was not a specific one [1; 9]. Also degree of reliability was not determined for such tests as jerk of weight rod, toss kernel (4 kg) by two arms from below, ten - times' jump from the spot from one foot to other and many other. There was not detected degree of reliability for sprinter exercises (60, 80, 100 meters' run) [2; 8; 12; 6].

Purpose, tasks of the work, material and methods

The purpose of the research is to determine advantages of power, speed, speed-power skills of high jumpers, considering specificities of competition exercise.

The methods and organization of the research: experiments embraced 87 sportsmen – high jumpers of different qualification. As a result of questioning of known coaches we selected tests for special physical fitness. We selected tests with the highest degree of correlation with indicators of power, speed and speed-power skills of sportsmen. They were: high jump, standing on jerking foot, by wave of free leg; high jump from three step run.

Results of the research

As a result of conducted research we determined close correlation dependence of these jumps' indicators between them at all levels of sport fitness: from III grade to international master of sports (correlation coefficients from $r = 0.635$ to $r = 0.735$ accordingly). With it in every grade group certain indicator of percentage correlation has connection with power, speed and speed power exercises (see table 1). For example at level of III grade numerical expression of percent correlation between two jumps from 65% to 70% has high correlation coefficient with indicator of speed exercise (30 meters' run - $r = 0.738$). Analogous picture is from 71% to 78% – with indicators of speed-power exercises (triple jump from the spot– $r = 0.912$) and from 79% to 85% – with indicator of power exercise (relative strength of muscle flexor of jerk foot– $r = 0.921$). It should be noted that with increasing of sportsman's qualification ranges of this correlation change to certain extent. At level of candidates masters of sports and masters of sports high correlation coefficient was detected with speed parameter (30 meters' run – $r = 0.824$) in the range of from 72% to 75% and power parameter – from 82% to 87% (relative strength of muscle flexor of jerk foot – $r = 0.836$). At level of international masters of sports high correlation coefficient was found with 30 meters' run – $r = 0.908$ in the range from 73% to 76% and power parameter from 83% to 88% ($r = 0.854$). In this connection it was assumed that indicator of percent correlation between these jumps can be the test for determination of prevalence of power or speed-power components of special physical fitness of different qualification high jumpers.

Thus, we determined the test, with the help of which it became possible to find out prevalence of power, speed or speed-power components in special physical fitness of sportsman at different stages of sport perfection (see table 1).

Table 1

Correlation of indicators of high jump, standing on jerk foot and high jump from three steps run with indicators of power, speed-power and speed fitness of different qualification high jumpers (%)

Qualification, sport result	Indicator of percent correlation between two jumps	30 meters' run from high start	Triple run from the spot from foot to foot	High jump from the spot by two feet	Relative strength of muscle flexor of jerk foot
III grade 1.55-1.74 m	79-85%	0.392	0.310	0.317	0.921
	71-78%	0.612	0.912	0.886	0.476
	65-70%	0.738	0.594	0.488	0.547
II grade 1.75-1.89 m	81-86%	0.216	0.114	0.436	0.708
	76-80%	0.765	0.419	0.584	0.814
	71-75%	0.900	0.401	0.727	0.442
I grade 1.90-2.04 m	81-87%	0.378	0.412	0.693	0.746
	76-81%	0.413	0.680	0.723	0.562
	72-75%	0.736	0.459	0.671	0.419
CMS, MS, 2.05-2.20 m	82-87%	0.216	0.642	0.687	0.836
	76-81%	0.468	0.492	0.926	0.362
	72-75%	0.824	0.236	0.342	0.244
IMS 2.24-2.41 м	83-88%	0.413	0.451	0.574	0.854
	77-82%	0.524	0.563	0.698	0.610
	73-76%	0.908	0.406	0.381	0.298

Notes: the most significant coefficients: IMS, MS, CMS – $r = 0.470$; $P = 0.05$; other grades – $r = 0.410$; $P = 0.05$.

Further course of the researches was oriented on testing and substantiation of the received by us test for checking up its reliability and informative character (validity). Reliability means degree of coincidence of many times' results. Role of reliability coefficient was played by correlation coefficient , which was calculated between to masses of results with testing of one and the same group of sportsmen . The obtained coefficients ŕ in the range from $r = 0.957$ to $r = 0.993$ witness about high reliability of the test and are applicable in groups of sportsmen from iii grade to international masters of sports.

Analysis of interconnection of physical skills and parameters of different qualification high jumpers was conducted with consideration of sportsmen's individual features. Distribution into sub-groups with prevailing of power, speed and speed-power special fitness' components at all levels of sport qualification was fulfilled with the help of test, received in our researches (see table 2).

Table 2

Results of determination of individual special physical fitness of different qualification high jumpers

Qualification, sport result	Indicator of percent correlation between two jumps	Prevalence of components of sportsman physical fitness's components
III grade 1.55-1.74 m	79-85%	Power
	71-78%	Speed-power
	65-70%	Speed
II grade 1.75-1.89 m	81-86%	Power
	76-80%	Speed-power
	71-75%	Speed

Qualification, sport result	Indicator of percent correlation between two jumps	Prevalence of components of sportsman physical fitness's components
I grade 1.90-2.04 m	81-87%	Power
	76-80%	Speed-power
	72-75%	Speed
CMS, MS, 2.05-2.20 m	81-87%	Power
	76-80%	Speed-power
	72-75%	Speed
IMS 2.24-2.41 м	83-88%	Power
	77-82%	Speed-power
	73-76%	Speed

Notes: as test we used percent correlation between high jumps standing on jerk foot by waving of free leg and indicators of high jump from three steps' run.

Discussion

Analysis of scientific literature, questioning of known coaches proved demand in working out of new, more effective, more reliable and informative tests in trainings of sportsmen, specializing in speed-power kinds of track and field events [1; 3; 8; 9; 16].

Results of the conducted researches supplement existing pedagogic tests, which permit to assess sport fitness depending on prevalence of power, speed and speed power components in jumpers' special physical fitness [1; 3; 12; 18; 19].

In our research we also received new data, which permitted to determine test - percent correlation between high jumps standing on jerk foot by waving of free leg and indicators of high jump from three steps' run, with the help of which it became possible to find out level of special physical fitness of sportsman at different stages of sport perfection. Informative character and reliability of this test was proved by factorial, correlation and dispersion analysis [7] and indeed can be applied for optimizing of system of training monitoring on the base of systemic control and prognostication. Besides, the main in determination of training process content shall be speed-power fitness.

Conclusions

The received results of the research permit to make conclusion that the offered test meets the requirements to informative character and reliability and can be used in practical work for assessment of special physical fitness of elite high jumpers from run and for training process's correction at different stages of sport perfection. We think that the most important condition of training programs content's determination shall be speed-power fitness's components.

The prospects of further researches are connected with seeking of informative and reliable tests for sportsmen of all speed-power kinds of track and field events.

Acknowledgement

The research was conducted in compliance with topic 2.11 "Theoretical methodic principles of control over sportsmen's training system, who specialize in track and fields jumps" of combined plan of scientific and research works in sphere of physical culture and sports for 2011-2015 of Ministry of Ukraine of family, youth and sports. State registration number; 0111U003839.

Conflict of interests

Author declares absence of any conflict of interests.

References:

1. Akhmetov R.F. *Teoretiko-metodichni osnovi upravlinnia bagatorichnoiu pidgotovkoiu stribuniv u visotu visokogo klassu* [Theoretical and methodological foundations of long-term preparation jumpers tall high class], Zhitomir, 2005, 283 p. (in Ukrainian)
2. Akhmetov R. F. *Teoretiko-metodichni osnovi upravlinnia sistemoiu bagatorichnoi pidgotovki sportsmeniv shvidkisno-silovikh vidiv sportu. Dokt. Diss*. [Theoretical and methodological foundations of the system of long-term training athletes speed-power sports. Dokt. Diss.], Kiev, 2006, 39 p. (in Ukrainian)
3. Bobrovnik V. I. Racional'na sistema organizacii trenuval'nogo procesu v stribkakh u visotu na etapakh maksimal'noi realizacii individual'nikh spromozhnostej ta zberezhennia dosiagnen' [The rational system of training process in the high jump on stage to realize individual capacity and conservation achievements]. *Teoriia i metodika fizichnogo vikhovannia i sportu*, 2002, vol.1, pp. 3–11. (in Ukrainian)
4. Verkhoshanskij Iu.V. *Osnovy special'noj fizicheskoj podgotovki sportsmenov* [Fundamentals of special physical preparation of athletes], Moscow, Physical Culture and Sport, 1988, 331 p. (in Russian)

5. Gamalij V.V. Modelirovanie tekhniki dvigatel'nykh dejstvij v sporte [Modeling technique of motor actions in sport]. *Nauka v olimpijskom sporte,* 2005, vol.2, pp. 108–116. (in Russian)
6. Kuznecov V.V., Shustin B.N. Metodologiia postroeniia model'nykh kharakteristik sil'nejshikh sportsmenov [Methodology of model characteristics of the strongest athletes]. *Sovershenstvovanie upravleniia sistemoj podgotovki kvalificirovannykh sportsmenov* [Improving the management of the system of training of qualified athletes], Moscow, 1980, pp. 68-69. (in Russian)
7. Kutek T.B. *Teoretiko-metodichni osnovi upravlinnia bagatorichnoiu pidgotovkoiu kvalifikovanikh sportsmenok, iaki specializuiut'sia v legkoatletichnikh stribkakh. Dokt. Diss*. [Theoretical and methodological foundations of long-term training of qualified athletes who specialize in athletics jump. Dokt. Diss.], Lviv, 2014, pp. 36 p. (in Ukrainian)
8. Laputin A. N., Bobrovnik V. I. *Olimpijskomu sportu – vysokie tekhnologii* [Olympic sports – high techniques], Kiev, Knowledge, 1999, 164 p. (in Russian)
9. Maksimenko G. N. *Teoretiko-metodicheskie osnovy podgotovki iunykh legkoatletov* [Theoretical and methodological foundations of training young athletes], Lugansk, Alma Mater, 2007, 394 p. (in Russian)
10. Ogandzhanov A.L. *Upravlenie podgotovkoj kvalificirovannykh legkoatletov-prygunov* [Management training of qualified athletes-jumpers], Moscow, Physical Culture and Sport, 2005, 200 p. (in Russian)
11. Platonov V.N. *Sistema podgotovki sportsmenov v olimpijskom sporte* [The system of preparation of sportsmen in Olympic sport], Kiev, Olympic Literature, 2004, 808 p. (in Russian)
12. Popov G. I. *Biomekhanicheskie osnovy sozdaniia predmetnoj sredy dlia formirovaniia i sovershenstvovaniia dvizhenij. Dokt. Diss*. [Biomechanical basis for the creation of the subject environment for the development and perfection of movements. Dokt. Diss.], 1992, Moscow, 626 p. (in Russian)
13. Popov G.I. *Biomekhanika* [Biomechanics], Moscow, Academy, 2005, 254 p. (in Russian)
14. Ratov I.P., Popov G.I. *Biomekhanicheskie tekhnologii podgotovki sportsmenov* [Biomechanical technology training athletes], 2007, Moscow, Physical Culture and Sport, 120 p. (in Russian)
15. Selivanova T.G. *Issledovaniia vozmozhnostej korrekcii dvizheniia sportsmenov pri ispol'zovanii stimuliacionnykh i programmiruiushchikh ustrojstv* [Research the possibility of correcting movement of athletes using stimulus and programming devices], Moscow, Physical Culture and Sport, 2005, 127 p. (in Russian)
16. Strizhak A.P. *Nauchno-metodicheskie osnovy upravleniia trenirovochnym processom vysokokvalificirovannykh legkoatletov-prygunov. Dokt. Diss*. [Scientific and methodical bases of management training process of highly skilled athletes-jumpers. Dokt. Diss.], Moscow, 1992, 32 p.
17. Khmel'nic'ka I. V. Programne zabezpechennia biomekhanichnogo videokomp'iuternogo analizu sportivnikh rukhiv [Software biomechanical analysis of computer video athletic movements]. *Olimpijs'kij sport i sport dlia vsikh* [Olympic sport and sport for all], Kiev, 2010, p. 568. (in Ukrainian)
18. Shestakov M. P. Upravlenie tekhnicheskoj podgotovkoj v legkoj atletike na osnove komp'iuternogo modelirovaniia [Management of technical training in athletics on based computer simulation], *Nauka v olimpijskom sporte,* 2005, vol.2, pp. 187–196. (in Russian)
19. Shustin B. N. *Model'nye kharakteristiki sorevnovatel'noj deiatel'nosti* [Model characteristics of competitive activity], Moscow, SAAM, 1995, pp. 50–73. (in Russian)
20. Kutek T.B. Application of hardwares in the process of training of skilled sportswomen. *Physical Education of Students*, 2013, vol.5, pp. 60-64. doi:10.6084/m9.figshare.771086
21. Kutek T.B., Impact on the effectiveness of rehabilitation funds qualified athletes specializing in the long jump with a running start. *Pedagogics, psychology, medical-biological problems of physical training and sports*, 2013, vol.12, pp. 37-41. doi:10.6084/m9.figshare.879680
22. Kutek T.B., Stimulation of regenerative processes of qualified athletes specializing in the high jump with a running start. *Pedagogics, psychology, medical-biological problems of physical training and sports*, 2013, vol.11, pp. 57-61. doi:10.6084/m9.figshare.815875
23. Moreno-Aranda J., Sierag A. Force response to electrical stimulation of canine skeletal muscles. *Journal of Biomechanics*, 1991, vol.2, pp. 595–599.

THE ASSESSMENT OF DIFFICULTY OF YACHT SAILING CLASSES AND STUDENTS' GLOBAL SELF-ESTEEM

Romanowska-Tołłoczko Anna, Piwowarczyk Piotr
University School of Physical Education in Wrocław

Abstract. *Purpose:* determination of relationship between the level of students' global self-esteem and their perception of the degree of difficulty sailing yacht classes. *Material and methods:* Study consisted of 178 students of University School of Physical Education in Wrocław. The study used two tools: Polish adaptation of SES M. Rosenberg Self-Esteem Scale and a questionnaire designed by the authors of the study. *Results:* men were characterized by a higher self-esteem than women. Distribution of the results obtained by women was closer to a normal distribution, but it was not completely compatible with it. The relationship was noted between the level of global self-esteem of the students and their perception of the degree of difficulty of the course. People with higher self-esteem assessed the knowledge and skills of sailing as easier. For people with lower levels of self-esteem sailing it was a more difficult. *Conclusions:* self-acceptance and self-esteem have a substantial impact on goal setting and the perception and taking various tasks. It is therefore important to help young people to build adequate self-esteem and positive self-image, because faith in its own strength and capabilities is a key element in achieving success in every area of life.
Keywords: students, self-esteem, sense of self-worth, yacht sailing, perception of classes difficulty.

Introduction

In the course of studies at the University School of Physical Education in Wroclaw students participate in summer camp, which is an integral part of the curriculum of universities in the fields of Physical Education and Tourism and Recreation. Subjects constituting the so-called "outdoor forms of physical activity", which include: canoeing, yachting, windsurfing, swimming in open water, games and recreation, and bicycling are realized during the camp [3].

The camp for full-time students lasts 10 days, during which yachting is conducted in two blocks of two and three hours. After the initial classes, students have the opportunity to choose the so called specialization of sailing and to hone their skills in this field for the next five days. However, for the purposes of this article, we deal only with people who undergo initial training. It includes a minimum basic knowledge of the construction of the yacht, sailing theory and safety rules. The first classes consist of a short presentation of the rules in sailing. The concept of wind and its types is explained Information about the construction of the yacht are presented in the process of preparing the boat to sail. These activities include: rigging the yacht and preparing the vessel for docks. The last part of the course is a cruise on the lake, during which students perform commands of instructor and work as a member of the crew maneuvering positions: in selecting, loosening, erecting and discharging of sails, at the helm, oars, on the moorings and the landing.

On the second day of classes, in the theoretical part, students learn about courses in relation to the wind, in which sailing boat can move, and basic information concerning the laws on the water. Then they have to independently prepare a boat to sail. After verifying the rigging, the crew together with an instructor comes to the lake. During the sailing students exchange the positions to perform activities such as working the sails and rudder. Tasks which they have to carry out are: keeping the course, sharpening and peeling from the wind, tacking and stern turning.

Sailing yacht belongs to difficult disciplines, requiring high knowledge and many skills and although the classes pass on only a small scope, it's for people who come into contact with this form of activity for the first time and for such a short time, it is a huge portion of the new material: vocabulary, theory and practice.

Sailing skills acquisition subjects to the same regularities that determine the process of learning and teaching each area. The effectiveness of this process consists of three basic elements: the properties of the learner, environmental conditions and course teaching situation and characteristics and competencies of the teachers [8.10].

In this study, we focused exclusively on the properties of the learner. The key features responsible for the acquisition of knowledge and skills include: intelligence, special abilities, interests, attitudes, motivation and self-esteem. These elements have been treated in a more selective and we focused exclusively on self-esteem. It may be understood in two ways, on the one hand as ambitions but also as an assessment of one's abilities within a certain range of activities and global activities [16,17].

Global self-esteem is the belief in the self value, which can be high or low, and affect the assessment of the different life situations and setting and achieving the objectives in a positive or negative manner [12].

Self-image is one of the largest "force" of a personality, governing the behavior of man. Man behaves in life the in way one pictures oneself. If someone sees itself as a bold, brave, one acts boldly and courageously. If he or she considers oneself as a loser while, unfortunate, someone unworthy, one will behave so as to reaffirm their self-esteem [11,18]. People with high self-esteem have a positive attitude to the tasks undertaken because they have much faith in your success.

Conversely, people with low self-esteem, for not believing in their own strengths, they recognize the many tasks too difficult. Fearing defeat, in advance doomed to failure and often do not even want to meet the demands for trial [13,14]. Empirical verification of the issues outlined above seems to be very interesting, and determining whether the correct discussed will also be visible in relation to the test group of students, the degree of difficulty involved in the assessment conducted by us sailing yacht classes.

Purpose

The purpose of the study was to determine relationship between the level of students' global self-esteem and their perception of the degree of difficulty of sailing yacht classes.

We hypothesized that individuals with higher levels of self-esteem recognize the knowledge and skills of sailing for easier and faster to their learning, while students with lower self-esteem classes will constitute more difficulties.

Material and methods of the research

The study was conducted in 2014 in Olejnica at the Centre for Sports and Teaching, during summer camps for full-time students. It was attended by 178 people, 72 women and 106 men.

The study used two tools: Polish adaptation of SES M. Rosenberg Self-Assessment Scale [7] and a questionnaire designed by the authors of the study. Self-assessment scale is composed of 10 claims, all are diagnostic. The result is the sum of points, which is a general indicator of the level of self-esteem. The range of possible points to obtain is between 10 to 40 points. Detailed interpretation of the received data is based on standards that can transform raw score on a scale sten.

Author's questionnaire contained 10 questions about attitudes of students to sailing, their assessment of the degree of difficulty of classes and self-esteem level of knowledge they have acquired skills and seamanship.

Students filled out questionnaires after the completion of the block of two classes. Statistical analysis was performed using Statistica 10.0.

Analysis of the results

Attitude of students to sailing and assessment of difficulty's degree of classes

The tested group of students consisted of people who came into contact with sailing for the first time in their life, so did not have any knowledge or experience in this field. Everyone began his contact with sailing with the same ceiling, which was the undoubted advantage of research.

The actions that a person undertakes for the first time are usually accompanied by emotions that are largely responsible for the attitude to the forms of activity. Depending on their type and strength, attitude can be positive or negative [6.20].

Sailing provides a lot of experiences that are somehow placed in the specifics of this discipline. Direct contact with nature, its beauty but also its dangers evokes different, often extreme emotions. At the outset, we asked students about their emotional state during yachting. Both women and men mostly felt pleasure (49%) and interest (36%), 10% of respondents said that swimming is boring for them, and for 5% it was exciting.

Attitude is also linked to the interests and motivation [5.19]; that is why we asked the students if they would like to train sailing? More than three-quarters of men and women would like to acquire sailing skills, although their motivation was slightly different - 60% is guided by pleasure, and in 18% of the students dominate theme pragmatic. Other people (6%) stated that they did not like sailing or it does nothing useful for them (16%).

Further issues related to theoretical knowledge transferred in the classroom and practical skills in demonstration. Students were asked to make a subjective assessment of the amount and degree of difficulty. Almost everyone agreed that the learning material was very extensive (63%) and extensive (32%), only a minority (5%) found that it was not extensive enough.

In the learning process, the scope of material is an important factor in its assimilation, but for the efficiency of acquiring knowledge and skills more important is the subjective perception degree of difficulty.

Theoretical knowledge, in the opinion of women, for the 25% was easy, for 64% of medium difficulty and for 11% it was difficult. Rating of men was similar - 19% considered it to be easy, 59% for medium difficult and 22% as difficult.

The perception of the degree of difficulty of practical classes a bit different. Practical skills proved to be more difficult to control for women than for men, which was confirmed in their assessment.

The level of students' self-esteem and their perception of the degree of difficulty of knowledge and skills of sailing

Using the standards for students, global self-esteem of subjects was determined. Men were characterized by a higher self-esteem than women and this difference is statistically significant ($p<0,05$). Distribution of the results obtained by women was closer to a normal distribution, but it was not completely compatible with it. Among women, a group of people with low self-esteem is much more numerous than the group with high self-esteem. While in men the size of groups from each level of self-esteem was similar, but among people with low self-esteem was until 1/3 of the students (table 1).

Table 1.

Global self-esteem of the students

Sex	Self-esteem level			Arithmetic average	Standard deviation
	LOW %	AVARAGE %	HIGH %		
Women n = 72	34,7	42,0	23,6	28,91	3,85
Men n = 106	31,1	33,1	35,8	30,43	4,29

The relationship was noted between the level of global self-esteem of the students and their perception of the degree of difficulty of the course. People with higher self-esteem assessed the knowledge and skills of sailing as easier. For people with lower levels of self-esteem sailing it was a more difficult (table 2 and 3). This regularity was observed in men and women, with the men's group differences in the mean result of self-esteem they were higher and statistically significant ($p<0,05$).

Table 2.

Perception of the level of difficulty of theoretical knowledge and the average of self-esteem

Sex	%	Difficulty level of theoretical knowledge	Average self-esteem	Standard deviation
Women n = 72	25,2	Easy	29,65	3,12
	63,8	Moderately difficult	27,66	4,01
	11,0	Difficult	27,50	3,74
Men n = 106	19,0	Easy	30,95	4,62
	59,4	Moderately difficult	30,44	4,16
	21,6	Difficult	29,95	4,51

Table 3.

Perception of the level of difficulty of practical activities and the average of self-esteem

Sex	%	Difficulty level of practical activities	Average self-esteem	Standard deviation
Women n = 72	2,7	Easy	29,25	1,41
	50,0	Moderately difficult	29,00	3,96
	47,3	Difficult	28,55	3,87
Men n = 106	17,0	Easy	32,33	4.05
	44,4	Moderately difficult	30,63	3,78
	38,6	Difficult	29,36	4,71

Discussion

The results are a confirmation of the results obtained by other researchers, who defined the relationship between self-esteem and functioning of people in various areas of life. Research in this field of studies show that people with high self-esteem perceive themselves as more gifted, intelligent, popular, attractive, despite the fact that objectively do not differ in this respect from others. Such an assessment of self results in greater drive for success, and forms belief in achieving success as more realistic. If success indeed happens, then they assign it to their abilities, that, in turn, causes the integration of further positive information to the image of oneself and motivation to achieve further emotional gratification [1]. Individuals with low self-esteem are uncertain picture of me. They approach the task so as to avoid failures, which they consider very likely. When you actually meet them failing, they consider that failures are due to their personal lack of ability than external circumstances. Uncertainty self-image and a tendency to protect I mean that is unlikely to believe in the possibility of achieving success, despite the fact that their desire [2].

Significant differences between individuals with high and low self-esteem are also noticeable in the levels of endurance and activity. High self-esteem has an impact on making more different activities and more persistent pursuit of the goal. It is closely related with the conviction of self-efficacy and internal placement of control. People with high self-esteem are committed to the objectives related to achievements and are willing to take risks, while low self-esteem primarily orients human behavior to avoid failures and preference for safe situation [9].

Conclusion

Analysis of the results confirmed the hypothesis, put forward by us, that people with higher levels of self-esteem recognize sailing skills and knowledge as easier and learn faster, while students with lower self-esteem, these activities account for a bigger difficulty.

Self-acceptance and self-esteem have a substantial impact on goal setting, on perception and taking of various tasks [4]. It is therefore important to help young people to build adequate self-esteem and positive self-image, because faith in its own strength and capabilities is a key element in achieving success in every area of life [15].

Participation in the classes of sailing is an important contribution to the study of one's own personality and the opportunity to disclose existing potentials and abilities. Sailing is a challenging area of activity, and mastery of skills associated with it, gives you a great sense of satisfaction and success. Both these elements constitute an important factor in the formation of human self-esteem.

Declaration of Conflicting Interests

The authors declared no potential conflicts of interest with respect to the research, authorship, and publication of this article.

References

1 Baumeister RF, Campbell JD, Kreuger JI, Vohs KD. Does high self-esteem cause better performance, interpersonal success, happiness, or healthier lifestyles? *Psychological Science in the Public Interest* 2003;4(1):1-44.
2 Blaine B, Cocker J. Self-esteem and self-serving biases In reactions to positive and negative events. An integrating review. In: R.F. Baumeister (ed.), *Self-esteem. The puzzle of low self-regard.* New York; 1993. p. 55-85.
3 Błacha R, Bigiel W, Wiesner W. (ed) *Summer camps*, Wrocław; 2011.
4 Branden N. *The Six Pillars of Self-Esteem*, Łódź; 2009.
5 Dryden G, Vos J. *Revolution in studying,* Warsaw; 2003.
6 Dubowik E. Regulatory processes. Emotions, In: E.Dubowik, R.Kościelak, H.Kulas, A.Tomczak-Witych, *Selected psychology issues,* Gdańsk; 2002. p. 49-96.
7 Dzwonkowska I, Lachowicz-Tabaczek K, Łaguna M. *Self-esteem and its measurement. Polish adaptation of M.Rosenberg's SES Scale. Textbook,* Warsaw; 2008.
8 Fontana D. *Psychology for teachers*, Poznań; 1998.
9 Heimpel SA, Elliot AJ, Wood JV. Basic personality dispositions self-esteem, and personal goals: An approach-avoidance analysis. *Journal of Personality* 2006;74:1293 -1319.
10 Kruszewski K. (ed) *The art of teaching. Teacher's tasks*, Warsaw; 2002.
11 Kulas H. *Youth's self-esteem*, Warsaw; 1986.
12 Niebrzydowski L, *About self-knowledge and self-esteem*, Warsaw; 1976.
13 Niebrzydowski L. *The psychology of human's needs, aspirations and possibilities,* Łódź 1999.
14 Niebrzydowski L. *Educational psychology. Self-consciousness, activity, interpersonal relations,* Warsaw; 1989.
15 Wegscheider-Crouse S. *Sense of self-worth*, Gdańsk, 2007.
16 Włodarski Z. *Psychological features of learnig and teachig process,* Warsaw; 1987.
17 Włodarski Z. (ed), *Psychology of studying,* Warsaw; 1998.
18 Siek S. *Autopsychoterapia,* Warsaw; 1985
19 Strelau J, Jurkowski A, Putkiewicz Z. *The basics of psychology for teachers,* Warsaw; 1997.
20 Zimbardo PhG. *Psychology and Life*, Warsaw; 1999.

STUDY OF BODY MASS INDEX (BMI), BODY FAT PERCENT (%BF), AND WAIST TO HIP RATIO (WHR) IN MALE PHYSICAL EDUCATION STUDENTS

Mehrzad Shabani[1], Saeid Shakerian[1], Rouholah Fatemi[2]
[1]Ahvaz Shahid Chamran University, Ahvaz, Iran.
[2]Ahvaz Jundishapur University of Medical Sciences, Ahvaz, Iran.

Abstract. *The purpose* of this study was to investigate body mass index (BMI), body fat percent (%BF) and waist-hip ratio (WHR) of physical education male students of Shahid Chamran University and comparison with national and international body composition standards. *Material*: Subjects were seventy five male students physical education male students of Shahid Chamran University of mean age (23.21±2.78), mean height (174±5.71) and mean weight (70.07±9.43) who were selected randomly. Some of body composition indices were determined with body composition analyzer apparatus (bioelectrical impedance apparatus). *Results*: Descriptive characteristics of subjects include: body fat percent (19.37±3.62), waist-hip ratio (0.80±0.037) and body mass index (23.18±2.68). To categorize and regulate data we used descriptive analyzes, to calculate Pearson correlation coefficient we used presumption analyzes and to compare the obtained data with national standards we used T-test statistical procedure. There are significant correlations between body mass index and waist-hip ratio (P=0.709, r=0.001), between body mass index and body fat percent (P=0.783, r=0.001) and between body fat percent and waist-hip ratio (P=0.809, r=0.001). There are significant differences between mean body mass index and its national standard (P=0.001), between mean waist-hip ratio and its national standard (P=0.001) and between mean body fat percentage and its national standard (P=0.001). *Conclusions*: Results revealed that according to national standards of body fat percentage and body mass index of subjects, they were assigned to more than intermediate limitation; it may be due to abnormal nutrition, unregulated exercise or physical activity and heredity.
Key words: Body composition, body fat percentage (%BF), body mass index (BMI), waist-hip ratio (WHR)

Introduction

Overweight and obesity are major, and increasing, public health concerns in all parts of the globe. Obesity increases the risk of chronic health consequences including hypertension, hypercholesteroaemia, hyperglycaemia, type II diabetes and cardiovascular diseases. In Australia, 19% of adult males and 22% of adult females are considered obese and the direct health care costs of obesity are estimated at approximately $830 million annually (Thorburn et al. 2005). To relate obesity directly to health risks, assessment of both total body fat deposition and distribution as subcutaneous or visceral fat are important. Methods frequently used to determine overall body fatness include Body Mass Index (BMI; body mass (kg)/stature $(m)^2$) and percentage body fat (%BF). However, a number of studies have shown that it is not appropriate to use a single BMI cut-off point to detect obesity as different BMI-%BF relationships have been observed in different ethnic groups (Deurenberg-Yap M et al. 2000; Deurenberg P et al. 2003). Using anthropometry, a previous study found that the BMI value of 23kg/m2 for young Japanese adults equates with a BMI value of 25kg/m2 for Australian Caucasians (Kagawa et al. 2006).

The use of BMI in this way has a number of limitations, including its inability to distinguish between fat mass and non-fat mass (Norgan & Ferro-Luzzi, 1982; Garn et al. 1986; Ross et al. 1988). These limitations may become an important issue when comparing ethnic groups with distinctively different body proportions or physiques. Several studies have suggested that the relationship between BMI and %BF (i.e. the BMI–%BF relationship) varies with age, gender and ethnicity (Schaefer et al. 1998; Deurenberg et al. 2002; Chang et al. 2003).

Longitudinal study which it performed in Hardward University during 27 years on 19292 students with mean age 46.6 years old had been shown that rate of mortality in men who had body mass index (BMI), 26 kg/m2 , 1.67 times is more than men who had body mass index, 22,5 kg/m^2 (Altan O. et al. 1999). Body mass index in male students of Thrtoww University is reported as 22.8 kg/m^2 (Jurimae.T et al. 1991), but by Clasey et al in Virginia University, it is reported as 24.7 kg/m^2 (Clasey. Jl. et al. 1999).

In this study, we investigated BMI, percent body fat, and waist - hip ratio in male students of physical education and sport sciences field and we compared them with Iran national and international standards.

Methodology

The study was approved by the Human Research Ethics Committees of Shahid Chamran University of Ahwaz. In this study, we measured body mass index (BMI), percent body fat (%BF), and waist to hip ratio (WHR) by using Bioelectrical Impedance apparatus

Subjects

Statistical population included 162 students of physical education and sport sciences field of Shahid Chamran University Ahwaz Iran and we selected simple randomly 75 students from statistical population.

Measurements

Test performed at 8 AM and subjects were fasting and they had not done any body activity before test. Test had been done through using Bioelectrical Impedance apparatus producted by GWON Corporation Korea, model Olympia.

Statistical analysis

To demonstrate means and standard deviation of study variables (BMI, %BF, and WHR) we used quantify statistical procedures and to determine relationships between measured variables - Pearson correlation coefficient; to determine difference between measured variables and Iran national and international standards we used independent T-test. Statistical analysis was done by using SPSS software version 17.

Results

In this research, students had height, 174 ± 5.71 Cm and weight, 23.18 ± 2.68. Total subjects' data are given in table 1, means and standard deviations of study variables (BMI, %BF, and WHR) are shown in table 2, percentage of BMI, BF, and WHR according to Iran national norm exhibit in table 3, percentage of BF, and WHR and percentage of BMI according to international standard are respectively given in table 4 and table 5, comparison between variables in this research (BMI, %BF, and WHR) with Iran national standard are presented in table 6, and relationships between study variables - in table 7. In this study, significant level was 0.05.

Table1.

Total subjects data

variable	Mean and standard deviation	Minimum	Maximum
Age	23.21 ± 2.78	18	26
Height	174 ± 2.78	165	193
Weight	70.07 ± 9.43	54.10	102.7

Table2.

Means and standard deviations of study variables (BMI, %BF, and WHR)

variable	Mean and standard deviation	Minimum	Maximum
%BF	19.37 ± 2.78	11.80	32.90
BMI	23.18 ± 5.71	18.30	33.90
WHR	0.80± 9.43	0.70	0.94

Table3.

Percentage of BMI, BF, and WHR according to Iran national standard

variable	Very low		Low		Moderate low		Moderate		Moderate to high		High		Very high	
	No	%	No	%	No	%	No	%	No	%	No	%	No	%
%BF	0	0	0	0	2	3	10	13	18	24	32	43	13	17
BMI	1	1	10	13	6	8	15	20	16	22	15	20	12	16
WHR	14	18	16	21	16	21	22	28	5	7	2	5	1	1

According to table 3, body fat percentage of most subjects in three age classifications assigned to in moderate to high and high classifications, body mass index of most subjects in three age groups assigned to in moderate, moderate to high and high classifications and waist-hip ratio of most subjects in three age classifications assigned to in moderate classification.

Table4.

Percentage of BF and WHR according to International national standard

Variable	Low		Excellent		Good		Moderate		Bad	
	No	%	No	%	No	%	No	%	No	%
%BF	0	0	4	5	25	34	29	39	17	22
WHR	0	0	71	94	3	4	1	2	0	0

In table 4 we can see that percentage of body fat of most subjects assigned to moderate and good classifications and waist - hip ratio of most subjects in three age groups assigned to excellent classification.

Table5.

Percentage of BMI according to International national standard

Variable	Thin		Normal		Overweight		Fat	
	No	%	No	%	No	%	No	%
BMI	0	0	60	80	12	16	2	3

Table 5 exhibits that body mass index of most subjects in three age groups are assigned to normal classification.

Table 6.

Comparison between variables in this research (BMI, %BF, and WHR) with Iran national norm

Variable	t	Significant levels
BMI	2.531	0.013*
%BF	9.724	0.001®
WHR	-6.301	0.001®

*: $P < 0.05$, ®: $P < 0.01$.

In table 6 we present comparison between variables in this research (BMI, %BF, and WHR) with Iran national standard. Obtained results from this table show that there are significant differences between subjects BMI, %BF, and WHR with theirs Iran national standard (respectively $P < 0.013$, $P < 0.001$, and $P < 0.001$).

Table7.

Relationships between study variables

Variable	BMI	%BF	WHR
BMI	1	r = 0.783 P = 0.001®	r = 0.709 P = 0.001®
%BF	r = 0.783 P = 0.001®	1	r = 0.809 P = 0.001®
WHR	r = 0.709 P = 0.001®	r = 0.809 P = 0.001®	1

®: $P < 0.01$.

Table 7 shows that there are relationships between BMI and %BF ($r = 0.783$, $P = 0.001$), between BMI and WHR ($r = 0.709$, $P = 0.001$), and between WHR and %BF ($r = 0.809$, $P = 0.001$).

Discussion

In the study it is reported that body mass index of male untrained athletics from Thrtoww university of Estonia was 22.8 kg/m^2 (Jurimae.T et al, 1991). Clasey. Jl. et al reported that body mass index of male trained students from Virginia University was 24.7 kg/m^2 (Clasey. Jl et al, 1999). Observed difference in results of this study can occur due to various economic, social, and cultural conditions which there are in different universities. Having compared results of this research with World Health Organization (WHO) standard, we determined that %79 male students of physical education filed of Shahid Chamran University of Ahwaz have optimal weights and they are healthy and can be assigned to minimum danger rate.

Mean body mass index of students, comparing with its national standard shows that they can be assigned to classification "moderate to high". Probable reason of current result can increase percentage of body fat. Also mean BMI of male physical education students of Shahid Chamran University of Ahwaz, compared with its national standard, shows that there is significant difference between their mean BMI (Masaharu Kagawa et al, 2007).

Waist - hip ratio in this study is in significant correlation with body mass index (r= 0.709, P=0.001). Current result is in accordance with Altan O. et al research's results that it likelihood was due to accumulating body fat in waist and hips (Altan O. et al, 1999).

Ninety four percent of male physical education students of Shahid Chamran University of Ahwaz located excellent WHR range, that is why they were put into minimum danger rate and they had low abdomen fat (Bray G.A., 1985).

In this research it is shown that there is positive significant correlation between percentage of body fat and waist - hip ratio (r = 0.809, P = 0.001). In general, body composition of students in this study, in comparison with Iran national standard, in better situation in respect to health. Body mass index of subjects was higher than Iran national standard that may be due to increased weight of subjects and can be as resulted from intake of additional kilo calories from food materials and also it possibly could be caused by irregular daily activities (Ronald K et al, 2006).

In general, in this research we determined suitable correlation between percentage of body fat, waist - hip ratio, and body mass index in subjects that could be caused by low daily activity and increased kilo calories intake through elevated food consumption, which can result in increasing of body fat in waist and hips and also can result in increased body mass index (Masaharu Kagawa et al, 2007).

Acknowledgment

This study was supported by Sport Physiology Department, Shahid Chamran University, Ahwaz, Iran. We submitted this article to my friends and we thank them.

References:

Altan O, Vedat S, Omer u. Waist circumference and waist to hip ratio in Turkish adults: interrelation with other risk factors and association with cardiovascular disease. *International journal of cardiology* 1999;70(1):43-50.

Bray GA Complications of obesity. *Annals of internal medicine* 1985;103:10-52.

Chang C-J, Wu C-H, Chang C-S, Yao W-J, Yang Y-C, Wu J-S & Lu F-H. Low body mass index but high percent body fat in Taiwanese subjects: implications of obesity cutoffs. *Int J Obes Relat Metab Disord* 2003;27:253–259.

Clasey Jl, Kanaley JA. Validity of methods of body composition assessment in young and older men and women. *J. Appl physio,* 1999;86(5):1728-1738.

Deurenberg P, Bhaskaran K, Lian PL. Singaporean Chinese adolescents have more subcutaneous adipose tissue than Dutch Caucasians of the same age and body mass index. *Asia Pacific J Clin Nutr* 2003;12:261-265.

Deurenberg P, Deurenberg-Yap M & Guricci S. Asians are different from Caucasians and from each other in their body mass index/body fat per cent relationship. *Obes Rev* 2002;3:141–146.

Deurenberg-Yap M, Schmidt G, van Staveren WA, Deurenberg P. The paradox of low body mass index and high body fat percentage among Chinese, Malays and Indians in Singapore. *Int J Obes* 2000;24:1011-1017.

Garn SM, Leonard WR & Hawthorne VM Three limitations of the body mass index. *Am J Clin Nutr* 1986;44:996–997.

Jurimae T, Jagomagi G, Lepp T. body composition of university students by hydrostatic weighing and skin fold measarment. *J. obesity* 1991;15:53-60.

Kagawa M, Kerr D, Uchida H, Binns CW. Differences in the relationship between BMI and percentage body fat between Japanese and Australian-Caucasian young men. *Br J Nutr* 2006;95:1002-1007.

Masaharu Kagawa, Colin W. Binns and Andrew P. Hills. Body composition and anthropometry in Japanese and Australian Caucasian males and Japanese females. *Asia Pac J Clin Nutr* 2007;16(1):31-36.

Norgan NG & Ferro-Luzzi A. Weight-height indices as estimators of fatness in men. *Human Nutrition* 1982;36:363–372.

Ronald K Hetzler, Iris F Kimura, Karin Haines, Michelle Labotz, Joseph Smith. A Comparison of Bioelectrical Impedance and Skinfold Measurement in Determining Minimum Wrestling Weights in High School Wrestlers. *Journal of Athletic Training* 2006;41(1):46–51.

Ross WD, Crawford SM, Kerr DA, & Ward R. Relationship of the body mass index with skinfolds, girths, and bone breadths in Canadian men and women aged 20–70 years. *Am J Phys Anthropol* 1988;77:169–173.

Schaefer F, Georgi M, Wiihl E & Scharer K. Body mass index and percentage fat mass in healthy German schoolchildren and adolescents. *Int J Obes* 1998;22:461–469.

Thorburn AW. Prevalence of obesity in Australia. *Obes Rev* 2005;6:187-189.

FORMATION OF STUDENT PERSONALITY'S PHYSICAL CULTURE AS SUBJECT OF PROFESSIONAL FUNCTIONING

Otravenko O.V.
Luhansk Taras Shevchenko National University

Abstract. *Purpose:* generalization of experience of higher educational establishments' future specialists' professional training, oriented on formation of students' personalities' physical culture. *Material:* we questioned students (n=50) and institute teachers (n=30). *Results:* it was found that for increase of future specialists' professional fitness effectiveness it was important to consider orientation of educational process on formation of student personality's physical culture. Besides, it was noticed that professional fitness of future specialists is greatly influenced by implementation of modern technologies of formation of students' physical culture in educational-learning process. Physical education means, oriented on aesthetic are of great health related and recreation significance. *Conclusions:* educational process shall be oriented on support of active motor functioning, motivation for physical exercises' and healthy life style practicing.
Key words: physical culture, teaching, students, means, professional, training, innovation, management.

Introduction

Entering of Ukraine in European educational and scientific space is conditioned by reformation of higher education and rising of requirements to professionalism of higher educational establishments' graduates in conditions of market competition [9, c. 1]. It should be stressed that at the stage of modern society's development in educational system modernization of educational teaching process, directed at personality oriented teaching is going. In this case organization of future specialists' professional training acquires the character of dialogue, cooperation, joint creation. Alongside with health problems of young generation more attention is paid to professional training of HEE specialists, in which wide opportunities are open for student to prepare for successful realization.

In modern society physical culture is regarded as the process and result of human purposeful functioning, directed at formation of person's physical and spiritual nature. In educational system of young generation physical culture is a mean of social formation of future teachers, active development of their individual and professionally significant qualities [1, pg. 32]. That is why formation of student personality's physical culture is an important component of future specialists' preparation for professional functioning.

Perfection of educational system and personality's development in educational process in sphere of physical culture has been paid attention to by such scientists as: L.P. Arefyeva [1], O.Ye. Aftimichuk [3], S.I. Belykh [2], I.M. Bykhovskaya [8], T.Yu. Krutsevich [4], L.I. Lubysheva [8], Ye.V. Otravenko [5], T.T. Roters [3], E. J. Savko [3], V.I. Stoliarov [8], S.O. Sychov [9], N.Yu. Shumakova [3]. Among other researches we can distinguish the works, oriented on problems of students' motivation for independent training [11, 13], formation of positive attitude to own health [10, 20, 27, 28], social-psychological adaptation to new conditions of learning [14, 23], professional-applied orientation of classes [21, 24-26], increase of health indicators [12, 15-19, 22].

In spite of significant quantity of researches the problem of student personality's physical culture is an urgent one. There are unsolved problems of increase of future specialists' professional training effectiveness.

Purpose, tasks of the work, material and methods

The purpose of the research is to analyze scientific methodic literature on the topic of the research; to study advanced experience of future specialists' professional training, oriented on formation of student personality's physical culture.

Material and methods: the methods of the research are analysis and generalization of scientific-methodic literature, questioning of Luhansk Taras Shevchenko National University students. In questioning 20 students of economic and business institute and 30 1st year students of physical education and sports faculty participated.

Results of the research

Continuous education ensures constant progressing, perfection and creative renewal of a specialist during all his (her) life. Objective content of education is determined by social order as well as by the tasks, which are set by society for education. Subjective content is expressed in individual-personality's sense and is bases on principles of active, systemic, individual and differentiated approaches [2].

In opinion of many authors [1-9], one of after effects of scientific-technical progress is increase of knowledge volume of mankind. The category of mental labor persons includes students as well. Recent years, the flow of scientific information has significantly increased that requires its processing in short terms. Besides, application of different means of education is being expanded. All these result in intensification of HEE educational process and set increased requirements to professional training of future specialists in sphere of physical culture and management.

The sense of ***"personality's physical culture"*** concept in context of future specialist's professional training is regarded by us in the following way:

- Combination of demands, motives, knowledge, oriented on formation of sound, successful personality and physical perfectness;
- Formation of professionally important qualities;
- Training of motor skills;
- Ability to realize learning, scientific, motor, health related-physical culture and sport functioning for ensuring healthy life style;
- Teaching of mobilization, relaxation, body perfection techniques.

In such context there is a demand in radical changes of HEE physical education system on the base of understanding the sense, purpose, tasks and content of pedagogic process, functioning of physical culture instructors. It is caused by understanding the fact that physical education shall not be reduced to compensation of motor functioning deficit. Motor functioning deficit results in lack of individuality of educational process, averaging of requirements to students' physical fitness. The ideas of personality's progress, student with his (her) individual features as the highest value shall be in the base of educational system. With it physical education system shall create maximally favorable conditions for students' complex development (spiritual, aesthetic, motor) for their conscious practicing healthy life style.

In modern conditions regular practicing of physical culture is undoubtedly an effective mean of health strengthening, diseases prophylaxis, increase of organism's resistance. Besides, it is a mean of favorable influence on formation of young generation's active life style, development of interest to social information, expansion of information contacts.

Analysis of economic and business students' attitude to physical culture classes showed that physical exercises, as mean of workability increasing is used by insignificant quantity of students (27.4%). Only 23.8% of students attend optional "physical education" classes. For 32.3% of students, physical culture is not a component of personality's general progress. The rest of students did not think about it.

In questioning of physical culture and sports faculty students we were interested in what means of physical education are preferred by them. The answers distributed in the following way. Girls prefer the following: fitness (35.2%), aerobics (28.6%), functional training (22.7%), health related gymnastic (12.5%), swimming (12.3%), sport dances (11.4%), badminton (10.9 %), light athletic (9.4%), volleyball (9.2%), hiking and orientation (8.2%). Boys prefer the following: bodybuilding (24.9 %), oriental martial arts (23.9 %), football (22.4 %), swimming (22.3%), light athletic (12.7 %), basketball (10.9%), ping pong (10.2%), street dances (8.1%), hiking and orientation (6.8%), handball (6.4%).

When questioning physical culture instructors we found that professional training of future specialists in marketing and management is influence to large extent by implementation of different innovative technologies of students' physical culture formation in educational process. In this case aerobics, fitness, bodybuilding and so on are the means of physical and aesthetic education.

Let us compare opinions of students and teachers and see what means of physical education are preferred by students (see table 1).

Table 1. Comparative analysis of students' attitude to and teachers' opinions about physical education means

Rank place	Girls' attitude to physical education means	Boys' attitude to physical education means	Teachers' opinion about physical education means
1	Fitness	Bodybuilding	Fitness, aerobics (girls)
2	Aerobics	Oriental martial arts	Power kinds (boys)
3	Functional training	Football	Game kinds
4	Health related gymnastic	Swimming	Health related gymnastic
5	Swimming	Light athletic	Functional training
6	Sport dances	Basketball	Oriental martial arts
7	Badminton	Ping pong	Light athletic
8	Light athletic	Street dances	Swimming
9	Volleyball	Hiking and orientation	Hiking and orientation
10	Hiking and orientation	Handball	Sport dances

As we can see in students' answers the most popular and interesting were those kinds of physical exercises, which are aesthetically oriented: aerobics, fitness, bodybuilding, oriental martial arts. Thus, present time sets requirement to implement interesting for students physical education means in educational process, as well as means, which facilitate formation of student personality's physical culture, oriented on interconnected physical and aesthetic training.

Observations over young specialists' social adaptation in working collective showed that the higher level of graduates' (providing they know foreign languages) physical culture-sport qualification facilitates better and more effective usage of their potentials in production activities.

In institute of physical education and sports in specialties "physical education", "human health", "physical rehabilitation", "Olympic and professional sports", "fitness and recreation" rather little class hour are allocated for foreign languages. Independent study of foreign languages does not attract students.

Studying this problem, employers pay special attention to high culture level and knowing of foreign languages (especially in management and marketing sphere).

Management is a system of rational managing of production activities, directed at achievement of planned results; it is a field of human knowledge, which helps to realize effective administration [5]. Innovative management is regarded by us as managing of innovative processes activity in physical culture – sport organization.

In opinion of many authors [3, 5, 6, 7], innovation is a final result of innovative activity. It is realized in the form of a new (perfected) product or technological process, or as new approach to rendering social-cultural services. It should be noted that spectrum of innovations in functioning of physical culture-sport organizations is rather various. It can be classified by different principles: technological parameters, type and degree of novelty, spheres of functioning and etc.

Discussion

Physical culture of higher educational establishments' students was researched through formation of future teachers' motivation for healthy life style and creation of the required educational medium in higher educational establishment. Such medium is directed at increase of students' interest in own health condition, student's development as personality, individuality, active subject of professional functioning.

Results of our research confirmed the data of other authors [2, 3, 4, 9], that achievement of high indicators in system of preparation of harmoniously developed specialists is impossible without scientific approach to organization of physical education at higher educational establishments. Humanistic, ethic and pedagogic ideas shall be in the base of such approach. Accordingly, humanistically oriented education shall not restrict personality's independence. Such education shall rest on internal, natural thirst of person for self-perfection and give him (her) opportunity of choice and independent solution of problems, connected with physical self-perfection.

For achievement of the above said it is necessary to change orientation of students' physical education, which is now oriented on physical training and physical fitness. Orientation of students' physical education shall imply formation of system of special knowledge, which would permit for students to consciously organize their life activity, to attach students to values of health related physical culture and recreation.

The results, received by us, also supplement our previous researches [5, 6, 7].

Conclusions

Analysis of theoretical researches and practical experience showed that formation of students' personality's physical culture, for them to be ready for creative interaction and successful self-realization envisages the following:

1) Its implementation in academic, scientific, health related-physical culture and sport functioning through independent choice of knowledge system:
    - Formation of moral, humanistic relations, development of pedagogic tact, mastering of administrative functions in sphere of physical culture and management;
    - Active participation in students' scientific practical conferences, Olympiads, competitions, master classes, forums, which create conditions for students' complex progress.
2) Teacher's and student's transition to technology of pedagogic cooperation for health strengthening, increase of workability. The system of curriculum, extra-curriculum and independent classes shall be oriented on the following:
    - Individualization and integral character of learning,
    - Proper mastering of foreign languages,
    - Implementation of modern informational and innovative technologies, means of health related physical culture and recreation.
3) Personal physical culture of a student is reflected in his (her) attitude to physical culture values. In this case main place is taken by active motor functioning, motivation for physical exercises' practicing and healthy life style. It was determined that the main methodological tools of personality's physical culture formation are physical education means, aesthetically oriented. They are the mechanisms of influence on inner essence of a man, his spirituality, emotionality, expressiveness. Such approach has great health related and recreation significance.

Conflict of interests

The author declares that there is no conflict of interests.

References:

1. Aref'ieva LP. Formuvannia fizichnoi kul'turi osobistosti studenta v umovakh vishchogo pedagogichnogo navchal'nogo zakladu [Formation of physical culture of student's personality in conditions of higher educational establishment]. *Naukovo-pedagogichni problemi fizichnoi kul'turi*, 2015;1(56):32-35. (in Ukrainian)
2. Bielikh SI. *Osobistisne oriientovane fizichne vikhovannia studentiv universitetiv* [Personality-oriented physical education of universities' students]. Donets'k; 2013. (in Ukrainian)
3. Roters TT, Aftimichuk O E, Zakolodnaia EE, Mazin VN, Otravenko EV, Savko EJ, Shumakova NIu. *Dukhovno-fizicheskoe vospitanie lichnosti v obrazovatel'nom prostranstve fizicheskoj kul'tury* [Spiritual-physical education of personality in educational space of physical culture]. Lugansk: LNU; 2013. (in Russian)
4. Krucevich TIu, Marchenko OA. Formuvannia fizichnoi kul'turi studentiv u sistemi fizichnoi osviti [Formation of students' physical culture in system of physical education]. *Teoriia i metodika fizichnogo vikhovannia i sportu*, 2009;2:78-81. (in Ukrainian)
5. Otravenko EV. Menedzhment rekreacionnoj i ozdorovitel'noj raboty [Management of recreational and health related work]. *Innovacionnye processy v fizicheskom vospitanii studentov*, 2012;2:201-204. (in Russian)
6. Otravenko EV. Sovremennye tendencii razvitiia sistemy fizicheskogo vospitaniia v usloviiakh nepreryvnogo obrazovaniia [Modern tendencies of physical education system's development in conditions of continuous education*]. IY nauchno-prakticheskaia konferenciia «Olimpijskaia ideia segodnia», IuFU* [4th scientific-practical conference "Olympic idea to day", IuFU], Rostov on Don; 2014. P. 368-375. (in Russian)
7. Otravenko OV. Organizaciia innovacijnoi navchal'noi diial'nosti majbutnikh fakhivciv z fizichnogo vikhovannia cherez intergraciiu zdorov'iazberezhuval'nikh tekhnologij [Organization of innovative teaching functioning of future physical education specialists through integration of health related technologies]. *Naukovo-pedagogichni problemi fizichnoi kul'turi*, 2014;3(45):249-253. (in Ukrainian)
8. Stoliarov VI, Bykhovskaia IM, Lubysheva LI. Koncepciia fizicheskoj kul'tury i fizicheskogo vospitaniia [Conception of physical culture and physical education]. *Teoriia i praktika fizicheskoj kul'tury*, 1998;5:15-20. (in Russian)
9. Sichov SO. *Teoretiko-metodichni zasadi priluchennia students'koi molodi do cinnostej fizichnoi kul'turi. Doct. Diss.* [Theoretical-methodic principles of students' attaching to physical culture values. Doct. Diss.], Kiev; 2011. (in Ukrainian)
10. Belykh SI, Chernigovskaia SA. About forming of personality physical culture of students in the process of physical education (in aspect of athletic activity). *Physical Education of Students*, 2013;2:18-24. http://dx.doi.org/10.6084/m9.figshare.156375
11. Boichy JC, Sarrazin PG, Grouzet FM. Pelletier L. G. Students' motivational profiles in physical education and achievement outcomes: A self-determination theory perspective. *Journal of Educational Psychology*, 2008;100:688-701.
12. David A. Birch, Michele Wallen, Elizabeth Chaney. Developing School Health Education Advocacy Skills Through College Personal Health Courses. *Health Education Teaching Techniques Journal*. 2011;1:70-86.
13. Dudnyk IO. Formation of positive motivation as the basis of students will qualities' perfection in physical culture practicing. *Physical Education of Students*. 2015;3:3-9. http://dx.doi.org/10.15561/20755279.2015.0301
14. Feuerman VV. Influence of socio-philosophical and spiritual values on the formation of social orientation and physical health specialists the sphere of physical culture and sports. *Physical Education of Students*, 2014;2:41-45. http://dx.doi.org/10.6084/m9.figshare.906859
15. Gorelov AA, Kondakov VL, Belikova ZhA. About necessity of use of Hatha Yoga exercises for correction of deformation of students' spine of special medical groups with violations of posture. *Physical Education of Students*, 2013;2:35-44. http://dx.doi.org/10.6084/m9.figshare.156378
16. Iermakova TS. Forming a health culture of future teachers in Polish educational establishments. *Physical Education of Students*, 2014;5:14-19. http://dx.doi.org/10.15561/20755279.2014.0503
17. Ivashchenko OV, Yermakova TS. Assessment of functional, coordination and power fitness of 7-8 form boys. *Pedagogics, psychology, medical-biological problems of physical training and sports*. 2015;9:20-25. http://dx.doi.org/10.15561/18189172.2015.0903
18. Ivashchenko OV, Yermakova TS. Structural model of in-group dynamic of 6-10 years old boys' motor fitness. *Pedagogics, psychology, medical-biological problems of physical training and sports*. 2015;10:24-32. http://dx.doi.org/10.15561/18189172.2015.1004
19. Kramida IE. Exercises for students of different medical groups as factors of the weakening bad habits at students. *Physical Education of Students*, 2013;4:46-50. http://dx.doi.org/10.6084/m9.figshare.669680
20. Kurmaeva EV. Fitness – programs as mean of forming of personality physical culture of students. *Physical Education of Students*, 2013;1:37-39. http://dx.doi.org/10.6084/m9.figshare.156355

21. Nizhevska TV. Results of experimental testing of system of future physical culture teachers' training for art pedagogic means' application in pedagogic functioning. *Pedagogics, psychology, medical-biological problems of physical training and sports.* 2015;10:51-55. http://dx.doi.org/10.15561/18189172.2015.1008
22. Prosvirina LN, Kolokoltsev MM, Kolchanova MA, Cieslicka Miroslawa, Stankiewicz Blazej. The characteristic of the engine qualities of the students of technical institute of III functional health group (special medical group). *Physical Education of Students*. 2015;1:43-49. http://dx.doi.org/10.15561/20755279.2015.0107
23. Prytula AL. Professional training of physical culture teachers for use in national martial arts career. *Pedagogics, psychology, medical-biological problems of physical training and sports.* 2015;1:62-67. http://dx.doi.org/10.15561/18189172.2015.0112
24. Semanyshyn TM, Popel SL. The professional valeological portrait of instructor of physical culture. *Pedagogics, psychology, medical-biological problems of physical training and sports*, 2014;10:41-44. http://dx.doi.org/10.5281/zenodo.10489
25. Sobyanin FI, Dudkina SG. About a competence and professional trade of specialists in the field of physical culture. *Physical Education of Students,* 2013;1:68-73. http://dx.doi.org/10.6084/m9.figshare.156361
26. Stone D, Deci EL, Ryan RM. Beyond talk: Creating autonomous motivation through self-determination theory. *Journal of General Management*, 2009;34:75-91.
27. Tikhonova NV. Sale leisure activities of children and youth in out of school educational establishments of physical culture and sports destinations. *Physical Education of Students,* 2014;5:38-42. http://dx.doi.org/10.15561/20755279.2014.0507
28. Yermakova TS. Individualization of forming health culture in schoolchildren of Polish schools. *Pedagogics, psychology, medical-biological problems of physical training and sports*. 2015;1:29-33. http://dx.doi.org/10.15561/18189172.2015.0106

PERMISSIONS

All chapters in this book were first published in PES, by Ukrainian Academy of Sciences/H.S. Skovoroda Kharkov National Pedagogical University; hereby published with permission under the Creative Commons Attribution License or equivalent. Every chapter published in this book has been scrutinized by our experts. Their significance has been extensively debated. The topics covered herein carry significant findings which will fuel the growth of the discipline. They may even be implemented as practical applications or may be referred to as a beginning point for another development.

The contributors of this book come from diverse backgrounds, making this book a truly international effort. This book will bring forth new frontiers with its revolutionizing research information and detailed analysis of the nascent developments around the world.

We would like to thank all the contributing authors for lending their expertise to make the book truly unique. They have played a crucial role in the development of this book. Without their invaluable contributions this book wouldn't have been possible. They have made vital efforts to compile up to date information on the varied aspects of this subject to make this book a valuable addition to the collection of many professionals and students.

This book was conceptualized with the vision of imparting up-to-date information and advanced data in this field. To ensure the same, a matchless editorial board was set up. Every individual on the board went through rigorous rounds of assessment to prove their worth. After which they invested a large part of their time researching and compiling the most relevant data for our readers.

The editorial board has been involved in producing this book since its inception. They have spent rigorous hours researching and exploring the diverse topics which have resulted in the successful publishing of this book. They have passed on their knowledge of decades through this book. To expedite this challenging task, the publisher supported the team at every step. A small team of assistant editors was also appointed to further simplify the editing procedure and attain best results for the readers.

Apart from the editorial board, the designing team has also invested a significant amount of their time in understanding the subject and creating the most relevant covers. They scrutinized every image to scout for the most suitable representation of the subject and create an appropriate cover for the book.

The publishing team has been an ardent support to the editorial, designing and production team. Their endless efforts to recruit the best for this project, has resulted in the accomplishment of this book. They are a veteran in the field of academics and their pool of knowledge is as vast as their experience in printing. Their expertise and guidance has proved useful at every step. Their uncompromising quality standards have made this book an exceptional effort. Their encouragement from time to time has been an inspiration for everyone.

The publisher and the editorial board hope that this book will prove to be a valuable piece of knowledge for researchers, students, practitioners and scholars across the globe.

LIST OF CONTRIBUTORS

Bondar A. A.
Kamenetz-Podolsk National University

Lopatenko G. O., Tumanova V. N. and Gatsko E. V.
Borys Grinchenko Kyiv University

Kolokoltsev M. M.
National Research Irkutsk State Technical University, Russia

Cieslicka Miroslawa and Muszkieta Radoslaw
Kazimierz Wielki University in Bydgoszcz, Poland

Mikhnov A. P.
National University of Physical Education and Sport of Ukraine

Shypulo I. P.
Chernihiv National Pedagogical University

Kubaj G. V.
Vasyl Stefanyk Precarpathian National University

Pichurin V. V.
Dnipropetrovsk National University of Railway Transport named after Academician V.Lazaryan

Singh Virendra Kumar
Shri Shankaracharya Mahavidyalaya, India

Agashe Chandrakant D.
Pt. Ravishankar Shukla University, India

Dzhym V. Yu.
Kharkov State Academy of Physical Culture

Skidan A. A. and Sevdalev S. V.
Francisk Skorina Gomel State University, Republic of Belarus

Vrublewskiy E. P.
Francisk Skorina Gomel State University, Republic of Belarus
University of Zielona Góra, Poland

Kirpenko V. N.
Kharkov Air Force University Kozhedub

Dudko M. V.
Kyiv National Economic University named after Vadym Hetman

Martsiv V. P.
Lviv State University of Physical Culture

Podrigalo L. V., Iermakov S. S., Alekseev A. F. and Rovnaya O. A.
Kharkov State Academy of Physical Culture

Masliak I. P.
Kharkiv State Academy of Physical Culture

Pryimakov A. A. and Eider E.
Szczecin University, Poland

Omelchuk E. V.
M.P. Dragomanov National Pedagogical University

Semanychyn T. M. and Popel' S. L.
Prikarpatskiy National University

Martinova N. P.
Luhansk Taras Shevchenko National University

Zhen Qiang San
Kharkov State Academy of Physical Culture

Podrigalo L. V., Galashko M. N. and Galashko N. I.
Kharkov State Academy of Physical Culture

Gaskov A. V.
Buryat state University, Russia

Kuzmin V. A. and Kudryavtsev M. D.
Siberian Federal University, Russia
Siberian State Aerospace University, Russia

Iermakov S. S.
Kazimierz Wielki University in Bydgoszcz, Poland

Bachinskaya N. V.
Oles Honchar Dnipropetrovsk National University

Michael Chia and Marcus Lee
Physical Education & Sports Science, National Institute of Education, Nanyang Technological University, Singapore

Liu Yong Qiang
Henan Polytechnic University, Republic of China

Kondakov V. L., Kopeikina E. N., Balysheva N. V., Usatov A. N. and Skrug D. A.
National Research University Belgorod State University, Russia

Kovalenko Y. O. and Boloban V. N.
National University of Physical Education and Sport of Ukraine

Olkhovy O. M., Petrenko Y. M., Temchenko V. A. and Timchenko A. N.
Kharkov National University

Kuzmin V. A.
Siberian Federal University (SibFU), Krasnoyarsk, Russia

Kopylov Yu. A.
The Federal State Scientific Institution of Russian Academy of education "The Institute of Age Physiology", Moscow, Russia

Kudryavtsev M. D.
Siberian Federal University (SibFU), Krasnoyarsk, Russia
Siberian State Aerospace University, Krasnoyarsk, Russia

Ionova O. M. and Yermakova T. S.
H.S. Skovoroda Kharkiv National Pedagogical University

Radzievskiy R. M. and Plisko V. I.
Chernigov National Pedagogical University

Kozina Z. L.
H.S. Skovoroda Kharkiv National Pedagogical University

Iermakov S. S.
Kazimierz Wielki University in Bydgoszcz

Tereshchenko I. A., Otsupok A. P., Krupenya S. V., Liauchuk T. M. and Boloban V. N.
National University of Physical Education and Sport of Ukraine

Iermakov S. S., Cieślicka Mirosława and Muszkieta Radosław
Kazimierz Wielki University in Bydgoszcz, Poland

Kutek T. B.
Zhytomyr Ivan Franko State University

Romanowska-Tołłoczko Anna and Piwowarczyk Piotr
University School of Physical Education in Wrocław

Mehrzad Shabani and Saeid Shakerian
Ahvaz Shahid Chamran University, Ahvaz, Iran

Rouholah Fatemi
Ahvaz Jundishapur University of Medical Sciences, Ahvaz, Iran

Otravenko O. V.
Luhansk Taras Shevchenko National University

Index